Date Due

THE PLAGUE OF THE SPANISH LADY

17.4

THE PLAGUE OF THE
SPANISH LADY

*The Influenza Pandemic
of 1918-1919*

RICHARD COLLIER

Atheneum   *New York*
1974

TO

THE

UNKNOWN DOCTOR

and

THE

FORGOTTEN NURSE

*who fought, who conquered, who died, in the
greatest epidemic known for six centuries*

THIS BOOK IS

DEDICATED

Much of a Race depends on what it thinks of
   death and how it stands personal anguish
   and sickness.

Walt Whitman
Memoranda During the War

Men who are occupied in the restoration of
   health to other men, by joint exertion
   of skill and humanity, are, above all,
   the great of the earth. They even
   partake of the Divinity, since to
   preserve and renew is almost as noble
   as to create.

Voltaire
Dictionnaire Philosophique

All men served their stricken brother, save
   those who deserved not the name of Man.
Guatama Buddha (attr.)

CONTENTS

ILLUSTRATIONS

Between pages 120-121

Top: Boy Scouts in twenty-seven countries carried soup and bland diets to flu-stricken households. *Bottom*: Hastily-converted transportation, from Model Ts to delivery vans, stood in as ambulances in Wellington, New Zealand.

Top: Futile emergency precautions abounded across five continents. Here zealous Harbour Board officials in Durban fumigate travellers' baggage. *Bottom*: For many, like these policemen in Seattle, Washington, medicated masks became compulsory.

Top: Business as usual for newsboys in Winnipeg, Manitoba. *Bottom*: Bank-tellers in Sydney, New South Wales.

Top: Placard worn by Parisian boulevardiers reads: "THE GERMANS ARE BEATEN BUT NOT THE FLU". *Bottom*: For 10,000 Australian travellers, border checks, long sojourns in cramped quarantine stations, became routine.

Top: Some law courts, as in San Francisco, transferred to the open-air. *Bottom*: In Copenhagen's *Politiken*, the Angel of Peace laments: 'They won't have anything to do with me, but that detestable Spanish woman can go anywhere'.

For newspaper cartoonists, the pandemic was a field-day: street arabs pictured in Joseph Pulitzer's *New York World*.

Top: Unfilial daughters as seen by Barcelona's *Esquella*. *Bottom*: Milan's *Avanti!* saw the killer virus as the new Napoleon, undisputed conqueror of Europe.

Tersilla Vicenzotto, seen in 1919 with (from L. to R.) Dora, one, Angelica, two, and Antonietta, four.

CHAPTER ONE

'My Friends, This is the First'

3 September—12 September 1918

She might have posed for a sculptor's statue of Grief. Under the muted blue glimmer of the single bulb lighting the cavernous booking-hall of Pisa Railway Station, at 3 a.m. on this autumn Tuesday, she sat motionless, her brown eyes alive yet unseeing, her face a mask of sorrow. All round her, on hard wooden benches, Italian soldiers in faded field-grey were slumped dead to the world, the harsh reality of the morning's return to the front curtained momentarily by sleep. Elsewhere in the gloom, the pinpoint lights of cigarettes glowed fitfully: the small hours solace of those whom sleep eluded.

Once, two soldiers seeking a resting-place, paused curiously before her: a dark petite figure in a black high-necked dress, a white crocheted shawl covering her shoulders, clutching tightly to her small wicker basket. 'Is it contraband, Signora?' one of them jeered, but she made no sign she had even heard, and, tiring of the jest, they moved on.

For twenty-three-year-old Tersilla Vicenzotto, the irony was bitter indeed. Inside her basket, wrapped carefully in scarce tissue paper, was a prize infinitely more precious than contraband: purple-black Regina grapes and soft yellow peaches, a luxury she could never have afforded had it not been for the generosity of the refugee committee. Now, somehow, she must transport this priceless fruit to Oscar, her husband of five years standing, mysteriously stricken with an unknown malady, 186 miles north in the war zone at Padua.

It was Tuesday, 3 September 1918. Once again, for the second time in twelve months, the hand of war had reached out to touch Tersilla Vicenzotto – a war which nineteen major nations had now waged with unceasing ferocity for four years, one month and two days. Yet already, it seemed, Tersilla had suffered enough. One year earlier, after the Austrian victory at Caporetto, she had been forced to flee the city of Udine at a moment's notice, along with her mother-in-law and her two small daughters, Antonietta, four, and Angelica, two; as they fought their way aboard the last train south, bombs were already raining on the outskirts. There hadn't even been time to find Oscar and say goodbye.

It was a nightmare journey which followed. Seven months pregnant with their third child, Dora, Tersilla had travelled on a train so crammed with 2000 soldiers and refugees that few could even reach the stinking brimming toilets – so tight-packed that when a peasant woman gave birth to a child, there among the benches, and the Red Cross man told them all to turn their backs, it was a physical impossibility, try as they might. Uneasy at intruding on a stranger's pain, they could still do no more than turn their heads.

Later had come the naked horror Tersilla would never forget: the halt at the wayside station near Florence, when a weeping soldier clung to his girl, refusing to board the train, and an officer drew his revolver, grinning like a dog, and shot him down.

Once outside the war zone, in the Villa Albini, the refugee committee's hostel on the sea-front, each day was long and lonely. A city-bred girl, who had never ventured beyond Udine, Tersilla found the restless surge of the sea at Marina di Pisa strange and disquieting. Time and again, to ease the pain of separation, she found herself re-reading the letters that Oscar had written her ever since their days as childhood sweethearts: 'I am going half-crazy after not seeing you for so long.'

Only once, on the very night of Dora's birth, Christmas Eve, 1917, had Oscar, a handsome, moustached thirty-one-year-old, joined her on a brief leave. He had thrilled, as Tersilla had done, to hold his new-born daughter in his arms and to the humble gifts the other refugees had borne like the Magi, to her bedside—linen, chemises, even a plump rooster. But all too soon he had returned to war duty, as a skilled mechanic in the railway workshops at Padua.

Now, from mutual friends in that city, had come a sudden postcard announcing Oscar's illness: 'He isn't too bad and you shouldn't worry – but come as soon as you can.' At once, filled with a strange foreboding, Tersilla had hastened to the Salvini brothers, who headed the committee. Could they prepare a declaration, to persuade the police to give her a travel visa north – and look after her daughters until she returned?

But earlier, on the night of 2 September, the police officials had quibbled: each man had ducked the ultimate responsibility of issuing a visa. She must return in the morning and see the officer in charge—though they held out little hope.

Now, alone and fearful in the gloom, Tersilla waited for dawn. There had been nowhere for her but the railway station to pass this night; the last tram back to the sea-front, eight miles away, had gone hours ago. And, absurdly, the very fact of being at the station seemed to bring her closer to Oscar.

Worse still, she did not even know why he was sick: it was an illness as inexplicable as the war itself. But in the morning she would go to Police Headquarters and try again. Ahead of her, even if God was good, stretched a gruelling three-day journey, but come what might she must reach the man she loved more than life itself before it was too late.

All over the world, the same sense of puzzlement gripped others, too. Even in an age when horror was commonplace, many felt a sudden sense of awe: something was wrong—yet no one could say what. Afterwards, many men and women would recall this first prickle of unease, beset by a fear they could not quite explain.

In the canteen of the Royal Dutch Cavalry Barracks, at Leeuwarden, Private Jelle Beintema, plying his broom, was humming a hit song of the day, 'World Peace'. Even in neutral Holland, there were lines to tug at any young soldier yearning for civilian life:

From now on there'll be peace,
They'll wage no war again

Still humming, he gave barely a second glance to the group of soldiers who now entered, in the blue-grey uniforms of the mounted police. By now, as canteen orderly, serving up mugs of hot chocolate, packets of Zodiak cigarettes, had become, for Beintema, an all-too-familiar routine. But suddenly, despite himself, he was wary. The men just stood before him dumbly, like visitors from another planet, no one uttering a word.

Then, as Beintema raised his eyebrows in silent interrogation, all of them, as if on cue, uttered a strange croaking sound, grimacing painfully. But no other coherent words would come. Plainly, as if spirited away, their voices had mysteriously gone.

And now, irked by Beintema's incomprehension, the group grew angry; faces suffused, they croaked and gestured and yammered as painfully as mutes. It was all so bizarre that Jelle Beintema, past patience, seized a slate and a stub of chalk: 'Here, write what you want on there.'

Soon enough he had filled their orders and his strange visitors had departed, mollified – but still the memory of those raucous croakings, though he didn't know why, perturbed Beintema.

Across the Atlantic, at Camp Devens, Ayer, Massachusetts, 40 miles north-west of Boston, the curious conduct of another group of soldiers was similarly puzzling Second Lieutenant Alfred Tennyson. At this stage of the war, Devens was typical of most Army camps across the United States; wrested from the forests only one year back, to train the Yankee Division,

it was now bursting at the seams with 45,000 men – 10,000
more than had been foreseen.

Yet despite the overcrowding, the drizzling October
weather, morale was razor-keen. Most were booked for France,
to backstop General John Pershing's great drive on the St
Mihiel salient of the mighty Hindenburg Line – and no man
among them would buck an order with impunity.

But now, halfway across the square, the Lieutenant saw
a callisthenics exercise come to an abrupt halt. An angry al-
tercation broke out in the ranks. Within minutes, a furious
Top Sergeant strode up to Tennyson, saluting smartly. Four
men in the company refused point-blank to do the 'bear crawl'
– a keep-your-head-down manœuvre essential for front-line
areas. The sergeant was adamant: court-martial charges
should be preferred.

But Tennyson, after one year as a private, had his own
reservations about sergeants. The men, he ventured, didn't
look like troublemakers. Before deciding, he would hear their
side of the story. Glowering dangerously, the sergeant still had
no option but to fall the offenders out.

Mincing no words, the enlisted men came straight to the
point. All of them were feeling off-colour – and the 'bear-
crawl' was entirely too strenuous to perform. They hadn't gone
to sick call because they'd hoped to stick it out; the drill had
just proved too much for them. To the Lieutenant, it was
plain that the men were coming down with some kind of
fever. Promptly, though the sergeant went pale with rage,
Tennyson ordered all four to report to the infirmary.

In truth, the men fared better than those at Västmanland
Regimental Barracks, Västeras, Sweden. Around this time,
Private Hjalmar Johansson felt more under the weather than
he'd ever thought possible, but though he duly reported sick
he didn't even rate 'Medicine and Duty' – only a tongue-lashing
from an M.O. who wrote him off as a scrimshanker. 'Don't
waste my time, Mother's Boy,' the doctor sneered, as he dismissed Johansson. 'You'll be fine after a month's hard drill.'

In these days, many actions took an eerie quality. At Kalkfontein, South-West Africa, a back-of-beyond railway junction, Stationmaster Charles Beard was crossing the tracks when an unusual sight stopped him cold. Emerging from the S.A.T. Government store was a group of black platelayers, every man of them armed with a large blue bottle. Instinctively, Beard feared the worst: the men were bent on a drunken shindig in working hours. Then, as he drew near, he recognised the bottles for what they were: castor oil.

Some strange instinct must have prompted the men to treat themselves against infection in advance – for solemnly, without even gagging, they were swigging down the laxative, there beside the tracks, with as much relish as if it was beer.

Another man, too, was sorely troubled. Almost 500 miles east of Kalkfontein, on the main street of Kimberley, Cape Province, sunlight sparkled, red, green and blue, from the tunbellied jars in William Cooper's pharmacy. The air was spicy with cardamom and menthol, but this morning, unusually, apprentice Joe Sperber felt no relish for the medieval mysteries of an apothecary's profession.

Try as he might, there were factors Sperber just couldn't reconcile in the latest prescription from the town's most noted physician, Dr Evelyn Oliver Ashe – senior surgeon to both Kimberley Hospital and De Beers Consolidated Diamond Mines.

Mystified, the youngster sought the guidance of manager Charles Austen. Days earlier, prescribing for a lad of eighteen, Dr Ashe had specified a compound of ten grains of phenazone (to bring down the temperature), seven grains of tincture of nux vomica (to stimulate the nervous system) and seven grains of digitalis (to strengthen the heart).

Now, out of the blue, a new prescription had arrived for the same patient. Poring over it, the two saw at a glance that it was completely at variance with the one they had so recently filled. This time, Ashe was calling for three grains of ammonium carbonate (to clear the bronchial tubes), fifteen grains of senna, (as a purgative) and twenty grains of camphor (used both for colic and to stimulate the heart by reflex).

Both men exchanged glances, not speaking: one factor, at least, was disturbingly plain. The celebrated Dr Ashe had no more concept than Austen or Sperber of the sickness that he was treating.

Ahead of them all stretched 120 days of such fear and uncertainty – the onset of a plague more devastating than war itself.

Three months had now passed since the Spanish wire-service Agencia Fabra had taken the unprecedented step of routing two cables from Madrid to Reuter's London headquarters in the space of a day. A STRANGE FORM OF DISEASE OF EPIDEMIC CHARACTER HAS APPEARED IN MADRID, the operator tapped out, though ending on a note of reassurance, THE EPIDEMIC IS OF A MILD NATURE, NO DEATHS HAVING BEEN REPORTED.

Mild or not, the sickness had hit the Iberian peninsula like the wake of a tornado. Soon eight million Spaniards were down with the 'three-day fever', and when King Alfonso XIII took to his bed, it was headline news in *El Sol*. In Madrid, with one-third of the citizens afflicted, some Government offices closed down, and trams ceased to run.

It began, undramatically, after a two-day incubation period, with a cough. Next there was pain – behind the eyes, in the ears, in the lumbar region. Soon a drowsy numbness invaded the body, and fever set in; often the temperature soared to 104°F. The pulse was thready and unstable; the victim's tongue was thickly coated, and solid food was now the most revolting sight on earth.

Every mortal fibre ached indescribably – the throat, the head, the naso-pharynx, which connects nose and throat. Yet, amazingly, within three days, the disease had run its course; the patient was up and about.

It was reported from other quarters, too. From April through May it hit France, Scotland, Greece, Macedonia, Egypt and Italy. By June it had taken hold in Germany, Austria, Norway and India. It rampaged through Canton, China, through Lima, Peru, and even smote tiny Costa Rica.

It was a sickness with a Marconi system, as intangible as a thought. In Denmark, doctors spotlit its two-fold invasion with clinical precision: on 10 July, it hit the market-town of Roskilde, via a negro roustabout in the Jack Joyce Circus, and one day earlier, the crew of the torpedo boat *Tumleren* had taken it to Copenhagen, twenty miles east. But such positive identification was rare. Most often, as at Manila, in the Philippines, it struck, without warning, overnight – so affecting one victim's diaphragm that he hiccoughed for forty hours.

It mowed down fighting men, too. For twelve days in May, King George V's Grand Fleet, counting 10,313 cases, couldn't even put to sea, and the King himself was stricken at the same time. On 22 June, at Etaples, France, what puzzled medics dubbed P.U.O. (Pyrexia of Unknown Origin) hospitalised 3000 men of the British First Army in three days flat; even at G.H.Q., 700 were out of action, only the aloof C-in-C, Field-Marshal Sir Douglas Haig, escaping. And all through the summer weeks, when General Erich von Ludendorff's final thrusts into French territory were being turned back at Château Thierry, Compiègne, and Hazebrouck, and Maréchal Ferdinand Foch was beginning the counterattack which would never stop until the war ended, some hard-hit German units were down to fifty rifles.

At first, not surprisingly, the blame was placed squarely on Spain. As early as February, the sickness was reported from San Sebastian, on the northern coast, but the town's leading citizens, fearing a boycott by summer visitors, did their best to hush it up. And in Madrid, Dr Martin Salazar, Inspector-General of Public Health, even hinted that the epidemic had been spread through the capital by infected tourists.

At Almeria, on the southern coast, the provincial governor, Don Esteban García, went further still. When the prison's medical officer, Dr Gómez Casas, reported a severe outbreak among the convicts, the governor was determined to nip such a dangerous rumour in the bud. Summoning Dr Casas to his palace, he ordered him to publish a written statement denying the existence of the disease.

When Casas indignantly refused, Don Esteban fined him 100 *pesetas* (about £4) – a tyranny which so outraged the local *Colegio Médico* they not only paid the fine but sent a furious protest to Madrid's Sanitary Council.

In truth, Spain bore no real blame. Months before the sickness hit Madrid, a kindred disease had been rife throughout the world – above all, on Monday, 11 March, at Fort Riley, Kansas, a sprawling 20,000-acre outpost near Junction City, where 1100 men had gone down. Nor was this surprising. Since April 1917, when the United States declared war on the Central Powers, her peacetime army of 190,000 men had swelled to more than two million – most with less than four months service.

This problem of susceptible raw recruits had troubled many an Army medic – not least among them Major Victor Vaughan, a renowned epidemiologist attached to the U.S. Council of National Defence in Washington, D. C. Studying the pneumonia incidence and mortality rate among young soldiers through the latter half of 1917, Vaughan was struck by one factor: many camps with a high pneumonia incidence had strikingly few deaths. Puzzled, Vaughan next drew up charts analysing the soldiers' immunity by home-states – and the key to the situation was revealed.

Almost every man who had escaped scot-free came from densely populated cities like Chicago and New York – while the men who fell sick and even died hailed from the wide-open spaces, the Iowa corn belt or the cattle country of Montana. Though smog-bound city dwellers had acquired some immunity to respiratory diseases, country boys had no such resistance. Vaughan had been on the brink of boosting that resistance, by vaccinating every countryman with dead bacterial cultures when the epidemic, like a spent candle, petered out.

Yet despite the mildness of this first wave, which barely affected mortality rates across the globe, there had been complications that many doctors, even now, in September, recalled with wonder and dread.

In the village schoolhouse at Cittadella, Italy, hastily converted to Camp Hospital 020, beneath the ice-bound slopes of Monte Grappa, Second Lieutenant Giuseppe Agostoni had been appalled by the 'terrifying phenomenon' that had decimated his regiment, the 53rd Infantry. Never has the twenty-five-year-old medic seen anything like this: men literally choking to death with pulmonary oedema, the lungs so swamped with blood, foam and mucus that the faces were grey and the lips purple and each desperate breath was like the quacking of a duck.

To relieve the congestion, Agostoni had time and again taken a 23 c.c. syringe, attempting to draw blood from a vein in the arm – but as fast as he tried, the blood, dark through lack of oxygen, clotted in the syringe, black and viscous like cooling tar. After withdrawing 10 c.c. he had to give up: the syringe was blocked solid.

At Monts-en-Ternois, on the western front, Captain Lucien Montel, surgeon to the 12th Battalion of the Chasseurs Alpins, had seen no such comparable horror – yet a sickness which could fell 1200 battle-hardened veterans like a gas attack still perturbed him deeply.

The C.O., Commandant Nabias, an officer of the old school, had been perturbed too: his text-book brain just could not grasp a man being so ill that he disobeyed an order to march. Worriedly, tilting his kepi backwards from his forehead as he surveyed the groaning prostrate shapes, he asked Montel: 'Do you think they are going to mutiny?'

Few had been so prescient as the Reverend Jan van Boven, military chaplain to the barracks in Ede, Holland. Halfway through the burial, with full military honours, of the first soldier-victim, the bugler playing the Last Post had collapsed beside the open grave, smitten by the same unseen force. 'My friends,' van Boven had warned the assembled mourners, 'this is the first. Which of us will be the next?'

But for the most part the people had viewed it all light-heartedly. In this fifth year of war, any excuse for a laugh was better than none – and the nicknames they gave the disease bore this out. To Spaniards, it was 'The Naples Soldier', after the

title-song of a long-running show at Madrid's Teatro Martín
that had at length become a bore. Hong Kong wits, mimick-
ing the pidgin-English of the bazaars, called it 'the-too-muchee-
hot-inside sickness'. It was 'blitz katarrh' to the Germans,
'wrestler's fever' to the Japanese, and 'Flanders Grippe' to
Field-Marshal Haig's Tommies. Few, in these early days, ad-
vanced causation theories, though the Persians, blaming the
boisterous west wind that romped through Tehran's streets,
named it 'the disease of the wind'.

It was especially hard on the Spanish that a score of nations
would always hold them entirely responsible for the epidemic.
From Murom, Russia, *Pravda* early on reported: 'Ispanka (the
Spanish Lady) is in town', and despite the appointment of a
Spanish medical commission to prove conclusively that the
disease stemmed from Russian Turkestan, for much of the
world it was 'the Spanish Lady' until the very end.

There was precedent for this. As far back as 412 B.C., the
father of medicine, Hippocrates, had described a respiratory
disease which 'broke out about Solstice' (22 December) and
was preceded by marked changes of winds. There was a great
tendency to relapses, 'further complicated by pneumonia affec-
tions'. But always, through every recorded epidemic and pandemic (world-wide epidemic) that had scourged the world since
1510, the names men had given the fever had placed the blame
on another nation: the 'Russian fever', the 'Chinese sickness'.

Then, in 1580, two Italian historians, Domenico and Pietro
Buoninsegni, convinced of the baneful influence of the stars on
men's health, had first called it by a name which was to endure
for more than three centuries: influenza.

In those centuries, influenza had struck hard and surely
twenty-one times – almost always between September and
March. Highly contagious, it was spread, mostly, through
coughs and sneezes, in droplets borne on the air; one unguarded sneeze alone could distribute more than 85 million
bacteria. Such a sneeze could hurl 4600 particles into the air
at a 'muzzle velocity' of 152 feet a second; often particles would
be hurled a distance of twelve feet, to remain suspended in the

air for more than half an hour thereafter. One droplet alone might create 19,000 colonies of bacteria.

Yet as a cause of death, influenza ranked a lowly tenth in magnitude, ending the lives of no more than five people, usually the old and infirm, in every hundred. For most doctors it had become little more than a lugubrious winter commonplace.

Thus the first complications of the summer epidemic had taken the authorities almost completely unawares. Fifteen miles outside London, in the Hertfordshire countryside, 100 lads of the Bushey Cadet Battalion who went down with it never even saw a doctor; their sole treatment was a daily dosage of no. 9 pills and cascara tablets administered by two stalwart officers of the Irish Guards, both of whom kept going on a bottle of champagne a day. Though all pulled through, it was a memorable and unhappy week: each hut had only one commode.

For Second Lieutenant Stefan Westman, of the German Army Medical Corps, it had been an experience both chastening and revealing. Only recently commissioned, Westman had barely commenced his medical studies when war broke out; at his first base hospital, the orderlies had even to teach him such elementary skills as how to operate a catheter or administer an anaesthetic.

Now, at Cappy airfield, in the valley of the Somme, as M.O. to the famous von Richthofen Squadron, Westman was confronted by symptoms as rare as plague itself: an officer-pilot, near-delirious, with a raging and inexplicable fever. Hastily, seeking superior wisdom, he sped his patient by ambulance to the nearest military hospital.

Three hours later, the near-empty building was overflowing with identical cases – yet though Westman stayed on until late that evening the specialist in charge was as baffled as his would-be pupil. Thumbing through text-book after text-book, neither man could find trace of any such symptoms.

Most doctors, in any case, ascribed the sickness to malnutrition pure and simple. 'You haven't heard of our doughboys getting it, have you?' New York's Health Commissioner, Dr Royal Copeland, one advocate of this theory, challenged a press conference as late as 14 August, 'You bet you haven't, and you won't...'

Thus, it was human, in the fifth year of war, to brush memories of that spring epidemic aside. To be sure, some cases had presented alarming symptoms, but they were unlikely to recur, and it was only natural to try and forget complications so horrible and inexplicable that the mind recoiled.

At 1 a.m. on 12 September, the tremendous almost unbearable roar of the guns of St Mihiel drove all such memories from the mind of Private John Lewis Barkley and his Cherokee Indian buddies, 'Jesse' James and 'Nigger' Floyd. In this moment, as the barrage split the dripping forest darkness along twenty-three miles of front, the stuttering doughboy from Holden, Missouri, a scout for Company K, 4th Infantry, 3rd Division, could almost forget one of the most traumatic moments he had ever experienced until now: the icy fingers in the night, gripping his left wrist in the hospital at Fort Riley, Kansas, when a Mexican in the next bunk, delirious with flu, had clutched him like a vice, his nose streaming blood – then died.

Somehow this, and the sight of the hospital train, moving slowly back from the Marne on a parallel track as they left Bricon for the front – a nightmare vision of blood and bandages and men shaking with pain – had come to make death seem as much an adversary as any German. Thus, in the face of death, Barkley had taken a conscious decision rare indeed for this shy introverted eighteen-year-old. He had come to accept these lithe raw-boned American Indians, with their coalblack hair and glittering eyes, as his friends.

Until the war had spurred him on to stammer his way past a draft board, Barkley had never, in his life, had a friend. Fear of incurring ridicule each time he opened his mouth had always driven him back to the woods round Scalybark Creek, a loner with his gun and his dogs, emulating his lifelong hero, Daniel Boone. He had spent more time in those woods, and nights too – learning to find his way in the dark, creeping up on his game without so much as the crackle of a twig – than ever he had spent in school.

From the first, a scout's life had seemed custom-built to him, and for eight months now he had lived night and day in a baggy burlap suit festooned with leaves, his face and hands smeared with clay, through the fighting at Troyes and Rozay and Belleville and Château Thierry, working unsuspected within yards of the German lines, signalling back their movements by morse and field telephone.

Yet now it was different from Scalybark Creek. Now there were, and always would be, the three of them – himself, Jesse and Floyd. The sight of that hospital train, the memory of the epidemic at Fort Riley, had decided that. All three had sworn a solemn oath to be on hand if the others were in trouble, never to let themselves be sent back from the front as long as they had legs to walk – but if one *had* to go, then all would go.

And thus far, though Barkley had stopped a glancing thrust from a German bayonet in his right side, near Le Charmel, and Jesse had caught a whiff of mustard gas and Floyd got a bullet in his left arm, they had patched each other up with iodine and bandages and stubbornly refused to report sick. Their solidarity would be proof enough against past memories, as they swore once again, on the night of St Mihiel: 'No pill-roller is going to put a tag on us.'

And others were as eager to forget. In the emergency hospital at the Château Gabriel, ten miles from Soissons, Nurse Shirley Millard, an attractive red-headed New Yorker, still found it hard to believe that the peaceful old castle, with its damask-panelled walls and massive chandeliers, had witnessed such horrors as recently as April. The men had run temperatures so high that often she had checked the thermometer twice, even three times, to make sure she wasn't dreaming – and the French doctors had made such use of the *ventouses*, or glass suction-cups, in an effort to prevent pneumonia, as she would never have believed possible.

Now all that was past. On this mellow autumn afternoon,

Shirley had other things on her mind. She was entertaining her favourite doctor, Dr Le Brun, the handsome young specialist from Lyons, to afternoon tea. Always she found his presence both delightful and disturbing: he was so much a man of the world and the way he coolly chain-smoked his way through an operation never ceased to fascinate her. Only one problem troubled her, and as yet she didn't know the answer: if Le Brun asked her to go to Paris for a week-end, would she go or not? Somehow the answer would have been simpler in New York than here in the war zone at Soissons.

As usual, it was an improvised tea-party: a Sterno lamp stood in for a stove, and she had had to use a German helmet to brew the tea. There had been a shortage of tea-cups, too, but the practical Shirley had solved this easily – pressing into service the now-despised *ventouses*.

Afterwards, looking back to that time, the epidemiologists would say that few ages had been so attuned to the climate of disaster as the autumn of 1918, the fifth year of war.

To be sure, it was a world in transition, and in many ways for the better. Doomed to extinction were the gold sovereign, the stereoscope, the muffin-man, the chaperon, the lamplighter, the living-in domestic servant and the divine right of private enterprise. On the way in were British summertime, the aspirin, the automobile, the fox-trot, the hand-cranked phonograph, the cafeteria, or 'one-arm Ritz', State control, and a wary scepticism and distrust of established authority. It was a world of transients, too; almost two million refugees were on the move.

It was a world irrevocably in dissolution. Four empires had toppled, spawning ten new republics, and the lives of ten million fighting men had come to dust. In this crucial week, as the German Army were forced to cede 175 square miles of territory in the St Mihiel salient, and many prisoners and guns, the words of the British Premier, David Lloyd George, would later take on a new significance as he spoke of 'empires and kingdoms, kings and crowns, falling like withered leaves'.

It was a patriotic world, that hated the Germans with a fervour which later generations would find hard to comprehend. On the streets of every American city, Liberty Bond posters exhorted the people: 'Take Hold of the Big Bond Broom – Sweep Hohenzollern and Hapsburg into the Offal Heap'. In Rio de Janeiro, it was mandatory, since the sinking of the *Lusitania*, to spit ostentatiously when passing the German Consulate. King George V had adopted the family name of Windsor, renouncing all connection with 'the unspeakable Hun', and Britain's First Lord of the Admiralty, Sir Eric Geddes, would announce his country's intention of 'squeezing Germany till the pips squeak'.

Even a French soldier who slashed his wife to death with a razor for praising the courtesy of the German invader was acquitted automatically – with the court breaking into spontaneous applause.

For all that, it was a world grown war-weary. One sight was common to the streets of every British city: the mutilated men creeping painfully along the pavements in hospital blue. Rousing hit tunes like 'Tipperary' belonged to the forgotten past; now it was 'God Send You Back To Me', and 'There's a Long Long Trail a-Winding'. On every lip, in a dozen tongues, the current phrases were, 'When our boys come back ...' and 'It must never happen again'. At least one German had stated frankly: 'We are too exhausted even to hate' – the Burgermeister of Cologne, Konrad Adenauer.

For millions, from Cape Horn to Cape Chelyuskin, it was a world pivoting round the home. Few of these homes had electric power, or gas, running water, sewage or septic tanks; galvanised iron tubs, not baths, were the norm, and so, too, was the outdoor bucket-seat toilet, sited perhaps 100 yards from the house. On autumn nights, the parlour was lit by an old-fashioned kerosene or coal-oil lamp, and warmed by the shifting embers of a wood-stove. On Sundays, if the house boasted a piano, the younger ones gathered after tea to sing hymns: 'Oh, What a Friend We Have in Jesus' and 'All People That on Earth Do Dwell'.

All laundry was done at home, and children were also born there, for this was an age of large families – nine children to a household was commonplace. Most often on a farm the girls slept three to a bed, the boys with the hired men. Lacking buses, many of these children walked to school, three miles there and three miles back. In winter, thousands of families subsisted, without refrigerators, on cured ham, canned beef and pickles, potatoes, and root-vegetables stored in the cellar – a squirrel precaution like the stacks of cordwood piled in the outhouse. Winter was also the time when water froze in the pail each morning and breath fogged in the schoolroom – as much a part of the season as the swarms of flies in summer, the long sticky rolls of flypaper.

Contact with the outside world was limited, for often the nearest telephone was sixteen miles away, and mail was delivered no more than twice a week. Doctors wore tailcoats, used a horse and buggy to make house-calls and presented their bills once a year. Most were G.Ps who carried out even tonsillectomies at home, administering the anaesthetic themselves, though for many families doctors were an unheard-of luxury.

It was a man's world, but women were making gains. As machine-operators, munitions workers, bank clerks, even tramdrivers, they had shown that most things a man could do, they could do as well, and on industrial Tyneside, observers noted, factory girls earning £5 a week now sported smart tailormades, with hats, blouses, gloves and silk stockings to match. Not only were British women over 30 due to vote in an election for the first time in history, but sixteen women candidates had obtained nomination. For their American sisters, the vote throughout the United States was still two years distant – though Montana's Jeannette Rankin had become the first woman elected to Congress in 1917.

It was a world of industrial strife. Spanish postal workers, 12,000 London bobbies, Zurich bank-clerks, Argentine dockers, Australian firemen and American boot and shoe workers, all had one thing in common – they were, or would be, striking in the autumn of 1918.

It was a world of pinching shortage. Even for a German officer, a complete uniform was a luxury; men shivered into action wearing rags or scraps of underwear. Often leather was stripped from railway carriage seats to fashion shoes, hotels kept their soap under lock and key, and on Berlin's Unter den Linden the street-walkers were using beetroot juice in place of non-existent rouge. At one French hospital, the doctors' request for fuel was met with the only wood the authorities could provide: 400 pairs of crutches. And in Cartier's window, on the Rue de la Paix, the jewellers offered their own silent comment on priorities: a frieze of diamonds surrounding one shining lump of coal.

Above all, it was a hungry world – sometimes from patriotic choice. Americans, stirred by the exhortations of Food Controller Herbert Hoover, had learned to 'Hooverise', observing 'the gospel of the clean plate'. Londoners, too, obeyed to the letter the injunction that loomed everywhere: 'Eat Less Bread – Let the Menu Beat the U-Men'. But millions had no choice. Italians were bartering their wedding rings for maize flour and sausage; mutton fat mixed with honey was the rancid Norwegian substitute for butter. One meagre slice of bread was a Berlin office worker's dinner, and in England one factor alone showed how near the bone things were. To conserve precious poultry, they were shooting foxes.

As the weeks drew on, this hunger would only intensify, so that for millions, weakened and emaciated by four years of privation, the dreaded face of the Spanish Lady was the last thing their eyes would ever see.

High above the needle spires of Cologne's mighty Gothic cathedral, it seemed that snowflakes were drifting. But below, watching expectantly from the broad paved expanse of the *Domplatz*, young Fritz Roth and his schoolfellows knew better. Once more, a shower of propaganda leaflets was drifting across the city: the latest attempt of the *Tommis* to undermine morale with what the disgruntled High Command called 'poison raining down from God's clear sky'.

The ethics didn't bother Fritz and his comrades. Always when the leaflets came there was a scramble to seize them and compare impressions before the police could impound them. Sometimes they were clever, like the specially-prepared postcards for German soldiers to send in event of capture, assuring their families they were well-treated and fed. But often they went wide of the mark.

Today, Fritz was one of the first to reach them as they fluttered limply to earth. A brief scuffle, then in growing wonderment they read:

> Betet tüchtig Vaterunser,
> Nach zwei Monat seit ihr unser,
> Dann bekommit ihr tüchtig Fleisch und Speck,
> Dann geht euch auch die Grippe weck!

Translated, it meant:

> Say your Our Father nicely,
> Because in two months' time you'll be ours;
> Then you'll get good meat and bacon,
> And the flu will leave you alone.

All of them exchanged troubled glances. Until this moment they had thought of hunger and flu as a closely-guarded family secret. Now it seemed the British shared it too. Somehow they felt strangely vulnerable.

The patient had lost consciousness by the time the eminent physician reached the bedside. But at this stage it would have made little difference. For hours now he had been slipping into the coma which preceded death, twitching as convulsively as a man with strychnine poisoning, the fingers plucking restlessly at the coverlet: an anonymous British Tommie, too moribund to realise that a man whose verdicts were sought by kings and statesmen now stood beside his bed.

'What is your diagnosis?'

A whole generation of London Hospital students had come to anticipate that question, posed by the tall dark courteous man in the immaculate white gown. And tonight, though the setting was a lamp-lit military hospital near Boulogne and the speaker wore the red tabs of a Major-General, the question did not vary. But somehow neither the ward physician or the great man's close associates, Dr Sam Bedson and Professor William Hume could find a ready answer.

Frowning, the senior man studied the chart. The soldier had been ill for four days—seemingly comfortable enough when lying flat, not propped by pillows, always mildly delirious, never fully conscious of his surroundings. Yet his breathing was rapid, deep painful 'air-hunger' breathing, and his nostrils dilated; often the respiration was 40 to the minute as against the average 20. The heart was rapid, too: 120, like that of a newly-born child, as against a normal adult's 72.

But what baffled the assembled physicians was the curious tinge that suffused the man's whole body. It was a strange shade of heliotrope that to experienced eyes betokened only cyanosis – the blood was hungry for oxygen. There were raised purple blisters, like a scurvy victim's, all over the man's back and face and chest, which suggested not the influenza which had first been diagnosed but acute septicaemia.

On the right side of the man's neck, above the clavicle, was another strange factor: a pronounced inexplicable lump. Despite marked subcutaneous emphysema (an enlargement of the air sacs of the lungs) the patient wasn't coughing. There was the rapid pulse of fever – yet no dilatation of the heart.

It had begun three days ago with nothing more remarkable than a sore throat, and now, despite all that had been done, the soldier was going to die. Now, in frustration and despair, every man present hung on the great man's verdict. After long moments it came.

'I fail,' confessed Major-General Sir Bertrand (later Lord) Dawson, Physician-in-Ordinary to His Majesty King George V, Consulting Physician to the British Armies in France, 'to see any explanation.'

CHAPTER TWO

'Now it's Five a Day'
13 September—30 September 1918

Above the roar of the guns in the night, her rapid footfalls
were barely audible on Padua's cobbled time-worn streets. Soon
she had quickened her pace and was running. On this fateful
September night, it seemed to Tersilla Vicenzotto that all her
life had now become a race against time.

Since her lonely vigil in Pisa's railway station, she had
known one bitter-sweet triumph: the moment when her angry
tears had finally shamed the officer in charge of Police Headquarters into signing her visa and speeding her on her way.
Yet the journey north had been desperately slow, and her sole
comfort was that every reluctant revolution of the old train's
wheels was carrying her nearer to Oscar.

No sooner had she reached the city that night than an air-
raid siren wailed. At this stage of the war, outright bombard-
ments had died away, but often lone bombers cruised above the
city and the guns would open up to turn night into day. As
she ducked through the gloomy stone colonnades, shrapnel
was pattering like spring hail, and to sustain her in this time
of fear, she held on to a thought from one of Oscar's most
precious letters: 'Dearest wife, without you I feel as powerless
as if I had no arms, so please have courage.' As always, he had
ended: 'A thousand kisses on your lips.'

Strangely, Tersilla Vicenzotto was not making directly for
the Ospedale Civile, where Oscar was a patient. A devoutly
religious wife and mother, she had decided that one vital and

determinant act of worship must first be performed. The thought had been with her for all the three weary days of the train journey, and it was steadfast inside her now while she ran, as a flare dripped beautifully and dangerously down over the Bacchiglione river and a Gotha throbbed somewhere above like a witch in a child's dream.

Passing beneath Donatello's mighty equestrian statue, she now entered the Piazza del Santo. There before her, enormous against the night sky, stood the building that she sought: the Romanesque rose-red façade of the thirteenth-century Basilica of San Antonio, patron saint of the city, friend of the poor and outcast. It was to this man, his sanctity embodied by these slender Gothic belfries and minarets, that she would appeal to save Oscar's life.

Noiselessly, she slipped through the porch entrance, her right hand automatically seeking the Holy Water stoup within. At this hour, Evensong was long over; the nave was shadowy and deserted, a perfume of incense lingering on the chill air. Swiftly, she crossed the shining marble floor, her eyes fixed on the true heart of the Basilica: the Renaissance chapel of San Antonio, where the saint's mortal remains lay beneath the altar, symbolised by the golden statue, flanked by candles and dim red votive lights, that towered above her.

Tersilla knelt at the altar's foot. Aloud in the silence, she prayed: 'San Antonio, do me the grace of letting my husband live because of the children.' Then, as swiftly, she rose and was gone, the darkness swallowing up her small slight figure.

Dimly she realised she still didn't know what sickness was afflicting Oscar.

Others were more fortunate: the strange illness now manifesting itself was as yet only a vague disquieting rumour, heard at second-hand. For some few people, even in four years, neither war nor epidemic had touched their lives.

In the pitch-pine mission house at Hopedale, Labrador, for more than 160 years a settlement of the Moravian Brotherhood, the Reverend Walter Perrett had other occasions to ponder:

his forty-ninth birthday on Friday, 13 September, his twenty-third wedding anniversary one day earlier.

As usual, Ellen had given him sealskin boots and mittens, but the gifts made rock-ribbed sense. Often enough, in a Labrador winter, the thermometer's indicator stuck at minus forty; ice on the river was eight feet thick and the breakfast milk stretched from the can in a sticky white skein like caoutchouc. A missionary had need of stout boots and mittens above all.

It was a simple enough joint celebration the Perretts planned – a coffee party, with cigars for the men of the mission, much good-natured small talk, with the women's needles never still – but Perrett, a burly moustached Englishman from Malmesbury, in Wiltshire, who had never quite lost his West Country burr, was content with simple ways. A one-time cobbler's apprentice, who had given twenty-six years of his life to the Eskimos of Labrador, his greatest pride was the total absence of crime and violence in the stations he superintended: Okak, secretly his favourite, where he had begun his ordainment, Nain, Hebron, Ramah, many of them ninety miles distant over lonely mountain passes and frozen bays.

His promotion to Superintendent of Missions had come one year earlier, but Perrett hadn't welcomed it at all. In truth, he had agreed to accept the post on one condition only: that he did not remain in office for long. 'May the time soon come when the Board will be able to find a more capable man,' ran the letter he penned, in genuine humility, to the Mission's London headquarters.

His true strength was drawn from the homespun virtues of his people; from time immemorial they had been teetotallers, and though outsiders had taught them to brew a dubious rotgut from treacle and mouldy biscuits, the village elders had smashed the kegs and all had voluntarily agreed that the drinking must cease. And every wooden hut, too, had its own Gudib A Glangit, The Writings of God – though a Bible printed in several volumes because of the polysyllabic Eskimo language.

Now, in his maturity, Perrett was as content as any of his flock with the ritual of the seasons: the spring migration, when whole villages loaded up their sledges with bedding and stores, trekking off to set up their reindeer-skin tents for the cod-fishing season on Cut-Throat Island; the autumn seal-hunt, with every household honing up its walrus-tusk harpoon heads; the stunned silence of a Labrador winter, when Attuarnek, the north wind, stifled the world with a blinding blanket of snow.

But soon Christmas came, the most cherished season of Perrett's year, when a lighted tree bulked in the schoolroom and the stove glowed ruddily, and all the children were attired in neat white smocks. Then the polished white turnips which Perrett, a jovial 'Fader Karismas' with cotton-wool whiskers, doled out were as much prized a treat to the youngsters as any apple or orange.

But after a quarter of a century, Perrett had come to look on them all as his children, old as well as young: Little John, greatest of all the pathfinders in that Arctic region; Big Josef, a legendary hunter; the schoolmistress, Juliana; her father, Old Abia, who drove the mail sledge; the crippled girl, Ernestina, who played the harmonium. He had become part of this sombre land, its rocks brightened only by tawny mosses and lichens and the silver filigree of streams, and for him a joint of seal meat or a plump eider duck with cranberries was as choice a delicacy as any round of English beef.

Day by day through autumn and winter he would make his pastoral round – again a ritual that never varied. Clad in a hooded Eskimo smock of mottled grey sealskin, he stooped from hut to hut, threading cautiously through the snow tunnel among the sleepy huskies, who stirred to show wolfish teeth. At the far end of that tunnel was the main door, at which no man, Eskimo or missionary, ever knocked: all were welcome as brothers.

'Aksusé' (Be strong, all of you), he would say as he entered, pushing back his hood, and from all the family – the father, in his shirtsleeves, mending nets, the mother, scraping a sealskin, the children, playing with tiny wide-eyed firewood dolls – would come the greeting: 'Ahaila' (And you, too).

Then, as custom decreed, the father would hand Perrett

some section of the Bible and he would read aloud until it was time for farewells and handshakes and the missionary passed on to the next household.

Sometimes, sickness was a problem, even in this icy Eden, for the Eskimos were particularly susceptible to infections like smallpox, measles, and, above all, influenza; in 1907 and again in 1908 there had been severe influenza epidemics, though with few fatalities. For now, thanks to Perrett's efforts, even tiny settlements like Okak, with no more than 266 inhabitants, boasted their own hospitals to tend the sick.

Only one problem, at first near insoluble, had caused Perrett endless mental turmoil in the past four years, but it was one he had been forced to face and resolve. Inevitably, the mission's barque, the 220-ton *Harmony*, had brought word to the Eskimos of the world-wide conflict – a conflict that Perrett had never once discussed in all this time with his German colleague at Hopedale, the Reverend Stefan Bohlmann.

But since the implications were infinitely puzzling to the Eskimos, who never fired a shot or struck a blow in anger, Perrett and Bohlmann had put their heads together to coin one new word for their long-standing Eskimo dictionary. The word was 'Sorsuktuksak', and its meaning was 'soldier'.

'Ia-ora-na!'

As ever, the traditional greeting of the islands came sweetly to the ears of Lieutenant Hector MacQuarrie. Lounging at his ease on the broad verandah of the Hotel Tiare, fringed by a vivid purple curtain of bougainvillaea, he watched, intrigued, for the hundredth time, by the colourful mid-morning bustle along the Rue Colette, main street of Tahiti's capital, Papeete. And as ever, the young New Zealander was conscious of living in a Paradise as remote from the everyday concerns of men as the Reverend Walter Perrett.

Beside him, resplendent in one of her sixty bright gowns, the proprietress, Louisa Chapman, whom the islanders called 'Lovaina', sat enthroned on a couch piled with cushions, 300 pounds of Junoesque auburn-haired majesty, hazel eyes sparkling as she told, in a mixture of broken English, salty French and sibilant Tahitian, of the long-ago night of her wedding.

'My God, you just should seen that!' she was exclaiming, her plump hands outspread, 'Bands playing from warship, all merry, drinking, dancing. Nobody walk barefoot one week, so much broken glass in the garden.'

It was a recital MacQuarrie had heard a score of times before – as had the audience now sprawled before Lovaina on the communal camphorwood chest, a motley group of schooner captains, traders and beachcombers. But this daily exchange of sleepy gossip, in an atmosphere hazy-blue with pipe tobacco, was a ritual as unchanging as Tahiti's way of life. Cats scurried past, chickens fluttered and squawked beneath the table, and all the scandals of the South Seas – a lucky deal in pearls, a new brown and white liaison – were brought out and aired yet again.

Yet MacQuarrie himself was no lotus-eating expatriate. A blue-eyed bantam-weight of twenty-nine, with a puckish amused smile, the New Zealander, as a Royal Field Artillery officer on the western front, had known the hells of both Ypres and Loos. Since then, wounded and invalided from the line, his war had been both lively and unconventional. Seconded to the United States, to liaise with the war plant manufacturers of Bethlehem, Pennsylvania, he had proved a public speaker both likeable and infectious – a discovery which had led to a six-month 12,000-mile tour of the States, publicising Britain's war effort.

Then, in Portland, Oregon, the doctors had made a discovery of their own: as grave as it seemed final. The ominous cough which for days had plagued MacQuarrie was caused by a spot on his left lung.

Seven weeks later, invalided out for good and all, MacQuarrie had arrived in Papeete, capital of the French Society Islands, seeking both to regain his health and to plumb the elusive magic of the South Seas: a 'white shadow', as the Tahitians called all such Europeans. Life was cheap and the rhythm as languorous as the surf off nearby Moorea; in a thatched beach house, at Taunoa, up the coast, MacQuarrie, with only his Chinese servant, Wong, as living companion had managed well on eleven dollars a week – four dollars for rent, plus a dollar a day for marketing.

He had explored, too, the wonder cures that the islanders could effect with massage, and every day, at 4 p.m., old Tina, a friend of his landlady, Ti-Ti, had massaged his back and chest for almost an hour with perfumed coconut oil. Miraculously, within six months, MacQuarrie knew that he was cured – his cough vanished, his wiry body, as brown as any islander's, now turning the scales at 154 lbs. Yet in part, he knew, the age-old routine of the islands, a life as simple and proscribed as Walter Perrett's, had done much to bring about his recovery: the leisurely 6 a.m. swim in the milk-warm lagoon at Taunoa, the peaceful mornings in his canoe with the fishermen beyond the reef, to bed by 9.30 p.m., like any Tahitian.

Yet this morning a recent memory had returned to disquiet him. It was prompted by a remark that Lovaina had meant only kindly: 'Johnnie says that party was the best ever – no one drunk, altogether jolly and nice.'

But MacQuarrie was less sure. The party was one that he had thrown himself, in his beach-house, ostensibly so that some local girls could demonstrate a true Tahitian *hula-hula* dance. At first it had all promised so well, with the candles twinkling among blood-red hibiscus blossoms and soft lemon-coloured lamps shining on baskets of green ferns and the traditional island feast Wong had prepared – cold sucking-pig, breadfruit, pineapple tarts. But when the Hotel Tiare's trap, driven by Vava, Lovaina's sullen deaf and dumb hired man, arrived with the dancing girls, the party had palpably hung fire. All six girls were as solemn as funeral guests.

It was Johnnie, Lovaina's nephew, who had persuaded MacQuarrie that a truly fearsome punch – a potent brew of gin, grenadine and white wine – would help break the ice. 'You've got to work 'em up,' he had encouraged the host, as glass after glass circulated.

MacQuarrie didn't like it. It dawned on him now that there

would be no dancing until every guest and every girl was tipsy, and as the evening wore on he watched with mingled shame and dismay as the soft sweet faces, framed in masses of coal-black hair, grew stupid with drink. Now they were capering and staggering in mad abandon, but MacQuarrie had sensed that in truth it was a dance of death he was watching: each girl irrevocably doomed to a slow decay through drink, disease, and the bought embraces of seamen. The memory he held fast of this night was of two of the girls finally collapsed in nausea on his verandah railing, moaning, 'Water – gimme water.'

Now, with an effort, he wrenched his attention back to Lovaina's chatter – the sullen Vava hovering jealously near, worshipping her as a mother, resenting that others should laugh and banter with her. Somehow Lovaina seemed as indestructibly part of Tahiti as the amphitheatre of mountains that cradled the lagoon: Lovaina, who had known Gauguin and the poet Rupert Brooke, the woman whom William Somerset Maugham was to immortalise one year later, as Tiaré Johnson, in his novel *The Moon and Sixpence*. But unlike Lovaina, the other Tahitians were defenceless: they needed help.

For MacQuarrie, the war was over, but he realised that it was to this gentle and vulnerable race that he owed his very life. Someday, he vowed, to cancel that debt – and to wipe out the shame of that party – he would find a way to repay them.

One man, reluctantly, had to acknowledge the truth: for him, the war was over before it had even begun. Under the clock at New York's Biltmore Hotel, a rendezvous legendary in the annals of courtship, twenty-year-old Lieutenant Charles Clapp Junior, of the Army Air Service, loitered impatiently. Only that morning the handsome young aviator had checked into town from Wilbur Wright Field, Dayton, Ohio, for the first time in months. Now, as the clock's hands moved towards 1 p.m., he was awaiting his lunch date, Margaret Macdonald, whom he had met first at a dance in Hotchkiss, Connecticut.

It was a date made on impulse earlier that morning, when they collided by chance in the Biltmore's lobby, as impulsively as Clapp did most things these days.

Despite his immaculately pressed uniform, his highly-polished cordovan boots, Clapp acknowledged that he was already slightly drunk, and for this he blamed the influenza entirely.

It had been the earlier wave of the epidemic – the one that hit John Lewis Barkley at Fort Riley, Kansas – that had been Clapp's undoing. The scion of a wealthy but teetotal New York family, living down the shame of a drunken grandfather, Clapp had never, as a Yale freshman, ventured more than a furtive glass of beer – but nine months back, in the A.A.S. Ground School, at Cornell University, he had found himself coming down with flu.

Now a wiseacre counselled a good shot of whisky as a pre-ventive, and the guilty curiosity that all Clapp's life had sur-rounded drinking would not be denied. Locked in the men's room of Ithaca's main hotel, along with a pint of rye, he had taken his first-ever gingerly sip of hard liquor.

The taste was truly appalling, yet somehow he was mes-merised from the start by the insidious larger-than-life effect. Gagging and heaving, the tears streaming down his face, Clapp had still gone on to down the whole pint.

From this moment on, Charles Clapp Junior had been irrevocably hooked and he knew it.

Now, in the past nine months, it had become plain that the war was too far gone for much hope of seeing action in France, and that at times Clapp was too consumed by liquor even to care. Instead he charted his travels through the training camps of the United States by the magnitude of his 'benders' ... San Diego, where the M.P.s had arrested him for drunkeness and Clapp, groping through a haze of hangover, had vomited in the lap of a provost lieutenant ... Dayton, where every night for four weeks had been given over to steady soaking, with Clapp and his buddies normally too drunk to be of any service to the women laid on by the bellhop ... Cincinatti, where a few of them, on a weekend, had managed to get through a whole suitcase of rye.

Already, braced hard on his heels beneath the Biltmore's clock, a dangerous little glow in his solar plexus told Clapp that he would be well and truly plastered by the cocktail hour, but he didn't worry. All that was on his mind was lunch – and more drinks – with Margaret at Sherry's at 45th and 5th.

If the flu came around again this fall, it didn't look like being serious; only this morning, *The New York Times*, quoting Health Commissioner Royal Copeland, had assured its readers: 'City is Not in Danger from Spanish Grip' – though the Commissioner did advise that any fellow kissing a girl would be wiser to do it through a handkerchief.

In any case, Clapp had no fears of catching it again. An old friend called White Rock would see to that.

As far as many fearful citizens were concerned, the epidemic was due to assume such dire proportions that nothing could stop it. Already they had observed signs and portents that told them the worst.

In Belém, on the Brazilian Amazon, a sailor praying before the statue of Our Lady of Consolation in the Basilica of Nazaré swore that the image shed a tear.

In Bangkok, Thailand, the British Embassy's doctor, T. Heyward Heys, noted with dismay that almost all his prize roses had withered and died, the blooms just wilting away. Something, he said, was in the air which would affect humans, too.

Over Montreal, the sky darkened, as with a thunderhead, but no storm followed, and a faith healer predicted a time of pestilence, when all the churches would close. Five months earlier, in the Breton village of Rétiers, a white mildew cloaked the leaves of the roadside trees, and the villagers had been convinced that they, too, would soon suffer. Overnight, owls came mysteriously to Paranhos da Beira, Portugal, hooting and screeching on every windowsill, in a mountain village which had never known owls before.

In a sickroom at Auckland, New Zealand, Nurse Alice Whittaker, keeping night watch at the bedside of an old and dying woman, glanced backwards at the window. Beyond the glass, she later testified, the Sign of the Cross lit up the sky.

At Sierra Leone, on the Gold Coast, there was merriment in the bar of the exclusive Freetown Club. A coloured labourer, recovering from a strange two-week coma, had told a preposterous story of being transported to another world, where a man claiming to be 'The Sword of the Archangel Gabriel' had bidden him read his Bible – above all, Joel, chapter II. Over their evening whisky-pegs, the bosses, in their trim white ducks, laughed uproariously; the man couldn't even read.

Finally, to crown the joke, someone fetched a Bible from the club's library, to trace the exact reference. And little by little, as he read aloud, the laughter died along the bar: 'Let all the inhabitants of the land tremble: for the day of the Lord cometh ... a day of clouds and of thick darkness ... nothing shall escape.

'The people shall be much pained: all faces shall gather blackness.'

Pale morning sunlight flooded through the shutters, and Dr Juan Zamora came suddenly awake in the big brass bedstead. For a moment he wondered if he had dreamed that irruption of noise, then it came again – a thunderous knocking at the door of the schoolmaster's house where he lodged, on the Calle de la Escuela, in the little Spanish town of Bijuesca. Someone was early abroad and wanting the doctor.

Knuckling sleep from his eyes, the twenty-three-year-old Zamora craned from the window. Below, in the sun-drenched canyon of the street, a peasant in rusty black, mounted on a sturdy mule, was peering anxiously upwards. 'Doctor, you must come at once,' he hailed the sleepy Zamora, 'we need help.'

He had come, the man explained, from Malanquilla, two and a half miles distant. Many were sick with a strange malady, and the parish priest could not bury the dead, for he was stricken, too. Beside the man, Zamora's eyes now took in

Don Mosen Buenaventura, the thin kindly old priest of Bijuesca. He would ride behind Zamora, the priest called up, to administer the last rites to those too far gone to need a doctor's help.

Hastily Zamora dressed as befitted a country doctor whose journeys were made at best on horseback, at worst on foot: corduroy jacket and trousers, with stout leather leggings, a hooded cape, the black beret known as a 'gorra', hastily adjusted over his dark sleek hair.

Next he checked the heavy black valise that would be stowed within his saddle-bag. Inside that valise were items as vital to his calling as the consecrated hosts and vial of holy oil that Don Mosen carried in his leather satchel; a hypodermic syringe, sterilised bandages and cotton wool, scalpel and surgical scissors, disinfectant, caffeine injections to stimulate the heart, ergot to arrest haemorrhage. In a moment he heard hoofs clatter on the cobbles. A servant, alerted by the priest, was bringing round his Arab from the stable.

In truth, the summons had come as no surprise. As a graduate of Madrid's top hospitals, the San Carlos and the Hospital Provincial, Zamora had followed the earlier milder epidemic that had swept the capital with more than passing interest – and only days earlier, the recurrence of the sickness had touched him in a painfully personal way.

Out of the blue, a telegram had summoned him to Siles, his home-town, 230 miles away; his twenty-four-year-old brother, Angel, the lawyer, was dangerously ill. It had been a wearisome three-day journey, but what had shocked Zamora profoundly was the fierce onslaught of this supposedly harmless infection. His brother had been dead long before he ever reached home.

The son of a small-town pharmacist, who had solved the costly problem of educating ten children by founding the local school, Zamora had at first chosen medicine as a career to help repay his father. Unlike a lawyer, who in Spain needed influence to obtain court work, a doctor was sure of an immediate job and was thus no longer a burden to his family. But now the disease had claimed Angel, the brother to whom he had been closest, Zamora felt more deeply involved than he cared to admit – warning himself that a doctor, must, above all, preserve detachment.

Yet on this warm September morning of 1918, Zamora was among the first to realise that this was no ordinary epidemic and that from this moment on he was as much in the front line as any Allied soldier fighting in France.

By 8 a.m. his Arab was tit-tupping lightly up the steep stony slope towards the plateau where Malanquilla lay. Behind him, Don Mosen clung tight to the horse's crupper; to the rear, the messenger on his mule kept silence, perhaps oppressed by the sights he had seen. In the early morning, the cold dry air of the Aragon region fretted their faces. Far away on the horizon loomed Mount Moncayo, capped with snow so white that it hurt the eyes.

Briefly, Zamora reflected on the irony of his presence here – to fight, of all things, an epidemic. When the year began he had spent four months as a clinical assistant in Valencia – at the same time carrying out his military service by standing in as night doctor at the Military Hospital. Near to breakdown from over-work he had opted for a tranquil spell as a country doctor in the medical district centring round Malanquilla. Then, days earlier, his colleague in Bijuesca had departed to look after a sick father. As of now, the young Zamora had sole charge of two medical districts, five small townships, scattered over twelve square miles.

It was lucky, he thought, that he knew the countryside as if he had memorised a relief map. Times without number, his horse had crossed the main Calatayud–Soria road, as it did now, on the outskirts of Malanquilla. He knew the town as intimately as he did Clares de Ribota and Torrelapaja.

Or so he had thought. As the riders entered the town's cobbled main street, a gasp was wrung from him. At this hour, Malanquilla was always vibrant with the colourful life of a close-knit Spanish community: women haggling over piles of tomatoes and lemons, donkeys laden with sacks of grain, children playing a clamorous game of *pelota* against the white-washed wall of the Plaza Marín.

Now the street was deserted. On housefront after housefront, the window-frames were boarded up, the homes abandoned. In the breathless mountain silence, Zamora could hear but one sound: the clatter of the Arab's hooves striking on the cobbles.

Then, by degrees, another sound took precedence – as persistent as the knocking that had earlier aroused him from slumber, echoing in grim counterpoint to the noise of the hoofbeats.

A moment, and then the realisation sank in. The hammer-blows of the local carpenter were fashioning rough plank coffins for the dead of Malanquilla.

It echoed across the world like a knell. The hammering that smote the ears of Juan Zamora in Malanquilla reverberated now in a thousand villages, a hundred cities. In the week that General Pershing's doughboys swept triumphantly through the St Mihiel salient, simultaneously, in a score of countries, the disease struck as remorselessly as a prowler in the night. It was in Freetown, Sierra Leone, where 500 stevedores on the water-front came down almost as one – and, in the same instant, was ravaging Budapest. It flared through every diamond mine on South Africa's Rand – and struck so hard at Rio Maior, Portugal, that the alarmed townsfolk barred their gates against frightened holidaymakers returning from the coast.

This was against all medical tradition, for always before influenza had travelled on a slow east-west axis, often taking months before making its presence felt.

In Leeuwarden, Holland, Private Jelle Beintema's canteen was now as cheerless as a darkened theatre; only six men in the entire barracks were still on their feet. Six hundred men had joined the four reluctant to do the 'bear-crawl' in Camp Devens' infirmary; six hundred sailors would soon follow suit in the Naval Hospital at League Island, Pennsylvania. By Thursday, 19 September it was in nine U.S. army camps – as far apart in location as Camp Dix, New Jersey, and Camp Gordon, Georgia.

It was in the *jhuggis* of Bombay, the infamous tar-paper and corrugated-iron slums infesting the Grant Road quarter, the bodies stacked like timber beside the burning ghats; by bitter irony, only the city's Untouchables – peóns, road-workers – condemned by a cruel caste system to exist as pariahs escaped the epidemic, for none would venture near them. It was in the narrow warren of streets stretching south of Rome's Piazza di Spagna, spawning 500 fresh cases a day, so that Deputy-Mayor Cremonesi ordered desperately: 'Spend whatever is necessary to get this disease under control.'

But which disease? All over the world, doctors were noting symptoms so at variance with the spring epidemic – and with any known form of influenza – that it might have been an unknown sickness. At Camp Sherman, Chillicothe, Ohio, it seemed to the Chief of Laboratory Service, Major Carey McCord, that every sufferer had been attacked by chlorine gas: each time a man so much as stirred on his pillow, serous fluid poured from his mouth and nostrils. In New York's Willard Parker Hospital, so many patients complained of 'a burning pain above the diaphragm' that Dr Henry Berg suspected the deep abdominal pain of Asiatic cholera – and in this same city, Dr Gedide Friedman, a veteran of Russian epidemics, had actually treated his first case as a cholera victim. Yet Dr Berg noted, too, the frontal headache that recalled typhoid fever.

What struck Dr Solomon Strouse, at Chicago's Michael Reese Hospital was the painfully congested conjunctivae – as if the patients, both men and women, had survived a sandstorm. One Swiss professor, seeing so many coated tongues with bright red tips, was convinced he was on to a scarlet fever epidemic. In Hammerfest, Norway, some doctors took the symptoms for a straightforward outbreak of food poisoning – and in many U.S. Army camps in France, scores of early cases were diagnosed as appendicitis.

At the United States Naval Hospital, Philadelphia, Lieutenant-Commander John Daland hit on another maverick symptom: what doctors term 'silent lungs', an absence of breath so total he was convinced his stethoscope had given out.

Indian doctors came down for sandfly fever, Irish doctors likened the illness to malignant typhus, and in Spain the symptoms varied so widely from region to region that many of Dr Juan Zamora's colleagues stood firmly by their own diagnoses, refusing to concede that the sickness was identical. It was, asserted Doctor Pittaluga, Professor of Tropical Diseases in Madrid's Medical School, an entirely new disease, unknown to science.

But not only Spanish doctors were flummoxed. Dr Rufus Cole, of New York's Rockefeller Institute, never forgot his visit to Camp Devens, along with Colonel William Welch, the dean of American medicine and one of the Institute's pioneers, at a time when cases at the camp totalled almost 11,000. In the autopsy room, as Welch inspected the blue swollen lungs of the first victims, with their wet foamy surfaces, Cole saw that he was 'quite excited, obviously very nervous'. 'This must be some new kind of infection or plague,' Welch ventured shakily, but to Cole the most shocking discovery was that the situation, momentarily at least, was too much even for the veteran sixty-eight-year-old Welch.

More puzzling still, the Institute's Dr O. T. Avery, using the crucial Gram test to probe the lung sections for influenza germs, could find no reaction at all – even after using every bottle marked 'alcohol' in the laboratory. Only when he sent to the store-room for a fresh supply did the long-awaited reaction appear. Someone had drunk all the alcohol in the first batch and refilled them with water.

It wasn't surprising Colonel Welch was alarmed. In hundreds of clinics and laboratories, doctors were now discovering that the true cause of death was asphyxia, as in a gas attack: an albuminous exudate in the alveoli (air sacs) of the lungs was checking the ability of the capillary blood vessels to supply oxygen. Worse, they were noting complications that no medical man had ever remotely connected with that winter perennial, influenza.

At Camp Lewis, Washington, Major William Kerr detected case after case of leucopenia – a kind of leukaemia in reverse, where the white corpuscles of the blood are strangely reduced in numbers. At Aldershot's Connaught Hospital, Major (later Sir) Adolphe Abrahams found that some victims had temporarily gone stone-deaf.

In Perth, Western Australia, twelve-year-old Mary Josephine Parsons lost her sight within six days, first developing cataracts, then total blindness; within weeks, she was learning Braille. From Waldeck, Germany, doctors reported gangrene of the sexual organs; in Chile, pathologists found the spleens of many autopsy subjects weighed over a pound as against the normal half-pound or less. One Italian teenager, Claudio Grezler, of Trento, was afflicted by diarrhoea so intense he endured twenty movements a day – yet Major Alexander Macklin, Royal Army Medical Corps, investigating the epidemic among the Russian Lapps, found most of the victims so constipated they had passed nothing for ten days.

On one factor, at least, all doctors were agreed: only in cholera did the collapse come so suddenly that most victims could fix the precise moment when they fell. Sometimes the first intimations were mundane – a man staggering home at a run, handkerchief clapped to a bleeding nose – but most often this killer-virus struck like a lightning-bolt.

North of Vestre Gausdal, Norway, twenty-three-year-old Tor Bådshaug swung his axe and the white splinters flew; one hundred feet above his head there was a creaking then a rustling as the great spruce fir bent slowly forward. As it fell, gathering momentum, striking at other trees, the rushing sound grew enormously and Tor realised it was no longer the sound of the fir that he heard but a terrifying vertigo inside his head, and he, too, fell forward, bathed in icy sweat.

By the Galeria Cruzeiro, in the heart of Rio de Janeiro, a man accosted Ciro Vieira Da Cunha, a young medical student:

'Excuse me, does the tram for Praia Vermelha stop here?'

'Yes, it does.'

'I am much obliged to you.'

With this banal exchange, the man fell dead. Fifty-five years later, Dr Da Cunha still recalls with awe: 'I saw a man take a street-car to death.'

One man literally took that journey. Off-duty in Cape Town, Driver Charles Lewis, of the Transport Corps, boarded a tram for his parents' home in Sea Point, three miles distant – but barely had the conductor signalled the start than the man collapsed on the platform, dead. It was Lewis himself who acted as starter – but within minutes a passenger had fallen dead, then another. Five times the tram was stopped to place the still-warm bodies on the pavement, for collection by municipal carts – but three-quarters of the way to Sea Point the driver, too, slumped forward and died. Absurdly glad to be still alive, Lewis walked home.

Some saved their lives by sheer chance. Near Amiens, Driver Albert Baker, of the British Army's Road Construction Company, was carefully manoeuvring his steam-roller along a shell-torn road when something felled him like a sandbag. With his last conscious thought, Baker toppled backwards from the roller – missing by inches the awful pressure of the wheel, 120 lb. to the square inch, as the monster lumbered on.

Acrobat Bertil Leman blessed the profession that had made falling from a dizzy height second nature. Just then unemployed, he was filling in time painting the proscenium arch of the Roda Kvarn Cinema in Umeå, Sweden, when, without warning, the attack came. Somehow, as the paint-pots sprayed outwards into space, expertise enabled Leman to ricochet down his ladder as effortlessly as a tumbler – landing shaken and unconscious where another would have broken his back.

For others it was a blessing in disguise. At the Collège Louis Léard, Falaise, France, seventeen-year-old Roger Dubois was profoundly relieved when the first symptoms hit him. A student teacher, he found his rowdy gibing pupils, some of them older than himself, a near-insupportable burden – the onset of flu would allow time for the moustache he was cultivating to lend him an air of authority.

Near Mount Kemmel, on the western front, Captain Albert Thorn, a company commander of the 30th Machine Gun Battalion, was *en route* to locate mule lines with his transport officer, Lieutenant John Parkin, when a terrifying weakness overtook him. Fearful that he would topple from his horse, Thorn dismounted at the medical centre in search of a pick-me-up – then, as the doctor was concocting it, passed out.

Next day, the horrified Thorn learned that at the cost of two other lives, the flu had spared his own. Rather than delay, Parkin had ridden on towards the front with Thorn's deputy, Captain Andrew Craig – and a mile along the road a shell had blown both of them to pieces.

In the hospitals, the doctors scarcely knew what to think. At the Middlesex Hospital, London, the resident Medical Officer, Dr Robert Parry, did little more now than 'direct the traffic' – speeding people who had collapsed in the street to the emergency wards or even the mortuary, so that B.I.D. (Brought in Dead) was now a routine entry in the Administration Book. At New York's Columbia Presbyterian Hospital, Dr Albert Lamb, Physician-in-Chief of the Outpatients' Department, phoned Acting Director Walter Palmer with grim intelligence on some new arrivals: 'They're as blue as huckleberries and spitting blood.'

And Major Victor Vaughan's earlier fears for the newly-enlisted doughboys were swiftly borne out – for none had experienced the years of trench warfare, of stress and privation, which seemed to guarantee Field-Marshal Haig's front-line Tommies almost total immunity from this second wave. Almost without exception, the first to succumb, as at Camp Sevier, South Carolina, were husky farmers, few of whom had ever known the city-bred infections of childhood. At Camp Dix, New Jersey, it was the men of the 'Sandstorm Division' – cowboys from Arizona and New Mexico – who fell as if pole-axed, while the pale-faced ghetto boys from Brooklyn stayed immune. As Dr Pierre Nolf, of the Belgian Army Medical Corps saw it, men with well-developed chests breathed more deeply – and thus more germs penetrated their lower respiratory passages. It was the same with their German adversaries: the body cells of stronger men, offering staunch resistance, killed the invading organisms too rapidly, flooding the body with lethal toxins.

By contrast, on tiny Pitcairn Island, midway between Australia and South America, the descendants of the *Bounty* mutineers logged only five fatalities among 174 islanders. Yet every man among them – including Parkins, great-great-grandson of the famous Fletcher Christian – had been rated too puny to pass an Army physical.

And whether Bombay coolie or Wall Street broker, Italian sharecropper or Russian commissar, it was always the same age-group – from 15 to 40 – that knew the greatest fatalities. This was unprecedented, for in past centuries influenza had slain only the aged and the sickly, and those with a poor pulmonary record. Now, for the first time, it was striking against the world's most vital and productive population group.

As yet unaware of the true gravity of the sickness, not everyone helped themselves as much as they might. In the fifth year of war, to keep up and about despite the odds had somehow become a way of life. In Naples, New York, packing-house Superintendent Leon Trembley had the most compelling of reasons not to give up: a wife, a small son and the best paid job he had ever had with New York Canners. Ignoring the first shivering fit, he carried on – and was dead within five days. Edna Brittingham, an auditor's clerk in Newport News, Virginia, had more frivolous reasons; she was determined to see the famous actress Maude Adams in *Madame X*, 'even if I have to be carried there on a stretcher'. Until an hour before the show she kept going, then collapsed – surviving to endure a headache that has persisted for fifty-five years.

And thousands who retired to bed disregarded the doctor's most vital caveat: don't get up until the temperature has been normal for four days. In Huntsville, Alabama, a premature urge to return to work, placed William Fanning in an embarrassing situation for a rural school principal; halfway to the schoolhouse he was reduced to crawling there on his hands and knees. One Lebanon, Indiana, farmer, Ermin Poer, recalls rising from bed then collapsing so regularly that his corn wasn't finally shucked until the following spring.

At first, the people's reaction was defensive: to treat the whole thing as a joke would somehow minimise the terror. Thus, when someone in the audience at Cape Town's Opera House coughed on the opening night of *The Pink Lady*, a long-forgotten musical comedy, the heavy at once ad-libbed: 'Ha! Spanish flu, I presume?' – and brought down the house.

A bizarre example of sick humour, 1918 style, went the rounds in Bergen, Norway: 'Mama, can I go out and play with Grandpa?' 'Be quiet, child, you've dug him up twice already.'

The Bright Young Things of Johannesburg flocked to a fancy dress ball at City Hall in Spanish dancing costume, with fans and tall starched head-dresses emblazoned 'Spanish Flu' – while their London counterparts held sneezing parties, with a bottle of champagne as a prize for the lustiest sneeze. And Gian Bino Quinto, a young Genoese factory worker, recovering from an early bout, patiently learned to play along when his workmates looked in each night to rib him: 'It's all right for you, you dirty pig, in bed with that Spanish tart.'

In a suite in Los Angeles' Alexandria Hotel, film producer Samuel Goldwyn paced the floor impatiently. Ten a.m. had come and gone, and still there was no sign of the three important bankers who had been due two hours earlier for a breakfast date – men of presumed integrity, coming all the way from New York to make a loan to his Culver City company.

Nor did the irate mogul ever learn that the shaken bankers had arrived and departed by the next train. Earlier, practical joker Sid Grauman, creator of the Chinese Theatre on Hollywood Boulevard, where film stars left their footprints in cement, had had the whimsical notion of placarding Goldwyn's door: 'STAY AWAY! PATIENT QUARANTINED.'

But soon enough the laughter died: a walk along any city

street became a terrifying experience for the most hardened observer. Newly-wed Alice Groves, arriving by train in Perth, Western Australia, was greeted by stretchers lining the entire length of the platform – and later, convalescing from a bout on her verandah she counted twenty-six funerals in three hours. Mrs Ida Evans, awaiting the lift in a Melbourne hotel lobby, instinctively recoiled when the gate slid back and a body on a stretcher was carried out. Dispassionately, the operator commented: 'Another flu victim.'

Even the professionals were taken unawares. In Phoenix, Arizona, the State Superintendent of Public Health, Dr Orville Harry Brown, was flabbergasted by one community doctor's telegram: 'Fifty cases of influenza, all mild, four deaths'. To Brown, the man's thinking was complacency itself: didn't he realise that his death rate was already eight per cent?

And ambulance attendant Perce Winter was never to forget one of the first cases he attended in Toowoomba, Queensland. Following an emergency call from the Ambulance Officer of a nearby town, Winter sped to the railway station to meet a patient off the 7 p.m. train – but though he searched every compartment he could find no one recumbent on a seat.

Suddenly a tall strapping young countryman hailed him: 'Are you looking for me?' Now Winter was more perplexed than ever: all the way to the hospital, the youngster sat bolt upright on the stretcher, chatting animatedly, the very picture of health. Convinced there had been some mistake, Winter waited until an intern had checked over the man and allotted him a bed then hurried off on another call.

It was a 140-mile round trip to collect a second patient, with time out for a bite of cold chicken and a pot of tea, but by 1 a.m. Winter was back in Toowoomba Hospital, helping his new patient to bed. Halfway across the ward, he stopped, aghast.

It had been exactly on the stroke of 7 p.m. when he picked up that husky young countryman at the station. But already his bed was ominously empty. He had gone so swiftly he might never have existed.

The thought worried Winter all that night: Did a man
know when he had just six hours to live?

In the old Butler Building, on Washington's New Jersey
Avenue, one man, in sombre silence, pondered the reports
spread before him on the wide mahogany desk. Early on the
morning of Wednesday, 18 September, Surgeon-General
Rupert Blue, Chief Public Health Officer of the world's most
powerful nation, had routed a cogent telegram to the Health
Officers of forty-eight states. The message had been as brief
as it was vital: 'Request all information regarding the pre-
valence of influenza in your State'.

Now, one day later, the reports that Blue studied made plain
that the Spanish Lady had not only passed through all of
New England but along the entire Atlantic Coast to the
Virginia Capes – and there were ominous foci, too, in the
States west of the Mississippi. The challenge facing Blue in
the days ahead was assuming tangible and frightening shape.

No man was better fitted to meet it. At 50, a genial heavily-
built native of North Carolina, Blue had sole command of
180 Health Officers and forty-four quarantine stations throughout the United States, and his easy charm of manner had in
times past smoothed over many an impasse. For twenty-six
years, since he first donned the royal-blue uniform of the PHS,
he had been respected as a front-line fighter, the man who had
triumphantly battled bubonic plague in San Francisco and
yellow fever in the Vieux Carré of New Orleans. He was no
desk-bound commander, retreating behind an aloof barrage of
memos; some of the most welcome visitors to Blue's Washington office were shabbily-dressed rat-catchers and ditch-diggers
with whom he had laboured in the past.

Yet on 19 September, Blue faced many problems unknown
in the free-wheeling days of the Barbary Coast and the French
Quarter. Only in a four-alarm emergency had the Surgeon-
General powers to override any State authority; for the most
part his role was to suggest tactfully, seeking rather than
enforcing cooperation, for many States had widely divergent

attitudes to the problem of influenza. In not every one was influenza reportable, and as many allowed public funerals as forbade them.

Nor was flu, in contrast to exotic plagues like cholera and typhus, even a quarantinable disease. When the second wave of infection first hit New York, at the moment on 12 August when the Norwegian liner *Bergensfjord* tied up at the sprawling Army Base in Brooklyn, and the first victim on the American Continent, passenger Jenine Olsen, died within hours, Health Commissioner Royal Copeland had to abide by the regulations as they stood. Neither Blue nor Copeland nor even President Wilson himself had any power to stop the liner docking.

There were other problems, too, and ones which Blue, on this day, shared with almost every Health Officer in the world. The First World War had proved a relentless siphon, drawing away thousands of officers and nurses to the fighting front. Out of 140,000 American doctors, fully 40,000 had enlisted; eleven days earlier, the Army School of Nursing had reported only 221 'green probationers' on duty in seven cantonment hospitals.

It was the same all over the world. In Paris, Minister of the Interior Jules Pams could not call on one doctor under sixty-five; with 19,000 French doctors under arms, many country districts were now in the valiant if shaky hands of octogenarians. The 366,000 square miles of British Columbia alone had ceded 200 doctors to the armed forces. Britain was down to one doctor for 5000 patients, a strain that had proved fatal to many older men, and in Hungary the villages round Lake Balaton had seen no doctor for more than five years.

As frustrating as the shortage of doctors was the hidebound lethargy of many authorities. Although eight years had elapsed since South Africa achieved Union, no steps had been taken towards the creation of an efficient central Department of Health – and in many rural areas of the Transvaal, Orange Free State and Natal, no health authority existed at all. Much the same problem hampered Australia's Director of Quarantine, Dr John Howard Cumpston, who hadn't even power to declare a State infected unless the State itself so requested.

In a second-floor Whitehall office, within the shadow of Big Ben, at the headquarters of Britain's sole medical authority, the Local Government Board, the Chief Medical Officer, Sir Arthur Newsholme, viewed the situation with mounting unease – as well he might. As far back as July, alerted by his experts, Newsholme had foreseen such an epidemic, and actually drawn up a warning memorandum to local authorities throughout Britain – then, incredibly, had taken no action whatsoever.

As Newsholme saw it, orders to local police to check overcrowding on trams and buses, or to factories to stagger working hours, might not only create panic but critically slow down Britain's momentous all-out war effort. On Newsholme's decision alone, this memo had been shelved – a decision which, in the weeks ahead, would be in part responsible for the loss of 228,000 British lives.

To do them justice, Britain's Medical Research Council had, as early as 10 August, forecast a second more serious epidemic by autumn – and had urged bacteriologists everywhere to collate their findings and forward them as early as possible. Yet the newly-formed Council, allotted a meagre budget of only £50,000 a year, carried little clout. As one of the Army's top brass had put it to the Council's Secretary, Walter Fletcher: 'Damn research, sir – we've got to get on with the war.'

As Newsholme later admitted, it was a pity more bacteriologists hadn't responded to that initial appeal, but they had his entire sympathy. He had quite neglected to read the Council's memorandum himself.

In this mounting hour of unease, Newsholme had no plan at all for coping with an emergency, should one arise. Though British regulations listed no less than nineteen notifiable diseases, influenza, despite the alarming death rate of 1890, when thousands of Britons perished, was not among them. In Britain, as elsewhere, the flu had always been undersold, a trivial case of the snuffles, a term so loosely-used, so widely and wrongly diagnosed, that Edinburgh's Local Government Officer, Thomas Finlayson Dewar, had found cases of mumps, smallpox, measles and cerebro-spinal fever – all of them pronounced as flu.

Thus, on 19 September, when Surgeon-General Blue alerted his officers across the United States, the 172 sovereign nations, republics, protectorates and Crown colonies that made up the world of 1918 had one thing in common: in none of them was influenza a notifiable disease, and no bill stood before any legislative assembly to see that it became so.

But if the central authorities almost everywhere were woefully unprepared, the men and women who would bear the brunt of the epidemic were ready. In Copenhagen, the Ministry of Justice, who oversaw public health, advised by a committee of doctors and chemists, had just complacently declared that it had 'no authority to legislate on influenza' – but 160 miles away, in the village of Ejstrup, Nurse Else Dahl was more than determined.

In the kitchen of the ground-floor flat attached to the Dahls' hardware store, Else, purposefully whipping egg-yolks in a basin, was preparing the evening meal and arguing about it yet again with Marius, her husband. 'I want to help,' she persisted, but just as before Marius shook a stubborn head. 'I will not allow it,' he told her curtly, 'The risk is too great.'

Else Dahl was not giving up. A dark forthright twenty-five-year-old, whose habit of smoking potent black cigars had long intrigued the little farming community, Else had always given as good as she got where menfolk were concerned. At first, her father, a border patrolman and a devout churchgoer, had been adamant that Else should accompany him regularly to church, but even he had met his match in the face of the child's implacable resistance. In the end, she had gone to church as often as he had wished – but only once the old man had substantially increased her allowance as a bribe. 'It's such a bore with all those old people,' Else explained cheerfully, 'but the money makes it bearable.'

Not that Else Dahl hadn't lived a good and useful life until now. At eighteen, fired by the example of her mother, the district midwife, she had undergone her nurse's training at Copenhagen's Kommunehospitalet, often studying for twenty-four hours at a stretch – the cigars, which helped keep her awake during the small-hours bookwork, were a legacy from that time. Then, holidaying with an uncle and aunt in Ejstrup, after her finals, she had met and liked young Marius Dahl, the ironmonger. Once again, Else had known her own mind. Promptly, to see as much of Marius as possible, she had signed on as the parish nurse.

Four years earlier, they had married in little Fellund church, where Else had been confirmed – and the changes that time had wrought since then were a salient part of Marius' objection. Now, he pointed out, as Else bustled from kitchen table to stove, they had three-year-old Kirsten, their daughter. Now he had a staff of four men and two girls, all of whom lived on the premises as a united family and took their meals with the Dahls.

'How would you feel?' he challenged Else, 'if Kirsten fell ill – and the staff?'

Else was unyielding. The Spanish flu was a fact now – no longer an uneasy rumour. The shoemaker had it, all the family at the inn had it, it was days since they had seen some of their neighbours. Meanwhile, since her marriage, no district nurse had replaced her – and the doctors were all too busy in the hospitals to spare time for rural Ejstrup.

'If we're supposed to get the Spanish flu, we'll get it,' Else countered. 'We can't be sure it'll be *I* who'll bring it in.'

'We cannot risk it,' said Marius sharply. 'We are responsible for our daughter and staff.'

Else made one last attempt. 'But we have so many customers coming to our shop each day. If one of them's infected with it, we'll get it anyway.'

Angrily Marius snatched up the newspaper – a clear indication that the discussion was at an end. 'I will not allow it,' he repeated yet again.

Else said no more just then – merely set saucepans to simmer, biding her time. Still there was an inner conviction that would not let her rest. Though by no means as devout as her father, she was yet, in a quietly undemonstrative way, a religious girl – and her family's whole life, moreover, had been a tradition of service. This conviction was as real as the husband who, one moment earlier, had stood angrily before her: a belief that God wanted her to play a part in this sickness which had been troubling Denmark without cease, ever since the summer.

If she was right, then nothing Marius or anyone else could say would ever stop her. When the time was ripe, she would know. God would send her the sign.

All that summer, on the plain below Stalag Josefstadt, the Russians had been dying, and the Italians, too. In another age, the grim eighteenth-century pile, forty-seven miles from Prague, built by the Emperor Josef II of Bohemia as a fortress against the Germans, had seemed proof not only against Teuton invaders but against pestilence itself. Now medical officers like Lieutenant Enrico Bedeschi saw it for what it was: a granite sham whose ramparts and bastions were breached time and again by the tireless onslaughts of death.

In the ten months since he had fallen prisoner to the Austrians at Caporetto, death, to the twenty-seven-year-old Bedeschi, had become an old familiar. Seconded as a medical officer to tend the Russian and Italian prisoners of Lager E, he had known it could not be otherwise. Supplies were so scarce that his tiny dispensary held little more than powdered digitalis, opium and bismuth cachets. Instruments were non-existent; aided by two fur-hatted Cossack orderlies, Bedeschi had even pared a shattered thigh-bone with a carpenter's plane, and trepanned a cranium with a hammer and chisel.

Thus, to Bedeschi and his colleagues, the distinction between the lagers on the plain below, where the prisoners were crammed on heaps of straw and shavings, 150 to a hut, and the cemetery beyond the barbed wire, had grown daily less defined.

Then, towards spring, the death rate among the Russians had soared alarmingly. Within hours of the first symptoms –

high fever, dyspnoea, cyanosis – men had breathed their last. No longer was there time to dig graves; in their threadbare grey overcoats, men were piled twenty at a time beneath tell-tale hummocks of snow. Once, tugged between compassion and a sense of his own unworthiness, Bedeschi, posing as a military chaplain, had even absolved a delirious Italian from confession.

The chaplain had been busy elsewhere, and the soldier had died so swiftly there had been no time to summon him.

Spurred to protest, Bedeschi, along with his fellow medicos, had stomped off to Oberst Koscario, the Russian commandant, to demand both drugs and instruments to combat the death rate. There followed weeks of irksome delay, until the hard-pressed Austrian High Command came up with the only sup-plies they could muster: for each doctor, a scalpel, scissors, pincers, a litre of alcohol, and, in place of bandages, corrugated paper.

Above all, Bedeschi prized the scalpel, for, mysteriously, all who survived this scourge broke out in purple-black abscesses on their arms and legs, which called for swift incision. Even so, he could disinfect his instrument only after every three operations. The alcohol, the Commandant had stressed, must last a year, for no more would be forthcoming.

At first Bedeschi had been puzzled that cases of dropsy, typhus and even dysentery should all develop the same alarm-ing symptoms of broncho-pneumonia. But rations were so sparse – bone-stock with pearl barley, bonemeal bread with a gram of margarine – that now, in the autumn of 1918, he knew well enough the cause of this soaring death-rate: malnu-trition.

As isolated from his homeland as any Russian, Dr Enrico Bedeschi was blissfully unaware that any epidemic even existed to challenge his medical skills.

One man knew all too well – and the knowledge had aroused in him a cold and deadly anger. At 3 p.m. on Tuesday, 24 September, more than 500 French Deputies, ranged tensely on the crimson velvet benches of the Salle des Séances, in the Palais Bourbon, Paris, saw the Deputy for the Côtes-du-Nord, fifty-year-old Gustave, Comte de Kerguézec, whose constituency embraced Brittany and its seaports, rise to confront Navy Minister Georges Leygues with a question that brooked no equivocation.

In the hushed autumn-hazy chamber, the Count's voice rang out, audible at the farthest points of the eighteenth-century hall. It was a shocking fact, he told the Minister, that he had to reveal. At Brest and Lorient, 450 young sailors had died in squalor and misery from this dread epidemic – deaths which need never have taken place. All had been fit men, yet they were drafted from the depot at Rochefort to coastal barracks more than 200 miles north, to be infected by men already down with flu.

Now De Kerguézec, a two-fisted crusader whose faith embraced such tenets as the abolition of the nobility and stringent lower-deck reforms, was calling on Leygues to justify those deaths – the first of many such challenges with which concerned men throughout the free world would harass authority from this time on.

A veteran politician, Leygues was, above all, a shrewd infighter when it came to debate. As such, he first sought to distract the Chamber by playing on nationalist sentiment. The epidemic, he charged, was entirely the fault of the Swiss, who had brought it across the frontier – and was gratified by the storm of anger that greeted his words.

More confidently, Leygues went on. The disease had been prevalent for six months – but not more so in the Atlantic ports than elsewhere. True, recruits were a favourable target for infection, but all prophylactic measures had been taken, and the sickness had shown every sign of dying down.

'We continue to fight the epidemic in every way possible,' he avowed, and a satisfied rumble of 'Good! Good!' greeted this assurance.

De Kerguézec was implacable. 'The men were mixed instead of isolated. Who was responsible for their deaths?'

Now Leygues shifted his ground. In many ways, the depots were to blame, though this could hardly be remedied. No Ministry in the height of a war could demolish and rebuild seventeenth-century barracks.

De Kerguézec would not yield. Then why had the men been transferred from the Lorient barracks to the filthy training ship *Caledonien*, 700 to a peak, in conditions so primitive they couldn't even wash. He knew this ship well, De Kerguézec said: the portholes didn't close, the bulwarks leaked water on to the trainees' hammocks, the heads were indescribable. And where 1500 men should have been quartered at most, there were now 4000. Again his voice echoed, as challenging as the conscience of France: 'Who is responsible?'

Minister Leygues squirmed with vexation. From the start, he insisted, everything possible had been done and *was* being done. No sooner had he heard of the deaths than he had ordered the barracks evacuated and tents set up along the beach, while recruiting and drafting had been suspended. In any case, he would remind the Deputy for the Côtes-du-Nord, the situation had been worse by far in April.

For answer, De Kerguézec flung back the cold irrefutable statistics that gave the Minister's words the lie. But in April, he protested, the men had been dying at the rate of five or six a month. 'Now,' he told the shocked and silent Chamber, 'it's five or six a day.'

Gustave, Comte de Kerguézec, might not have agreed, but in one way, at least, the French sailors had been lucky: on dry land they stood something of a sporting chance. For thousands cooped up on troopships throughout the world, there was little hope if the epidemic should gain ground. Twenty-one hours after the French Deputy's impassioned plea in the Chamber, at 12.30 on the cold raw noonday of 25 September, one such convoy, HX-50, sixteen strong, steamed past the fog-shrouded Statue of Liberty in New York Harbour: 20,000 American soldiers, bound for the United Kingdom ports of Liverpool and Glasgow.

As Corporal Harold Rath, of the 126th Field Artillery still recalls it, few men aboard the convoy's thirteen merchantmen were scared of being 'tinfished' – the doughboys' slang for 'torpedoed'. By now, the Atlantic route was well policed for submarines, and the freighters had a considerable escort, besides: two American cruisers, the U.S.S. *St Louis* and the U.S.S. *Louisiana*, and a destroyer, the U.S.S. *Dorsey*. Aboard Transport 641 – the 6000-ton *Otranto*, once an Orient Line mail steamer – the talk was all of the Spanish flu, and the British sailors who manned her had taken a ghoulish delight in recounting the ravages of the disease in Europe.

Nor could the medics derive much comfort from the memo which the Surgeon-General's Office of the Army had issued only one day earlier: 'No disease which the Army surgeon is likely to see in this war will tax more severely his judgement and initiative.'

There was scant comfort to be found below decks either. The cramped mess-tables, running crosswise beneath the hammock hooks, the sickening odour of phenol, like a hospital – it all added up to a death-trap, and to make matters worse, on the night of the 24th, with the ships still at the pierhead, many men had been coughing. That very morning, before sailing, Captain Charles Dickson, Medical Corps officer aboard *Otranto*, had rousted out nine sufferers and dispatched them to a New York hospital.

It was much the same aboard the 8900-ton *Kashmir*, where Corporal Rath and his artillery buddies were quartered. Their living-space was bounded by the sloping steep walls of the ship, at all times cold and sweating, and since the hammocks were slung lengthwise, the sleeping troops, if the ship pitched, would swing with each roll of the vessel. And most men griped loudly, too, at one of the first orders given out on embarkation: under penalty of the brig, each soldier must wear a heavy lifebelt athwart his body all through the voyage.

Almost every man in the convoy had travelled an infected road. Many, hailing from Fort Screven, Georgia, had come via Raleigh, North Carolina, Baltimore and Philadelphia – all

cities stricken with flu, at which they had detrained to stretch
their legs. Others, one week earlier, had journeyed from Fort
Sill, Oklahoma, to Camp Upton, Yaphank, Long Island, to
find 900 of its inmates down with pneumonia, but even this
hadn't halted the preparations for departure – trading in khaki
uniforms for winter O.D.S., hobnails for tan shoes, with every
man yielding his hair to the horse-clippers for an aseptic
'overseas hair-cut'.

To some, it seemed the convoy was jinxed from the start. At
Nantucket Lightship, word came that two German submarines
were lurking ahead – so the *Otranto*'s Captain Ernest Davidson, Convoy Commander of HX-50, decided on a northern
course, zig-zagging round the banks of Newfoundland. Ahead
lay rough weather, a sore trial for landlubbers who had never
seen the sea, but a preferable risk, Davidson thought, to German U-Boats.

Not all would have agreed. Within hours, the pitching of
the ships grew worse. Plunging and wallowing in the troughs,
the men found their sea-sickness more terrible than any fear
of the Germans; most were too sick to shave, let alone to eat.
Soon the greenish-yellow faces were coated with a harsh stubble
of beard; with the smell of phenol, stewed mutton and bitter
black tea, there mingled now the acrid smell of vomit. Worse,
everyone was now too ill for the medics to distinguish flu
victims from the others – though later reports suggested that
Otranto, for one, had 100 cases, *Kashmir*, 2068 troops aboard,
almost three times that number.

Seasick nights followed seasick days – nights in which Convoy HX-50 ran without lights, a habit of ships in war. Then
disaster struck. By sheer misfortune, the convoy's course now
crossed that of twenty-two fishing barques, also running without lights. With a bone-jarring thud, one of them, the barque
Croisine, scraped the whole length of the *Otranto*'s port side,
carrying away one of her life-boats, littering the *Otranto*'s
deck with broken spars. Then, helplessly, she drifted to the
stern of the transport, off to the port side.

Under the brilliant glare of a searchlight, the *Otranto*

lowered a boat, with Lieutenant F. R. O'Sullevan and a crew aboard her. As the oarsmen pulled through the light swell towards the barque, long anxious minutes followed, a silence broken only by the creaking of rowlocks. Though *Otranto*'s engines were throttled down, her searchlight bathed the whole sea with a white uncanny light – a perfect target for any German submarine. It went on for so long that finally Captain Davidson shouted a peremptory order : 'Transfer that barque's crew.'

At length, O'Sullevan returned with the *Croisine*'s survivors – Captain Jules Le Hoerff, a huge grizzled man, bearded like an old-time picture-book sailor, along with his sleek New-foundland dog and thirty-six of his crew. Now Captain Davidson lost no time in breaking the worst to them : the crippled *Croisine*, as a menace to navigation, must be sunk forthwith. Like it or not, the fishermen must travel with *Otranto* to England.

On *Otranto*'s bridge, the two Captains watched, motionless, as the gunners sought the correct range. Then, as they found it, twenty-five shells crashed into *Croisine*, and within minutes she was burning fiercely, the night sky dancing with the dull red glow. More shells found her three-inch gun and her am-munition hold, and as burning planks shot skywards like rockets, men stood silent all along *Otranto*'s deck, bereft of words.

Only later did Le Hoerff break it casually to Davidson that his barque, laden with dried cod, had been just then returning from the Grand Bank, south-east of Newfoundland – an area where the epidemic was to reap as deadly a toll as anywhere in the world.

Dr J. S. Koen bent forward and prodded the hog again, but it was useless. The beast merely sprawled on its flank in the pig-pen, sweating, eyes closed, breathing hard. Normally Koen, an Inspector for the Division of Hog Cholera Control of the Bureau of Animal Industry, was too wary a man to take liberties with three hundred pounds of mean-tempered boar, but this hog had no fight left in him. Even prodding and shouting wouldn't rouse him.

Amazingly, it was no lone example. At 8 p.m. on Monday, 30 September, the National Swine Breeders' Show was nearing the sorry end of its first day's exposition at Cedar Rapids, Iowa. Among the exhibition pens of the William Holland Building, literally hundreds of hogs were in the same plight as the one Koen now surveyed.

Poland China Junior Yearling Boars, Berkshire Grand Champion Sows, some of them priced at $15,000 apiece – all of them lay prostrate among the red cedar shavings, breathing painfully from the stomach, at times afflicted by a sharp hacking cough. Often there was muscular tenderness, too – the lightest touch and the hog cried out pitifully.

Within five days, the National Swine Show would come to a disastrous close. Totting up untold losses, the breeders would move out for their home farms, along with all those hogs fit enough to travel back with them. Soon, to their dismay, millions of hogs that had remained in the droves back home were down with it, too – not only in Iowa but all over the middle west.

It was less surprising to Koen. All week he nourished the lone theory that this was a disease a long way removed from any other he had ever seen afflicting hogs – yet strangely akin to the so-called 'Spanish influenza' that had recently hit the citizens of Cedar Rapids.

Other veterinarians to whom Koen had voiced the theory were cautious, and most breeders were downright indignant – didn't Koen realise that talk like that could ruin the pork market once for all? But Koen was unrepentant. From what he had seen, the diseases were one and the same, and by this reckoning a new disease rated a new name. When the Bureau of Animal Industry, back in Washington, got his report, he'd identify it as 'hog flu'.

For the first time he wondered. Were the humans giving it to the hogs – or were the hogs maybe giving it to the humans?

CHAPTER THREE

'Are We Going to be Wiped Out?'

1 October—8 October 1918

Of all the crises in the life of Dr Frederick Willmot, Cape Town's Assistant Medical Officer of Health, the phone-call that posed his city's dilemma in one anguished question was perhaps the worst. On the wire, his voice tight with emotion, was his old friend William Davies, a wealthy building society director, newly arrived from Groote Schuur, four miles distant.

'Will you answer a straightforward question,' Davies was asking. 'Are we going to be wiped out?'

No longer could Willmot temporise. 'I'll tell you what I wouldn't tell any other man in the Union,' he had to admit. 'For the first time in my life I'm panicky, and I believe we are.'

It was a daunting confession – yet none knew better than Willmot and his chief, Dr Jasper Anderson, that Cape Town was a stricken city. All along the Peninsula, from Sea Point, through the slums of Salt River and Woodstock, to the wooded retreats of the wealthy by False Bay, the plague was sparing neither man, woman nor child. Unspoken in the minds of Willmot and Anderson was the question only Davies had dared to ask: How long could Cape Town hold out?

For both doctors, too, there was the bitter realisation that the Union Government, based 960 miles away in Pretoria, had given no lead whatsoever in combating the disease now ravaging the Cape. As far back as 1 September, word had reached them that 500 black stevedores had been struck down in Sierra Leone – yet all along the Department of Health had stuffily insisted that local problems must be dealt with by local authorities. Cape Town must shift for itself.

What followed was shameful neglect. On 13 September, the s.s. *Jaroslav*, outward bound from Sierra Leone, steamed into Cape Town's Table Bay. Aboard were 1500 workers of the Native Labour Corps, returning from war service. In a nightmare nine-day voyage, ninety had already died from Spanish influenza – yet no one had thought to warn Anderson in advance. In any case, not until one month later – on 14 October – did the Union Government declare 'epidemic influenza' an illness 'for which isolation (quarantine) is necessary'.

Thus, as things then stood, neither Anderson nor Willmot had had power to prevent any man able to make a shaky progress down the *Jaroslav*'s gangway from entering Cape Town – or from entraining for cities, town and kraals all over South Africa.

Within days the horrified medics saw the pandemic for what it was: a Pale Horseman, outriding even war. On Cape Town's Main Street, Adderley Street, men and women stopped as suddenly as if stabbed, clutching desperately at lamp-posts or telegraph-poles – then slid, in agonising slow motion, to collapse unconscious at the base.

It was suddenly a desperate race against time. Above all, the sick must be fed: for the first time in history, the soup kitchen, by now a European commonplace, had reached more sheltered shores. Anderson and Willmot had sent out a city-wide call for women to make soup, but though volunteers weren't lacking, another problem arose: the butchers were all too sick to dismember the carcasses. In the nick of time, 100 medical students from the University of Cape Town filled the breach, trading in their scalpels for cleavers.

Soon City Hall more resembled a vast provision store: raw sides of beef piled higgledy-piggledy among crusty loaves of bread, sacks of potatoes, polished pyramids of carrots and onions, a veritable ossuary of bones for stock. Medicines, too, weren't lacking, for Anderson was currently faced with 8000 applications a day. But now another crisis became apparent. The disease was striking so hard and so fast that some households lacked even one member able to visit a depot and pick up supplies.

More volunteers had been the answer, but though Anderson and Willmot had a non-stop shuttle service of 150 private cars and twenty-seven trucks, they would need many more yet.

Hence Willmot's relief at William Davies' call, for though the business-man demanded the stark facts, he still had a course of positive action to propose. Now he urged: 'Can you get me Ellerslie Girls' High School at Sea Point?'

'But whatever for?'

'I'll turn it into a hospital at once.'

Willmot knew an overwhelming relief, for where Davies led, Cape Town's company directors, lawyers and other prominent citizens would surely follow as volunteers. Overjoyed, he shouted back: 'Then get on with it! And if anyone opposes you, break down the doors and refer them to me.'

Before cradling the phone, he recalled an old Bantu proverb, destined to become South Africa's watchword in the embattled days ahead: '*Ningadinwa nangomso.*' (Don't be tired, even tomorrow.)

Soon it would be dawn. Across the 1200 square miles of the Witwatersrand (the Ridge of the White Waters), the world's largest goldfields, soft yellow light would suffuse the sandy hummocks of the mine dumps. Engine-house chimneys, the huge spinning-wheels of the winding engines: all were etched, black and skeletal, against the paling sky. It was 3 a.m. 1 October 1918.

At Farrar Shaft, Driefontein Section, East Rand Proprietary Mines, 100 miles from Bloemfontein, Driver William Hill had still three hours to go before clocking off. Now, at the controls of the winding engine, he was engaged on one more routine assignment: hoisting the steel cage, packed with forty helmeted Basotho miners, 3000 feet from the bowels of the earth to ground level.

Momentarily his eye caught the notice: 'Spanish Influenza: In the event of a driver feeling indisposed, he is to stop hoisting immediately and inform the banksman.' A conscientious driver, nine years on the job, Hill fully understood the implications; for ten days now the sticker had been a fixture on the engine-house wall. Still he felt no premonition.

Without warning, icy sweat drenched his body. The strength seemed to be ebbing from his limbs, and he knew with sudden desperation that at all costs he must stop the engine. He rose, grasping the reversing lever and one of the brake levers.

'Powerless to act', Hill spun backwards to his seat. His brain was still diamond-clear, but 'a multitude of lights' was exploding before his eyes. He could no longer see his hands. Both, though he didn't know it, were resting impotently on the brake lever. The reversing lever was now unmanned.

On the built-up area surrounding the shaft as a precaution against storm water, banksman Carl Celitz stood transfixed. Swooping past the collar of the shaft, the cage was now ploughing upwards towards the headgear. Bells rang frantically in the darkness, the warning bell, the bank bell. Then, with a rending splintering crash the cage struck the headgear, the overwind ripping away the winding rope like a strand of twine.

Plummeting at 1000 feet a minute the cage left the rails and crashed backward, to smash with awful impact against the timbered rim of the shaft's mouth, 100 feet below.

Fireman William Ackerberg, the first on the scene, found an appalling sight: the overturned cage jammed across the collar of the shaft ... black sightless faces eerily illuminated by the light of a storm lantern ... picks, helmets, safety-lamps and lunch pails, all scattered in wild confusion among the dead and the dying.

In the engine-house, Hill, his senses now fully recovered, slammed on both brake levers.

Soon a doctor would certify William Hill as a Spanish influenza victim – and a court of enquiry would absolve him, accordingly, of all criminal neglect. Pale and shaken, he was just then descending from the engine-house in search of medical aid. Already, to the east, the sky was paling: a dawn that twenty-four Basotho miners would not now see.

For all those entrusted with the lives of others, these were anxious hours – not least among them Captain Edward Davidson of the *Otranto* and Captain Edmund Bartlett of the *Kashmir*.

Every since that fateful night near the Grand Banks, when the barque *Croisine* had struck the *Otranto*'s port side, disaster in the shape of Spanish flu, had dogged Convoy HX-50. And though the *Croisine*'s grizzled Jules Le Hoerff and his crew had come from flu-ridden Newfoundland, there is no doubting many cases had eluded the medics' expert scrutiny before the ships even left New York.

Then, on 2 October, while the *Otranto*, following the collision, was racing to overtake the convoy, death came upon the waters. Now the *Otranto*'s engines were throttled almost to stop, and to a volley of rifle fire, the first flu fatality, Pte Lonnie Smith of Fort Screven, was eased gently over the side, draped in the American flag.

By 3 October, almost every ship in the convoy was flying its flag at half mast.

Hardest hit of all were *Kashmir* and *Otranto*. By 5 October *Otranto* had reported a second victim – and aboard *Kashmir*, the hospital in the after-end was now so crowded the patients were stretched out on mess-tables, each man's legs straddling another's. Soon the medics had to allot their own priorities: no man with a temperature below 104°F was eligible for treatment. Faced with hundreds of sufferers and one crate of lemons, thought valuable as a febrifuge, the Chaplain of the 126th Field Artillery found only a razor-blade would yield enough wafer-thin slices.

Thus at 8.43 a.m. on Sunday, 6 October as a hurricane-strength Force 11 wind lashed the Atlantic off the coast of Northern Ireland, almost every man in the convoy was fighting just to keep going. And aboard *Otranto*, at least 100 men were so prostrate with flu none could have moved if their lives depended on it, which, tragically, they did.

By now, every ship was hopelessly lost; in the buffeting south-west gale, their cruiser escort had eluded them and they were proceeding by dead reckoning – at least twenty miles north of their true course and now within sight of the Scottish isle of Islay. It was black misfortune that Captain Davidson, on *Otranto*'s bridge, should only now have noticed that *Kashmir* was veering fatally close to him. Again too late, he ordered: 'Hard aport.'

Above the banshee fury of the storm, on *Kashmir*'s bridge, Bartlett heard the warning blasts from *Otranto*'s siren and ordered 'Hard astarboard.' But somehow, within seconds this order was reversed: *Kashmir*, too, went hard aport. By now the epidemic had taken such toll, it was hard for any man to comprehend orders, let alone obey.

Those few soldiers above decks on *Otranto* now saw a sight to send them scattering for their lives: the cruel black prow of the *Kashmir* looming through the mist and rain like a monstrous leviathan on the crest of a forty-foot wave. Then, with the inhuman screech of steel against steel, the *Kashmir* knifed eight feet into *Otranto*'s port side below the waterline ... slicing into the boiler-rooms below the forward and aft stokeholds ... drowning every stoker within seconds.

From *Kashmir*'s bridge, Captain Bartlett watched sick at heart: as the waters found *Otranto*'s fires, a vast geyser of steam shot skywards, pressing above the sea. The symbolism appalled him; it was as if the dying ship had gasped forth her last breath.

In a sense, it was true. Those 100 flu cases below decks had never stood a chance – but by 10 a.m., as the British destroyer *Mounsey* hastened to the scene, alerted by S.O.S. signals from an emergency wireless set, the epidemic was to cruelly impede even the work of rescue. As the *Mounsey*'s Captain, Lieutenant-

Commander Francis Craven, R.N., saw it, the survivors' sole hope was to leap from *Otranto*'s starboard side as the destroyer came alongside.

Seizing a loud-hailer, Captain Davidson protested: in the plunging seas, *Mounsey*'s risk was too great. But Craven – awarded one of the First World War's last Victoria Crosses for this exploit – proved both courteous and implacable: 'I am coming alongside. Please lower your lee boats to act as fenders.'

Time and again – eight times by some accounts, four by others – the 896-ton *Mounsey* lunged gallantly, perilously into *Otranto*. Yet time and again men groggy with flu just couldn't make the final effort and missed their footholds – to plummet fifteen feet to the boiling water or be sliced clean in two by the *Mounsey*'s razor-edged deck-plates.

One of the many who didn't make it was Captain Jules Le Hoerff. Falling short of the *Mounsey*, he was still battling the sea when his Newfoundland dog espied him; before any-one could restrain it, it had hurdled the rail. Le Hoerff's coat collar was at last firm in the dog's jaws when a giant wave washed them both from view.

Those who did survive made it by a hair's-breadth. The Y.M.C.A.'s T. L. Campbell owed his life to his yarn socks; landing on the slippery edge of *Mounsey*'s deck he was teeter-ing backwards until the thread gave him purchase enough to cling to a wire cable. Pte Robert Shawd, one of twenty washed ashore on Islay, blessed his brothers back in Lebanon, Penn-sylvania – survivors of an earlier shipwreck, they had never ceased to nag him until he had learned to swim.

By now the *Mounsey* was wallowing badly: both masts carried away, her port side 'like a concertina', water up to her engine-room floor-plates. She could take no more. But cramped beneath her hatches as she limped painfully towards the North Channel and Spencer's Basin, Belfast, were 577 *Otranto* survivors – a shining testament of defiance against the worst that the sea could do.

From the wreckage of the bridge, Craven caught one last glimpse of the doomed *Otranto* as *Mounsey* steamed away:

Captain Davidson smiling and waving unconcernedly ... a
bugler formally sounding the 'Abandon ship' before arcing the
bugle towards the waves ... a seaman, his mind unhinged by
the carnage sprawled on a pile of life-rafts, slapping his thigh
and laughing uproariously like a drunk at a stag party.

The end was mercifully brief. Half an hour after *Mounsey*'s
departure, the *Otranto* dashed against a reef at the very entrance of Islay's Machir Bay, snapping squarely in two like a
child's toy, catapulting all hands into the sea. Then wind and
waves savaged her with such malign fury that her wreckage
was carried more than half a mile to the shore, pounding
against cliffs 300 feet high.

What the epidemic had begun, the sea had ended within
hours: 431 lives had been lost in one of the greatest shipping
disasters America was to suffer in the First World War.

The newspapers were scattered everywhere in wild confusion: the *Daily Express* on the chest-of-drawers, the *Daily
Mail* on the bed, the sober *Morning Post* strewn across the
floor. It was as if, thought Lieutenant Arthur Lapointe bitterly,
tossing aside sheet after sheet, Canada just didn't exist. The
influenza epidemic was raging again in Spain – but who cared
whether King Alfonso's temperature was 102°F? In Bombay,
deaths had topped 700 in twenty-four hours – a tragedy to be
sure.

But in Canada, apart from one brief mention in *The Times*
six days back – 350 engineers were down with it in Lac St
Jean, Quebec – there was resolute silence. Yet Lac St Jean was
only 200 miles from Lapointe's native village, St Léandre.

And today, Monday, 7 October, Lapointe had special need
of links with home. Four days earlier, after two months officer
training, the dark impetuous twenty-year-old had put up a
Lieutenant's burnished stars for the first time, and his pride
knew no bounds. The tanned confident face staring back from
the bedroom mirror in Bexhill-on-Sea's Metropole Hotel was
a far cry from the shy homesick farmer's son who two years
back had sailed with his regiment from France, the tears of

loneliness stinging his eyes as the band played 'Il est parti mon soldat'.

But slowly, from two years of combat at Ypres and Neuville Vitasse a new Lapointe had emerged: the orderly who would have died under bombardment rather than return with empty water-cans from the well at Petit Vimy; the signaller pinned down without food by mortar-fire for two days at Lens; the Corporal who had vowed grimly: 'We shall reach the German trenches or gain a simple cross of wood.'

Fighting fear and diffidence, he had gained an inner steel, an alien self-reliance – yet this new Lapointe was all too conscious of his status as a hardened soldier. What marred his triumph on this autumn Monday was that the whole family – Papa, Mama, Alphonse, Guillaume, the girls – weren't here *now* to pay their tributes to his triumph.

It was weeks since they had even written, and the English newspapers were no help at all in discovering how the parish of Rivière Blanche was faring.

From his bedroom window he could see the flower-beds on the promenade, bright with dahlias and chrysanthemums; the tawny crescent of the beach thronged with officers and their smartly-dressed girl-friends. It was a world away from the mud and torment of Flanders, but suddenly Arthur Lapointe's triumph seemed hollow. He felt alone.

Private John Lewis Barkley felt alone, too – more alone and more scared than he had ever been in all his months of combat with Company K, 4th Infantry, 3rd Division.

Just as he and his Indian friends, 'Nigger' Floyd and 'Jesse' James had feared, the war had at last contrived to separate them – for a spell at least. Worse, Barkley was at this moment closer to the Germans than to any fellow-American. He was literally within yards of them, behind the 65-mile redoubt that all the world knew as the Hindenburg Line.

It was 10 a.m., Monday, 7 October. Knee-deep in the mud of a shell-hole, screened from view by the branches of a fallen tree, Barkley was crouched over a field-telephone on the north-east slope of Hill 253, hard by the village of Cunel. He could see all too well why Sergeant Nayhone of Intelligence had assigned him to this vantage-point. From the German-held hill to his right, troops would be forced to march down the valley, straight across his front and up the slope of Hill 253 before they could make contact with the U.S. 7th Division.

'The aviators haven't been able to find out a damned thing,' Sergeant Nayhone had said. 'Somebody's got to go.' Barkley had replied sombrely, 'If you want to bump me off, for God's sake do it here' – knowing he had no choice but to obey.

Already it had been an eerie all-night vigil. Barkley's watch had showed 2.30 a.m. by the time the signal corps men had inched away into darkness, after fixing his phone so that the bell would just buzz instead of ringing. At intervals Nayhone would ring to check that the connexion wasn't broken, but with nothing to report Barkley wasn't permitted the luxury of speech. The scratching of his fingernail on the mouthpiece was his sole acknowledgment that he heard and understood.

At first, the sick-sweet smell of death from the corpses in the dripping Argonne forest around him, the German voices, uncannily loud to his rear, fretted Barkley's nerves to snapping-point. Then, as the hours crawled, hunger and fatigue anaes-thetised his body like a shot of morphine and he nodded off.

He awoke to the sound of thunder: the sullen rumble of German artillery, pounding up through the afternoon from Cunel, the answering crack of American 155s. Away to Bark-ley's right, among the oak trees, grey-clad figures were flitting: the Germans were readying for an attack. Simultaneously his phone buzzed. It was Sergeant Nayhone.

'Be on your toes,' Nayhone warned. 'Stay with it as long as you can. And take care. If anything . . .' Then the phone went dead.

Barkley thought fast. Shell-fire had cut the line – so his role as observer was ended. But how to warn Headquarters of the impending attack? Should he make his way back through the forest, running the risk of snipers? Then, before he had reached any concrete decision, he saw Germans emerging from the wood half a mile away – Jägers, by the look of them, thick heavy-set men in good fighting trim. At this moment he saw the tank.

It was a light French-built Renault, abandoned some days back, seventy-five yards away on the ridge. All around it was strewn the wreckage of war: the silent bloated bodies of Germans and doughboys, canteens, bread, bayonets, bloody helmets, ammunition boxes. And now Barkley remembered. Back in the forest, not far from his shell-hole, he had spotted a light Maxim machine-gun and more boxes of ammo. If he could reach it, he thought, he might check the advance long enough for Headquarters to get wind of it, and even 'make things interesting for the Germans'. Cautiously he began to inch back among the saplings.

He had reached the Maxim and his hand was on its breech when suddenly the whole Argonne trembled with explosions: the Americans were firing smoke-shells. Within thirty seconds, a billowing grey-white curtain of smoke had screened Barkley from the Germans on the opposite hill.

Grabbing the Maxim and all the ammo he could carry, the Missourian sprinted for the tank. Piling in head first, he examined his booty. The Maxim was minus a breech-block and the water-jacket was almost empty, but by a miracle Barkley had hoarded a breech-block, for so many weeks now that it was worn bright, in his hip pocket. He snapped it in and tested it. It worked.

This was good, but better still, the firing compartment of the Renault, large enough for two men, a machine-gun and ammunition, was conveniently minus its gun.

With one eye on the smoke-screen, Barkley foraged the battlefield. For siege rations he had only a loaf of French bread, filched from a dead American, and four inches of water in his canteen – but soon he had more than 4000 rounds of ammo inside the tank, and yet more boxes piled up outside within reach of the door.

The smoke-screen was lighter now, thinning to a bonfire swirl. Shoving the gun from the firing-port, he inserted a belt of shells, then swung the turret. Clinically he noted that his legs were giving out. Was it the good old-fashioned jitters or Spanish *grippe*?

The Germans were massing now, grey-clad figures marching boldly into the open, moving diagonally across his front. A rapid calculation suggested five or six hundred men – a battalion made up of four companies. The nearest column was less than 200 yards from his tank. He swung the turret slowly, keeping pace, gun port five feet above ground level, carefully picking the direction of fire which promised the best results all the way to the farthest flank. Then he eased down on the trigger.

The first burst seemed to paralyse the Jägers. Huddled together, they were craning desperately in all directions. It was minutes before they spotted the tank and spilled for cover, but in these open fields there was little cover for most, and everywhere men fell dying.

As fast as he could reload the Maxim, Barkley fired, burst after fifteen-shot burst, finishing one belt, jamming in another. But now the Germans were hitting back, and rifle-bullets were beating a devil's tattoo on the Renault's sides – every bullet a ton blow. German machine-guns, light and heavy, fanned him with a hail of fire.

Already the Maxim was beginning to boil and smoke. Uncaring, Barkley dashed the last of his canteen into the jacket. Near-scalding water hissed back into his face and over his hands.

Strangely, no machine-gun fire sounded from the American lines, but somewhere, 1000 yards to the left, a sniper was backstopping him, deliberately picking off German after German. All afternoon that methodical firing went on – a lone ally whom Barkley couldn't even see.

Shells from a German 77 were probing for him now – too distant, at first, to trouble him. The gun was maybe 600 yards away, in the woods at the far edge of the valley. But now, minute by minute, the shells came closer; the gunners had raised their elevation. A third shell, falling short, screaming and splintering among the oaks. A fourth, clean overhead. Then a ringing in Barkley's ears, a blackness, and, to his naked horror, blood gushing from his nose.

He knew well enough what this could signify, from his memories of the epidemic at Fort Riley, Kansas: the nasal haemorrhage that marked the crisis-point in an attack of Spanish influenza.

One day prior to Barkley's collapse, 900 miles north-east in Porsgrunn, Norway, fourteen-year-old Andrea Kristoffersen had never been so excited. Even the fever that had set in two days earlier and started this violent shivering, couldn't wholly dim the splendour of the occasion. This morning, Sunday, 6 October, was her confirmation day.

In all her life, Andrea had never owned a dress like this: a snow-white confirmation dress of finest cotton that in a way was an emblem of the dedication she felt. In this dress, after six months intensive preparation, she was to be confirmed by the Bishop in the Lutheran Church nearby. Now, even though Elise, her mother, had to prop her in the rocking-chair to attire her, Andrea was determined to pass off her fever as no more than a bad head-cold. Whatever happened, she must go through with it.

As the old horse-drawn cart creaked towards the church, Andrea knew how a princess must feel; all along the street she caught the envious sidelong glances of other girls. Beside her sat Halvor, her father, visibly proud at the sight of his lovely young daughter. Halvor was a labourer, and work was scarce, but somehow he had scrimped and stinted to find the cost of that material.

What followed was stark humiliation: a moment so traumatic that even fifty-five years have not erased it from Andrea's mind. At the very moment that the Bishop laid his hands upon her, invoking the strength and comfort of the Holy Ghost, it was like a dam breaking. Abruptly something seemed to snap inside her head. Blood as black as ink gushed from her nostrils, spurting on to the close-fitting white bodice, defiling forever the memory of this day. All over the church she could hear the startled murmurs of alarm and consternation.

Sobbing bitterly, Andrea was hurried down the aisle and back home – but even the local doctor's contention that the haemorrhage had saved her life could never quite reconcile her to that moment of pure and abject humiliation.

In Mayen, Germany, Käthe Nattermann, aged five, was as yet too young to appreciate the mysteries of confirmation – or even to comprehend why a strange fire consumed her whole body yet filled her veins with ice. It was two days since she had taken solids, so Maria, her mother, had carried her from her bedroom to the apartment's main salon to sponge her face with lukewarm water and coax her to eat – 'if only a *butterbrot*, *liebchen*'.

Suddenly Käthe screamed in terror. One moment she could see her face, mirrored opaquely in the bowl of water that her mother held. Next instant it had vanished, blotted from view by the blood pouring from her mouth and nose. Summoned by telephone, old Dr Hennewig arrived in a hurry. His verdict confirmed that of the doctor at Porsgrunn: 'I have seen many such cases – without the haemorrhage she would not have recovered.'

There seems no doubting the doctors were right. Later, Germany's Public Health Administration was to report that in many areas epistaxis (bleeding from the nose) affected up to half of all influenza victims – often as much as a pint of blood at a time. Though some doctors viewed this as no more than the tendency to haemorrhage attending any septic infection, at least one American medic, Major Charles Mix, of the Army Medical Corps, saw a greater significance.

Among doughboys at Camp Mills, New York, Mix noted, interference with the passage of blood from the heart's right ventricle to the lungs caused enough damming back of venous blood 'to make possible nasal haemorrhage on the slightest occasion'. Many were even then cyanotic, and some, despite this haemorrhage, developed pneumonia – yet hundreds lived to attest that this severe nose-bleed vented enough poisoned blood to mark the turning-point.

Somehow, sixteen-year-old Laura Riva, in Valdagno, Italy, couldn't convey to Dr Papesso how very ill she felt: for two days her head had been clenched by a migraine so intense she couldn't even open her eyes or bear to be touched. She was sweating and near-delirious, and when Papesso bade her sit up in bed, she refused. Convinced this was mere teenage caprice, the hard-pressed doctor grasped her arms and shook her like a rag doll – at once provoking a massive nose-bleed and a strong menstrual period. Within the day, Laura's headache had eased and the fever had abated.

Propped up in bed against pillows, above the family café, in Toul, France, thirteen-year-old Gilberte Boulanger scarcely dared to move: the slightest turn of her head brought on another nasal haemorrhage. Blood would jet from her nostrils as if at high pressure, spraying as far as the foot of the bed – a terrifying phenomenon which had been in evidence up to thirty times a day for more than a week.

Once Dr Brûlard, the military doctor, had tried to stem the flow by means of cotton-wool tampons, then had to give up. The blood only flowed into Gilberte's throat, threatening to choke her.

In despair, Marie Boulanger decided to give her daughter a spoonful of castor-oil, and to the terror of epistaxis was added now the miseries of diarrhoea. Weak beyond belief, Gilberte fainted.

Next morning, she woke, in wonder, to realise her fever had dropped. Her pillows were as clean as when her mother had changed them the night before – there had been no more haemorrhage. At the foot of the bed stood Dr Brûlard, in solemn consultation with her mother. 'It has saved her,' she recalls him saying, 'it has all acted like a purge.'

As he spoke he was tucking a sober-looking document back into his tunic pocket: the death-certificate that was no longer needed for Gilberte Boulanger.

*　　*　　*

The fragrance of a Romeo y Julieta cigar hovered above the orangery, pungent in the damp autumn evening. On the terrace of the Château of Chaumont-en-Bassigny, 160 miles southeast of Paris, a man was pacing, lost in thought. Briefly, light filtering from a shuttered window caught the square jaw and clipped moustache of the four-star General two million Americans in France knew affectionately as 'Black Jack'. His name was John Joseph Pershing.

Tonight the fifty-eight-year-old Commander-in-Chief of the American Army in France was a worried man. By day he was now so tense that he continually paced his office floor, unable to relax – 'grey with lack of sleep and unceasing strain', an aide had noted. Yet the reasons were as much medical as military. In thirty-six years as a soldier, John Pershing had faced adversaries as formidable as Geronimo, Sitting Bull, Pancho Villa and General Erich von Ludendorff. Now he faced defeat from an enemy no man had ever seen: the phantom figure American cartoonists delighted in portraying as 'Old Man Grippe'.

On 3 October, four days before John Lewis Barkley's lone stand in the Argonne Forest, Pershing had sent a peremptory cable winging to Adjutant General Peter C. Harris in Washington: 'Influenza exists in epidemic form amongst our troops in many localities in France, accompanied by many serious cases of pneumonia. Request 1500 members of Army Nurse Corps at earliest practicable date.'

Five days later, he followed up: 'Request information ... as to present status of influenza and pneumonia at embarkation ports.'

As always with important cables, Pershing had set on both his own seal of priority, scribbling: 'RUSH RUSH RUSH RUSH. J.J.P.'

The situation was desperate indeed. At this week's end, 16,000 doughboys were down with flu in the Argonne Forest alone. Only Haig's Tommies, advancing from St Quentin to the Scarpe, remained unscathed – as if the virulence of that spring attack, to which almost every man had succumbed, had created antibodies to resist the deadlier onslaught of the autumn. All over France, the pandemic had cut down so many American troops that newcomers from the States were being sped to frontline divisions within five days of their arrival. Under constant pressure from Maréchal Foch, Generalissimo of the Allied striking force, to smash the Hindenburg Line, Pershing now faced but two choices.

Either he must at this critical hour withdraw veteran divisions from the Argonne forest or incoming divisions high in morale must be immediately skeletonised to secure replacements. Unless, somehow, from some unknown source, Pershing could gain more troops.

Six thousand miles from Washington, Pershing could not know that the epidemic had just then forced a crucial decision on the Army's Provost Marshal, General Enoch Crowder.

On 7 October, draft calls for 142,000 new recruits due to entrain for Army camps throughout the United States had been cancelled until further notice.

The polished rosewood door swung back, and the Army's Chief of Staff, General Peyton March, came face to face with the President of the United States. Immaculate, in a light grey single-breasted suit, grey tie secured with a pearl stickpin, the President, as always, was smiling and imperturbable.

Taken unawares, the abrupt ruthless March was momentarily less sure of himself. The hour of 9.40 p.m. on Tuesday, 8 October seemed late for Thomas Woodrow Wilson to pay a routine call, but with the influenza epidemic at its height, dropping in when least expected had become the President's way. Time and again, at any hour up to midnight, the White House Pierce-Arrow slid away unannounced from the pillared portico, bound for one or other of Washington's war bureaus.

And in this first week of October, Wilson had especial cause for concern. Only two days earlier, on 6 October, Max, Prince of Baden, Imperial Chancellor of Germany, had appealed to the President for an armistice that would truly end 'the war to end all wars'. All Wilson's instincts, like those of General

John Pershing, were strong against a negotiated peace; to treat
with the imperial ruler of Germany rather than a government
controlled by the people was, to him, anathema. Yet any pro-
longation of the war, Wilson knew, was to expose American
lives to an enemy as deadly as any German bullet.

Now, in the office of Assistant Secretary for War, William
M. Ingraham, Wilson was spelling out that dilemma to the
fire-eating Chief of Staff.

'General March,' he said, 'I have had representations made
to me, by men whose ability and patriotism are unquestioned,
that I should stop the shipment of men to France until the
epidemic of influenza is under control.'

March knew well enough whom the President meant. Only
that week, the famed sanitarian, Dr Victor Heiser, who almost
single-handed had revolutionised hygiene in the Philippines,
had gone on record: 'It is more dangerous to be a soldier in
peaceful United States than to have been on the firing-line in
France.' And Heiser had challenged the wisdom of the War
Department: 'Is there a military or other emergency that
would justify so great a sacrifice of life?'

The statistics bore him out. All over the United States, from
Camp Devens, Massachusetts, to Camp Fremont, California,
stricken this very day, every fourth man was now down with
influenza – every twenty-fourth to contract pneumonia, every
sixty-seventh to die. At ports of embarkation, like Hoboken,
New Jersey, processing 300,000 troops a month, deaths from
pneumonia had reached a staggering twenty per cent. Troops
like Colonel E. W. Gibson's 57th Pioneer Infantry Regiment
from Vermont, marching by moonlight from their staging
area in Yonkers, New York, toppled, fell, and even died on
the dusty road to Hudson river ferry.

Now, eyes grave behind his rimless spectacles, the President's
challenge to the Army's Chief of Staff hung in the silent
panelled room high above Washington's 17th Street: 'They
tell me you decline to stop the shipments.'

Patiently, in much the same terms as France's Navy Minister
Georges Leygues had addressed the Chamber of Deputies,

March stated his case. All men slated for embarkation received an individual check at Army camps. Once at the port of embarkation, they were checked again, and all suspicious cases culled from the ranks. Aboard the troopship, yet one more check – the third.

Despite all, March admitted, cases had yet occurred *en route* to Europe: the ill-starred *Otranto* was proof of that. 'But,' he avowed, 'every such soldier who has died has just as surely played his part as his comrade who has died in France.'

Wilson listened in silence, his mind, as always while he weighed evidence, 'open and to let'. He was now never free from gastric pain, afflicted by neuritis which troubled his eye with a nervous tic, yet even for a man in rude health it was a cruel dilemma. An obstinate yet compassionate man, the former President of Princeton University spoke of his soldiers as he had spoken of his graduates – as 'our boys' – and it was an open Washington secret that his bedtime reading never varied: one chapter from a khaki-covered Y.M.C.A. Bible which a soldier bound for the front had pressed on him.

Seeing the sadness in the President's face, March yet pressed home his point. In the face of the German Chancellor's appeal, think of the effect on a weakening enemy if they learned that American divisions and replacements were no longer reaching Pershing. Because of the flu, shipments in October could total little more than 180,000 troops, as against 257,000 men in September, yet it was vital that every man who could bear arms should be shipped to Europe as a show of strength.

'The shipment of troops should not be stopped for any cause,' the General wound up.

Still Wilson was silent, yet instinct told March that his point was taken. While draft calls for new recruits remained suspended, there would be no reprieve for those already quartered in Army camps. Within forty-eight hours the President would authorise him to cable Pershing: 'If we are not stopped on account of influenza, which has passed the 200,000 mark, you will get replacements and all shortages of divisions up to date by 30 November.'

As March watched, the President swivelled in his chair. He gazed from the window into the Washington night. His face was care-worn, mirroring his decision; as he nodded slowly, irrevocably, a faint sigh came from him.

Then, to March's astonishment, his eyes twinkled. Oppressed by the gravity of the situation, the Chief of Staff had forgotten Wilson's insatiable love of limericks which had often startled staid Princeton dinner parties.

Lost for words, General Peyton March stood stiffly at attention while the President solemnly recited a jingle that was just then current in thousands of children's playgrounds across the United States:

> I had a little bird,
> Its name was Enza,
> I opened the window
> And in-flu-enza.

President Wilson, of course, had spoken in jest – but all over the world people were reacting as if the flu bug, possessed of wings, *could* fly through the window. Thus many were coming to embrace a dangerous fallacy: the one sure preventive was to blockade every door, window and crevice of their house or apartment as if for a siege.

In Hong Kong they had more reason than most; the coolies and street vendors in the teeming slums of Wanchai feared sneak-thieves, so that every window remained tight-shut and even ventilation windows were choked with bundles of old rags. But coolies weren't the only offenders. For almost an hour, in the dark of the night, Dr Dudley Deming, a Waterbury, Connecticut, physician, tried vainly to explain to one immigrant family: their little girl wasn't sick at all. It was the stifling room, the mound of blankets and quilts in which they had buried her which alone had induced a fever.

Thousands fell into the same trap, immuring themselves behind windows tight-shut or even nailed down, behind doors screened by heavy baize curtains, kerosene heaters that consumed every vestige of oxygen going at full blast. In Citerno,

Italy, one well-to-do woman, who had sealed every chink in her shutters with cotton-wool, died of suffocation as much as Spanish flu. Health workers on the sunny island of Jamaica told the same story; with even the key-holes blocked up, scores of blacks literally stifled to death.

And when people huddled together in an illusion of security it made matters worse still. Following one disastrous weekend, the disease struck Letterkenny, Ireland, like a cyclone; in six cottages mourners had held a two-day wake round the open coffin of a flu victim. A Sunderland sanitary inspector, arriving to escort a pneumonia victim to hospital, found fourteen women neighbours clustered in her over-heated bedroom, endeavouring to 'cheer her up'. Within the hour, every woman had carried the infection to her own home.

Even farm-folk viewed the air as an alien element, to be feared and distrusted. Near the little farming community of Max Meadows, Virginia, share-cropper John Brinkley had his wife Mary and four children down with the flu, but Brinkley, a devout country preacher, put his trust in both his Lord and his axe. Moving his sick to the main living-room, he chopped kindling for seven days as if his life depended on it, fuelling the old wood-burning stove day and night until the ironwork glowed red-hot. Doors and windows were tight-closed too. 'A little fresh air,' Brinkley warned his gasping invalids, 'could be fatal.'

On the eighth day, as luck had it, two relatives dropped by to pay a five-minute courtesy call – time enough to alert the horrified Brinkley that the roof of the old over-heated frame house had taken fire. Hastily they aided the farmer to carry his sick one by one to improvised beds in the vegetable patch. Never in his life would sixteen-year-old Roy Brinkley forget the first fresh air he had breathed in more than a week, the cabbages looming above him, 'seeming two feet off the ground and as big as wash tubs'.

Then came the crucial journey by horse-drawn wagon to a neighbour's house, and for twenty-four hours John Brinkley prayed as he had never prayed before. 'All that air,' he agonised to all who would listen, 'will surely hasten death.' On the ninth day, when the doctors had sworn that pneumonia must supervene, he knew his prayers had been answered, for all four invalids, to Brinkley's lifelong surprise, were now on the road to recovery.

Even many doctors saw a wide-open window as a true source of danger, though some, in a desperate attempt to save life, now cast old prejudices aside. In Halifax, Yorkshire, Dr Andrew Garvie found a sick woman and two children in an airless little one-room cottage; the window, encased in one frame, wasn't even made to open. Borrowing a rolling-pin and smashing the glass to smithereens, Garvie both defied a slum landlord and saved three lives; within a day his patients were out of danger. At Barons, Alberta, Dr Wesley Wallwin went farther still, treating every case in tents set up on hay-racks outside his house. Not one patient died.

Pioneer of this then revolutionary therapy was Britain's Dr (later Sir) Leonard Hill, a fifty-two-year-old zealot from the London Hospital's Medical School, who had urged that the entire population of Great Britain should sleep in the open air. Ceaseless experimentation had convinced Hill that cool dry air not only increased the flow of blood to the pleura, the double membrane lining the outside of the lungs, but stimulated the flow of cleansing lymph that washed away bacterial toxins. Many flu victims were literally dying of oedema of the lungs, drowning in their own secretions – yet cool air, as Hill pointed out, was beneficial, too, in increasing the pleura's rate of evaporation.

It was a theory other British doctors had cherished, too, among them Sir Thomas (later Lord) Horder, and Sir Hector Mackenzie, and now other authorities were swift to act upon it. At New York's Roosevelt Hospital, child sufferers under-went the 'roof treatment' – bedded down on the hospital's roof with hot-water bottles, screens shielding them from the north-west wind. The Chief Medical Officer for Frederiksberg, Den-mark, Dr Frants Djørup, urged all apartment dwellers to take their windows off the hinges until the epidemic was past. And doctors at Milan's Ospedale Maggiore found, even as late as November, that the sick quartered in tents in the courtyard fared better than those in the main wards.

Public sentiment wasn't easily allayed. Six Massachusetts hospitals who launched the scheme in the United States were condemned by Bostonians as 'barbarous and cruel' but State Commissioner of Health Eugene Kelley defended them hotly: a few hours of sunshine and fresh air had shown an almost universal drop in temperature, from 104 °F to a reassuring 97 °F.

Ironically, the greatest successes were registered by one hospital that was a true child of necessity. On Monday, 7 October, Dr Louis Croke, who had charge of all ships of the Recruiting Service of the Shipping Board, East Boston, found dozens of men supine in their bunks – or collapsed upon the open decks as if struck down by a boarding party. But enquiry revealed that every Boston hospital was too hard-pressed to admit them.

Along with Director of Recruiting Services Henry Howard, Croke now hit upon an emergency plan: why not call out the State Guard and establish a tent hospital on nearby Corey Hill, Brookline?

Events now moved swiftly. At 2.30 p.m. this same day, the State Guard's Colonel Emery received a call from his adjutant-general: tents and field equipment were needed urgently on Corey Hill. By 5.30 p.m. as truck-loads of tents rolled in from Framingham, 40 miles away, men of the State Guard were already standing by to erect them – along with labourers hired to make sewer and water connexions. Before midnight, Corey Hill's first thirty-eight patients were snug inside those tents.

All that week, rain curtained Boston's skyline, blotting out the Customs House, the gilt State House dome. For doctors and nurses scurrying from patient to patient, it was a week of mud and misery yet so thoroughly had the State Guard ditched the tents that the ground inside them all along remained dry. And from the first results were startling. Many were severe pneumonia cases, troops from those parts of the ships where the ventilation had been worst, but once on Corey Hill's breezy heights, almost all showed a lower temperature at night than in the morning.

It was a triumph of improvisation. Fire hydrants stood in as water-taps; for prophylactic masks, nurses and attendants wore wire gravy-strainers taped over their ears, padded with medicated gauze that was changed every two hours under the surveillance of a Superintendent of Masks. Where rubber hot water bags were lacking, the patients' feet were kept warm with hot bricks wrapped in newspapers.

Virtually only two drugs were used – Dover's powder and iodide of lime – for to Surgeon-General William Brooks the temperature charts told the story: fresh air, sunshine, a fruit and water diet were daily producing miraculous results. Almost four weeks later, when Corey Hill closed down, 351 serious cases had been treated, with no more than thirty-five deaths.

For the first time since the epidemic began there was hope that the unknown virus might yet be defeated with nature's own weapons.

CHAPTER FOUR

'But it's their Disease – the Brutes'

9 October–12 October 1918

Major Victor Vaughan checked his calculations yet again. It was an awesome conclusion – yet beyond the shadow of a doubt it was true. For days now, in his office in Washington's Butler Building, the lights had burned late while Vaughan grappled with the implications of statistics flooding in from all over the world: sober yet truly frightening tallies.

Today, Wednesday, 9 October, Vaughan saw all too plainly the shape of things to come. Time and again, epidemiologists had written of the Plague of Justinian, which from A.D. 542 had slain 100 million souls, and of the fourteenth-century's Black Death, which claimed 62 million victims. Now, for the third time in recorded history, the world's population, close to two billion men and women, faced a common crisis.

As Vaughan saw it, each man or woman infected might only shake hands or have close personal contact with ten people a day – but the day following each of those ten might themselves meet ten more. Thus, in one week's time, by 16 October, the infection could reach more than a million people.

Eight days earlier, the epidemic had reached its peak in places as far apart as Boston, where Lieutenant-Governor Calvin Coolidge had appealed for Federal aid, and Bombay, almost 8000 miles away on the Arabian Sea. Some 3000 miles north-west, 75,000 cases were reported in the Black Sea port of

Odessa – and trade was at a standstill in Rio de Janeiro and
Cape Town. The scourge had struck at five continents. No
longer was it an epidemic but a pandemic that was in force.

As if strewn from a giant Pandora's Box, the disease was
girdling the globe. In Rhodesia, it travelled at thirty-five miles
an hour, 384 miles up the railway line from Bulawayo to Salisbury. Across Somaliland, it progressed at a quarter that speed:
in the wake of a *dhow* on the Gulf of Aden or the plodding
gait of a camel caravan. On 6 October it had struck Damascus,
at the flanks of the victorious Australian Mounted Division,
sweeping down the Street called Straight, the dusty unshaven
troopers with drawn swords slumping in their saddles or crawling to hide like wounded animals in the shade of green gardens. It spared neither victor nor vanquished; within days,
8000 of Djemal Pasha's Turks, too sick to contest their city,
were down with it too.

From the northern ports of Liverpool and Glasgow, it
racketed at express-train speed down the spine of England, to
London, thence, at the sedate pace of a country bus, outwards
to the provinces. Somehow it reached outposts as isolated as
Maatsuyker Lighthouse, six miles off the Tasmanian coast,
where the keeper and his wife hadn't seen a soul for three
months. Even in remote Shansi province, China, far from the
trade routes, it dogged the steps of a wood-cutter who all unknowing carried it from village to village.

Across Canada, within days, it cut a 2600 mile swathe from
coast to coast, thanks largely to a dogged Canadian Pacific
Railways official named David Reid Kennedy. A dedicated
by-the-book passenger agent, Kennedy was assigned to escort
a train-load of repatriate soldiers from Quebec City to Vancouver, B.C., and an armed sentry outside Military Headquarters, insisting the building was quarantined, in no way
deterred him. Scaling the fire escape, Kennedy vaulted into
the C.O.'s office by way of the window. Despite the officer's
heated protests, his persistence won him the travel vouchers
he sought.

Cochrane ... Regina ... Winnipeg ... Calgary ... at every

junction point along the route, the implacable Kennedy found it necessary to cut out one or more cars, as men went down like ninepins with the strange disease. Still the skeleton of the troop train hurtled west towards Vancouver. Never in fourteen years had Kennedy allowed trifling obstacles to impede a C.P.R. operation.

Nearing Vancouver, Kennedy had a shock: word had come that the train was to be shunted into a siding and no man allowed to leave. Kennedy, though, had no intention of complying; back in Quebec he had yet more trains waiting to be moved to other points of the compass. As the troop train ground to a halt in the Vancouver yards, Kennedy hopped off and within minutes had leaped aboard another train heading east.

On the return journey, he learned the flu was now raging at every point where his cars had been disconnected, but he felt neither curiosity nor remorse: just as he had planned it, another C.P.R. operation had been brought to a successful close.

The names that people were calling the disease showed how far and how fast it had spread. In Cuba and the Philippines it was 'trancazo', meaning 'a blow from a heavy stick'; in Hungary it was 'The Black Whip'. To the Swiss, it was 'the coquette', giving its favours to everyone; to the Siamese, *Kai Wat Yai*, 'the Great Cold Fever'. The Poles, indulging in wishful thinking, named it 'The Bolshevik Disease'; both, they hoped, would soon go away. Other names were downright chauvinistic: it was 'Bombay Fever' in Ceylon and 'Singapore Fever' in Penang.

Only to Britain's august Royal College of Physicians was it now, for the first time, 'influenza' – a welcome advance on their previous high-flown designation, *catarrho epidemico*.

From naming it was but a short step to pointing an accusing finger – often at any ethnic group that differed from the norm. The Russians blamed the Kirghiz tribesmen, the nomadic fur-hatted cattle-breeders who roamed the steppes of Turkestan. Germany raged that the disease had been imported by the 100,000 strong Chinese Labour Corps serving behind the

British lines in France – though, ironically, while many German units were down to fifty rifles, the Tommies failed to contract it. In the Argentine, the Spanish were held so culpable that their national chicken rice and shellfish dish, *paella*, was banished from every menu.

And now, as national tempers rose dangerously, outright accusation became the order of the day. As caption to a photo of Spanish peasants in colourful fiesta costume, the Trondheim paper *Adresseavisen* charged: 'From these people we got the epidemic!' When London's Regents Park Zoo screened its chimpanzees with glass cages to protect them from infection, a woman visitor protested indignantly: 'But it's *their* disease – the nasty brutes!' Even Lieutenant Philip Doane, of the United States Emergency Fleet Corporation, went solemnly on record: the Spanish influenza was the Kaiser's secret weapon, spread by agents sent ashore on the eastern seaboard from German submarines.

Unexplained was one puzzling factor: the 'Secret weapon' was to end the lives of more than 225,000 Germans.

The mood wasn't altogether surprising. The onset of the pandemic had been too swift, too frightening, for people to adjust – and local authorities, even governments, had shown themselves pitifully unprepared. Lacking leadership and guidance, many, at first, reacted with callousness – as if each man refused resolutely to acknowledge that he was his brother's keeper.

In Freetown, Sierre Leone, out-of-town visitors callously decamped from one boarding-house without even settling their bill – leaving behind a comrade's dead body in lieu of payment. A hard-pressed British clergyman, seeking help from a workman's family for a stricken next-door neighbour, was told flatly: 'I reckon you're the parson – you should do your dirty work yourself.'

But even men of God were not immune. On the Samoan island of Upolu, ministers taking up a cash collection for one London based mission, spread the flu from Apia harbour sixty miles west to Mulifanua. On their return they found every village laid low. Now too sick to reach their plantations for food, the villagers begged for the return of at least some of their money, to help buy rice from the stores. But the reply was a stony refusal.

Not long after, Resident Commissioner John Gillespie, a towering (6 ft 4 in.) giant chanced by the Mission headquarters. How was it, he asked, that there were still corpses putrefying in the ditches close at hand? For reply, the ministers just shrugged: 'Oh, they're Catholics! We've buried our own dead.' Only when Gillespie sent to his truck for tins of petrol, proposing to burn the mission to the ground, did they arrange a hasty burial party.

In many cities, the sick were as isolated as in the Middle Ages, when plague-stricken houses were marked out by a red cross and the legend 'God have mercy upon us!' Now a red or a yellow flag, or a large white sticker marked 'I', prompted the same reactions; tradesmen left provisions only at the gate and many people instinctively crossed to the other side of the street. Some were marked out as pariahs: often a nurse couldn't get even a letter posted and the sight of a soldier in uniform was a signal to step into the nearest tree-lot until he had passed. One Knysna, Cape Province, hotelier, both anxious to keep in business and steer clear of infection, hit on a novel idea: what was perhaps the world's first drive-in dinner service.

There was blatant racism, too. Warsaw's anti-flu hygiene drive was limited to the Jewish ghetto – the race, ran a public proclamation, was 'a particular enemy of order and cleanliness'. Some West African hospitals refused point-blank to admit black patients, and the *Montreal Gazette*, reporting on the city's morale, unashamedly headlined 'NO PANIC EXCEPT AMONGST ORIENTALS'. A few were so prejudiced as to spite even themselves. Many Afrikaaners, with rankling memories of the Boer War and bitterly opposed to South Africa's alliance with Britain, died at home – refusing to accept any aid from a military hospital.

And many survivors still recall small acts of deliberate malice – as if the sickness had placed them, like faltering animals, at the mercy of the pack. In Namsos, Norway, ten-year-old Nancy Ramstad had been the butt of unfeeling schoolmates, ever since her sailor father walked out on the family, forcing her mother to win bread scrubbing out the houses of the wealthy. Hit suddenly by flu in school, Nancy got the teacher's permission to leave, but as she staggered homewards, vomiting along the gutter, she was followed by other children who taunted her: 'You don't have to mess up our town just because you've a bad father.'

Lieutenant Pietro Cignolini felt the same humiliation. The flu had struck him in the dead of night, on the banks of the River Piave, in Northern Italy, and he knew he couldn't go on. Running into a group of soldiers, he begged for help: was there a hospital close at hand? 'Of course,' they reassured him. 'The civil hospital. You'll see it at the end of the road.'

At the far end of a dirt road, Cignolini found it: a crumbling wall, bearing the fading legend, 'Ospedale Civile', only blackened silent ruins lying beyond. Faintly, as he slumped to its base, he heard their cruel derisive laughter receding into the night.

Consider, too, the case of sixteen-year-old Ilona Molnar. At lunchtime on 9 October, Ilona, a maidservant employed at no. 20, Maros-utca, Budapest, complained of feeling unwell. At once, Mrs Anna Németh, her employer, flew into a most unladylike panic; already there were 100,000 cases in the city. Her prompt reaction was to send the girl packing.

'You should go at once to your mother's, Ilona,' she instructed, 'or get admitted as a lying-in case in a public infirmary.' And Mrs Németh added a generous rider: in such an instance, she would, of course, defray Ilona's expenses.

It was now midday. Unsteadily, clutching her few belongings in a bundle, Ilona set off. Whether she was heading for her mother's or for the infirmary, no one ever knew. But suddenly, as she reached Krisztina-körút, halfway across the city, she could go no further. Exhausted, she sank down upon a wooden bench.

All afternoon, as the street-cars ground by, she huddled there, unremarked, frightened and alone. By 3.30 p.m., the curious blue tinge, the telltale sign the doctors had learned to dread, had suffused her lips and ears, and, at a discreet distance, a curious crowd had gathered to watch her.

Though everyone was careful to keep well away, someone, around 4 p.m., thought to send for Officer János Juhász, on point-duty nearby. One glance at Ilona's face and Juhász sent a rush call for an ambulance.

By 5 p.m., when the ambulance clanged to a halt, the crowd had assumed riot proportions; street vendors did a brisk trade with sweetmeats and roast chestnuts. Loud cheers rent the air, along with shouted scraps of advice and suggestions. But the ambulance attendants – again keeping their distance – shook their heads. The girl had Spanish influenza; she couldn't be transported to a hospital in a public ambulance. This was a case for the Disinfection Institute.

At 5.30 p.m. Juhász was again on the phone. But the Institute was non-committal. As of now they were rushed off their feet. They might be able to arrange a pick-up sometime that evening – perhaps between 8 and 9 p.m.

On Krisztina-körút, Ilona had now slumped to the pavement, not moving, her whole face suffused. Still the crowd grew – but still they kept their distance.

In fact, the Institute were as good as their word. Promptly at 8.30 p.m. their closed black van wheezed up the boulevard to halt opposite no. 8, by the public bench. By now the officials had to fight their way through the crowd, for even in Budapest, on the eve of the Revolution, it was rare to see a young girl lying dead on the public street.

It was a glorious autumn evening. You could see all the way across the Danube, to the lights sparkling on the Pesth shore, but not to where Ilona had gone.

Yet for many the epidemic's savage onslaught on all that they cherished most had but one result. By dawn on 10 October, thousands of men and women had just one resolve; the only thing that mattered now was the lives of others.

At Ellerslie Girls' High School, outside Cape Town, executive William Davies had been as good as his word. Following that urgent phone call to Dr Willmot, Davies had mustered a task-force of tycoons and company directors to work under his banner ... all of them toiling in their shirt-sleeves to launder towels, sheets and pillow-cases ... next enlisting the aid of 140 doctors and nurses ... caring for the sick on hastily-assembled beds in classrooms and dormitories ... setting up new centres in any building that became available ... speeding nurses on urgent calls ... taking in young babies bereft of their mothers.

Community after community met the same challenge. Most, like Massachusetts' State Commissioner for Health, Dr Eugene Kelley, swiftly learned that the first lesson was 'Centralise'; at the outset the frustrated Kelley realised that his state harboured no less than fifty-seven voluntary public health agencies, dealing with every aspect of health from child welfare to oral hygiene and all at odds with one another.

Paramount above all was the need to keep the public informed. In New York, a thicket of brightly coloured arrows pointed the way to newly-established health posts, where medical help and nursing services were available. Moscow, not to be outdone, set up flu advice centres throughout the city, staggering the doctors' hours so that they were manned round the clock.

Yet, as Bermuda's Chief Medical Officer, Dr Eldon Harvey, warned the House of Assembly : it was easy to advise families to stock up with nourishing food, but what if they lacked the money to buy it? The recognition of this plight early led cities like Lahore, India, to send seven dispensary vans patrolling the streets with free milk and medicine – and prompted Rio de Janeiro to seize all chickens and dairy produce reaching the city to be sold at controlled prices.

Nor were minority needs neglected. Bloemfontein, South Africa, undertook a novel census; a roster of all those bachelors and working girls likely to remain unattended in rooming-houses. Such unfortunates were the special concern of Chicago's City Prosecuting Attorney Harry Miller when, following fifty

complaints, he announced a decision that became a legal land-
mark: henceforth he would file suit against any landlord who
refused to heat an apartment housing an influenza victim.

Yet few communities could have made such headway without the true Christian compassion of private citizens. Often it
was an organisation long noted for its public-spiritedness; in
New Orleans, the Elks from the first offered to finance a free
medical service for the poor, and in two short weeks their
medical staff made 14,000 prescriptions. Sometimes a community's need was bizarre, but mostly the benefactors played
along. The Caribbean Oil Company freely donated gasoline
all over Venezuela – for bonfires to scare away the influenza
spirit.

It was the same all over the world. Norway's Automobile
Association not only laid on cars for over 100 doctors but threw
in 4000 litres of free petrol. Milan's Giannino's, world-famed
as a gourmet's paradise, donated all surplus food from its
kitchens to the flu-stricken. To aid Philadelphia's overburdened
Council of National Defense, the Strawbridge and Clothier
Department store gave over their switchboard to answer emergency calls – 'every need from soup to an undertaker'.

Some citizens seem to have operated what were virtually
unofficial one-man hospitals. Mining merchant Reuben Greer
of Cape Province took over the village school on his own
initiative, first dosing every patient with Epsom Salts 'to clear
the system', following up with a tot of brandy 'for Dutch
courage'. At Obidos, Portuguese landowner Luis da Gama
did things on a grander scale still ... stripping whole fields of
mustard and linseed for poultices ... even slaughtering an
entire herd of cattle to make soup for his bedridden tenants.

Almost without exception, neighbours and friends rallied in
the common cause. Twenty young married couples in Sherbrooke, Quebec, formed an unique mutual aid society, linking
their homes with telephone dry batteries, wires, and cow-bells
on clothes-lines, so that any who fell ill could at once avail
themselves of this primitive alarm system.

'White and coloured worked side by side then,' recalls one

survivor, Willard Bryan, of Monroe, Louisiana. 'Had we the cooperation between races today that we had during that epidemic it would be a blessing.'

Rarely in the history of mankind had so many volunteers toiled so long or so patiently in the service of humanity. To the constant shrilling of the emergency phone, workers at Winnipeg's Alexandra School daily whipped up quarts of lemonade and soup, gallons of orange juice, egg-nogs and soft puddings. At Wilkes-Barre, Pennsylvania, other volunteers from Red Cross classes worked like Furies to equip a chain of emergency hospitals ... cutting draw-sheets ... scrubbing hat-racks to serve as linen shelves ... partitioning off wards with beaverboard.

The entire Council Chamber of Ottawa's City Hall was now jampacked with 200 busy women, sewing each night until 11 p.m.; in one day alone they equipped a newly-opened emergency hospital with a complete change of linen. Soon, working twenty-four-hour staggered shifts, their flashing needles were turning out 1400 items – hospital shirts, towels, diapers – per day.

Sometimes the volunteers' zeal was their undoing. In Bloem-fontein, Orange Free State, one task force who found a man collapsed outside a garden gate bore him into the house and settled him comfortably beside the unconscious woman in the double bed upstairs. Long before the innocents returned with medical aid, two total strangers awoke to stare at one another in mutually speechless horror.

Another group, in Sea Point, Cape Town, obeyed a doctor's injunctions to deliver two coffins so speedily they didn't even check the address. Hours later, a mildly-afflicted householder and his wife, laid up two doors away, were hailed blithely by their schoolboy son with words which sent them groping for the brandy bottle: 'Hey, Dad! Two coffins downstairs for you and Mum!'

A few were hoodwinked into service. In the cantonment at Potchefstroom, Gunner Charles Eustace of the South African Heavy Artillery was one of many who stepped smartly from the ranks when a call came for volunteers; the 'special duty' promised, Eustace thought, would be a welcome change from parade-ground drill. Hours later, to their chagrin, Eustace and his fellow 'volunteers' realised that they had fallen for the oldest of all Army games. The 'special duty' was scouring bedpans for a ward of ailing flu victims.

Among all those who laboured in these nightmare days, Lydia Phillips somehow emerges as symbolic. A petite blue-eyed twenty-three-year-old with fair wavy hair, Lydia had yearned to be a nurse from as far back as she could remember; in her teens she had even applied, unsuccessfully, to St Thomas's Hospital, London. The daughter of a prosperous City umbrella manufacturer, Lydia had set her heart on St Thomas's – but in 1914, the outbreak of war had put paid to that ambition. On a holiday voyage to South Africa with her mother, Lydia found herself exiled in Johannesburg for the duration. All shipping had been commandeered.

A resourceful self-willed girl – once she had threatened to sell all her trinkets to pay the fees until her parents agreed to enrol her in business college – Lydia found a job as shorthand typist, with a firm of wholesale merchants, yet still that old dream would not be denied. True, life in the leafy suburb of Malvern, eight miles from the city, was pleasant and there was time enough to pursue her many hobbies; poetry, the piano, swimming. But often the closing words of the Florence Nightingale Pledge, which all nurses must affirm on gradua-tion, returned to haunt her: *With loyalty will I endeavour to aid the physician in his work and devote myself to the welfare of those committed to my care.*

Then in the first week of October, Lydia saw her chance. The *Rand Daily Mail* had announced that the need for help was now 'immediate and imperative'. Above all, volunteers were needed for four hours each day at Twist Street School Emergency Hospital, a red brick two-storey building in the suburb of Hillbrow, not far from Lydia's office.

Cannily, Lydia decided that she would volunteer first, only breaking it to her mother and employers once she was accepted.

Otherwise, she guessed shrewdly, they would bring all their guns to bear to dissuade her from this risky step.

Now, at 8 a.m. on an autumn morning, on the asphalt playground of Twist Street School, Lydia was more excited than she could ever remember. Along with a motley group of volunteers, she listened raptly as a Staff Nurse explained their duties; already, in her mind's eye, she saw herself administering to the sick and the dying, trusted by them as implicitly as Florence Nightingale herself at Scutari. Only one small detail clouded her happiness; she wouldn't be issued with a uniform, only an apron, with a piece of white cloth to be twisted into the semblance of a nurse's cap.

Suddenly she was puzzled. 'You are always,' the Staff Nurse was telling them, 'to give the men a bottle when they ask for it.' Before she had properly reflected, Lydia had piped up: 'Bottle? What kind of bottle?'

Suspecting a humorist, the Staff Nurse gave her a long hard stare. There was a ripple in the crowd, and abruptly the other volunteers were craning round, searching for the questioner, some convulsed with giggles at such ignorance. As the Staff Nurse patiently explained, Lydia felt her cheeks catch fire. She wanted to claw a hole in the asphalt, to hide from the mocking laughter.

Worse was to follow. Once inside the building, Lydia was assigned to a ward that was perhaps the school's main hall; it was long and narrow with beds lined closely against each wall. Here a further shock awaited her. The ward did not smell of carbolic and iodoform and starched linen, but of sweating bodies and human excrement and clothes that had been too often rained upon. All the patients were male, but few had the noble aspect of Crimean heroes. They were frightened and alone, made savage and resentful by fear and by pain.

Several smaller wards – former classrooms – led off this main hall. In one of these a man was slumped on a truckle bed, fully dressed, tossing and mumbling in the throes of a high fever. As the Staff Nurse led her briskly into the room, Lydia all but recoiled. The man was filthy and unkempt, typical of the many vagrants who haunted the gutters of the City of Gold.

'Kneel at the foot of the bed,' the Staff Nurse instructed her, 'and rub the soles of his feet until the doctor comes. And remember – watch his face for any change in his condition.'

Bustling away on her rounds, she did not pause to explain that this was a primitive attempt to promote circulation. Bending to her task, Lydia could see no reason for it; she knew only that the feet were hot, sweaty and sour-smelling, caked with a patina of grime. Chafing at the soles for dear life, she was engulfed by waves of stench. Only an hour previously she had breakfasted, and she had to fight down the desire to vomit with everything she knew.

Covertly, seeking some unknown miracle, she stole a glance at the patient's face. This, too, was clammy with sweat, but she could see no visible change. The feet again, rubbing and rubbing until her palms were sore and chapped. Then the face; still no change. Face to feet, feet to face, face to feet. The hard stone floor was a torment to her knees. She retched painfully, and kept on rubbing.

In the distance she could hear the doctor's footfalls; in minutes now her vigil would be over. I'll never make a nurse, she told herself, in shame and blind despair, never in a thousand years.

Despite the gallantry of countless thousands of citizens, one factor was becoming daily more apparent. In many communities, appalling defects in organisation were revealed as surely as in concrete flawed by frost.

If South Africa's Union Government had been derelict in their duty, ignoring all warnings from Freetown, the authorities in Sierra Leone were as much to blame. When flu arrived on the British troopship H.M.S. *Mantua*, Acting Colonial Secretary Edward Evelyn at once disclaimed all responsibility. Infectious passengers were permitted to land and the ship allowed to coal, since, Evelyn avowed, 'His Majesty's ships do not come under the control, sanitary or otherwise, of the authorities.'

In fact, no section of the Quarantine Ordinance excluded any class of ship from the laws written therein – but because of this laxity 2000 were to die in Freetown alone.

In Tangier – jointly ruled since 1912 by France, Spain and Morocco – the *Conseil Sanitaire* all along displayed a callous unconcern for the people's suffering. The epidemic had raged for three weeks before the Council even convened to announce that 'steps would be taken'. Yet although the Public Works Department, controlled by the Diplomatic Corps, had lavished public money on handsome boulevards in the Embassy quarter, in the hard-hit *souk* of Marsan, many streets to the Moorish cemetery were literally impassable, choked with liquid sewage. It was left to Mouley Yussef, Sultan of Morocco, to shame the Europeans, stepping in with a cash grant to purify the city.

Of all the sins of omission, few loomed larger in the world's headlines than the scandal of New Zealand and the s.s. *Niagara*.

At 11.50 a.m. on 11 October, Captain John Rolls, Commodore of New Zealand's Union Steamship Company, sent an urgent message from his cabin to the Admiralty's Naval Intelligence Officer at Wellington. It read: 'Please advise Health Department Spanish influenza cases aboard; increasing daily. Present time over 100 crew down. Urgently require hospital assistance and accommodation for 25 serious cases.'

The message called for swift action, as none knew better than Captain Rolls. At noon on Saturday, 12 October, the 13,000 ton *Niagara*, flagship of the Union Company's fleet, was due to berth at Queen's Wharf, Auckland Harbour. Prominent among her passengers were New Zealand's Prime Minister, the Right Honourable William Ferguson Massey, and his Minister of Finance, Sir Joseph Ward. But plainly, if the pandemic had the *Niagara* in its grip, absolute quarantine was a necessity – VIPs or no.

Promptly the Admiralty called the steamship company – who in turn called Dr Thomas Hughes, Auckland's District Health Officer. But Hughes, of his own volition, could do nothing. The Dominion Quarantine Act made no mention of Spanish influenza – and despite the holocaust of the past few weeks, no parliamentary motion had been put down for its amendment. In turn, Dr Hughes passed the problem to the Right Honourable George 'Rickety' Russell, New Zealand's Minister for Public Health.

Incredibly, Russell made no request for a general report from Auckland's health authorities. Instead, clearing all wires for a 'Take Precedence' telegram, he was content to pose two questions. How many deaths had occurred since the *Niagara* left Vancouver on 21 September? And was the disease not merely 'pure influenza'?

It was a monumental error of judgement – one which a Royal Commission was later to censure as 'either a non-recognition or a dis-regard of the gravity of the position' outlined in the Captain's message. As was later revealed, either Rolls or Prime Minister Massey himself could have told Russell that the voyage had been disastrous from the first.

As Steward William Ferguson recalled it later, the *Niagara* was only three days out of Vancouver when the first victim, a bell-boy, went down with it. By 9 October, when the liner berthed at Suva, Fiji, eighty-three had succumbed. The disease was now headline news throughout the world, yet the ship's doctor, Dr Arthur Latchmore, was treating every case as dengue fever, a painful virus disease of the joints transmitted by mosquitoes.

Among them was Steward Ferguson himself, fully convinced this was no bout of dengue. When Latchmore – who never personally examined him – sent quinine tablets to allay the fever, the steward was stubborn: he wanted castor-oil. Latchmore now lost his temper; a medical orderly appeared at Ferguson's bunk with an eight-ounce glass of the laxative. If Ferguson didn't drink it all, he would be reported as a malingerer. Knowing well enough that the normal dose was a tablespoon, Ferguson yet held his nose and gulped, and soon after his mates carried him unconscious from the head back to his bunk.

At first, those passengers still on their feet made a show-the-flag attempt to carry on. To the very end, most wore black ties for the customary seven-course dinner in the First-Class Saloon: caviare, consommé, sole with parsley sauce, roast lamb, curried prawns, apple pie, bloater toast. There were concerts in the Music Room, too, with stirring songs like 'I fear no foreign foe'; once Sir Joseph Ward auctioned some pen-and-ink sketches for charity and Massey gave a short patriotic address.

But soon it was a gong, not a bugle, that summoned the passengers to dinner; the entire ship's orchestra was down and the Music Room was now an emergency hospital lined with mattresses. Some passengers like chemical manufacturer John Blogg even did steward duty – beef tea at 11 a.m., doling out hymnbooks at church service – for by now eighty per cent of the crew were prostrate.

It wasn't entirely surprising. Regular passengers like Dame Nelly Melba and Prime Minister William Hughes of Australia knew the *Niagara*, built only five years earlier, as the most glamorous and up-to-date ship on the Canada-Australia run, but the crew, working a 70-hour minimum week, had their reservations. The stewards slept sixteen to a peak in the stern, and the tainted air below decks, the wormy bread and dish-water soup were common waterfront gossip. And many, not surprisingly, had fallen sick through carrying on long after they should have done – above all, the night-watch stewards, who answered cabin calls after 8 p.m. and netted the choicest tips.

Thus, at 1.25 p.m. on 12 October – the precise moment that the *Niagara*'s gangway came down and Dr Hughes, on the quayside received Russell's two-question telegram – the crew at least knew the liner for what she was: a floating hotbed of infection.

Afterwards, critics charged unfairly that Prime Minister Massey and Sir Joseph Ward had used their influence on the port authorities to obtain the *Niagara*'s absolution from quarantine. Both men, leaders of a Coalition government, had been absent for five months at a conference, and a split was said to have developed between them; as a result, both were anxious to rally their followers and the country at large.

Yet no valid evidence was ever produced to prove that either man pulled rank. A bluff homely farmer, who had typically received the telegram nominating him as an M.P. on a hayfork's prongs, while roofing an oatstack, the sixty-two-year-old Massey had never been a man to rock the boat. The true tragedy was that he made no attempt to intervene and insist on the ship's quarantine.

Plainly, though, every man involved was bent on minimising the pandemic as much as possible; to order a prime minister to remain in quarantine could be embarrassing indeed. Before Dr Hughes had even boarded the *Niagara*, Russell had personally cabled his premier: 'Sincerely hope answers will be satisfactory and that there will be no delay.'

It was unlikely to say the least. Once aboard, Dr Hughes did little more than go politely through the motions. While the first-class passengers got up a £278 whip-round for those 'noble stewards' who had carried on, Hughes conferred briefly with Dr Kenneth Mackenzie and a Dr Barnett. Though both were passengers, they had stood in as locums when Dr Latchmore himself fell ill.

Never at any time did Hughes approach Captain Rolls for elucidation of that wireless message – or seek further information from passengers or crew. All three doctors were agreed, however, that there were fifty-eight cases aboard, twenty-seven of them in the ship's hospital – as opposed to the 100 signalled by Rolls, the 130 reported in next day's *New Zealand Herald*. They agreed, too, that this was 'simple influenza', to adopt Russell's phrase – and thus of no danger to the community.

Later Dr Edwin Milsom, on duty at Auckland General Hospital, was to affirm that as early as the night of 12 October, he examined six influenza cases brought ashore from the *Niagara* and that he 'had never seen the like before'. Yet two factors alone make plain that Dr Hughes had already decided on his course of action before the gangway ever went down.

Despite bitter protests from the Waterside Workers' Union,

the *Niagara* was permitted to berth at Queen's Wharf, instead of lying off – and ambulances had been waiting on the quay-side since 10 a.m., with police constables in attendance to carry the invalids ashore.

It was thus a foregone conclusion that Dr Hughes would cable Russell: 'On *Niagara* one death last night, broncho-pneumonia after influenza. Disease purely "simple influenza".'

Promptly, again clearing all wires, Russell cabled back: 'Ship may be cleared.'

Shortly after 2 p.m., beaming broadly, with Sir Joseph Ward at his side, William Ferguson Massey rode in his landau through cheering crowds to the saluting base, his top hat raised to acknowledge the tributes of his people.

It was then too early for any of them to chart the stark cost of disembarkation: the lives of 6680 New Zealanders.

Wide awake, her eyes fixed on the shadowy ceiling, Tersilla Vicenzotto stared into the paling darkness. It was almost dawn, yet she could not sleep. It was as if a cruel fate was willing her to live, over and over again, here in the bedroom her husband had rented, the most terrible nights she had passed on earth.

Within minutes of her fervent prayer in the Basilica of San Antonio, Tersilla had arrived at Padua's Ospedale Civile, barely a block away. As a nun led her to the ward where Oscar lay, the air alarm was still on: guns were thudding dully over the Bacchiglione River. The long room was dim, lit only by wavering blue pilot lights, made dimmer by the sandbagged windows that blotted out the night.

From the first, Tersilla had been frightened. Oscar recog-nised her at once – this much she knew from the relief that showed in his eyes, the faint pressure of his fingers. But what alarmed her was the deathly pallor of his face, the painful rasping breath. Plainly he was far more sick than their friends had ever divulged.

He had hardly spoken at all, not even to ask about her journey or the children's health. It was only when she un-packed her basket of precious fruit, revealing the grapes and the peaches, that his eyes had clouded over with disappointment, like a little boy's. His whisper was quite distinct: 'I want an orange.'

Tears of mortification pricking her eyes, Tersilla sought the help of the nuns, but there wasn't an orange to be had in the hospital. Once more, despite the barrage overhead, she hastened into the night. She knew now that this strange sickness, the 'Spagnola', of which the nuns had spoken, had temporarily affected Oscar's mind.

The Oscar she had known and loved would never have consigned her to the streets on a dark night, in an unknown city, on the strength of a childish whim. Her Oscar was the husband who had never returned from a card game at the *osteria* without a small flask of wine for his true love. Her Oscar was the father who, when fuel grew scarce, often did without lunch to chop sleepers – three for a lira was the concession rate for railwaymen – for kindling that would keep his children warm.

Then, in the night, blundering and afraid, she had searched in vain through rows of deserted streets, past silent shuttered shops, until a thin bar of light from a hotel doorway suggested this might be her one chance. Somehow, pushing through dust-smelling black-out curtains, she found herself in the hotel's dining-room.

All conversation suddenly halted. Candlelight glowed on goblets and polished silver. She hung her head, abashed, before the curious unspeaking stares of officers and their elegant women.

To the head waiter, polished and impassive, she could only stammer out, as she pointed to the fruit trolley: 'Please … could I buy an orange? My husband is in the hospital, very sick.'

Momentarily, the *maître d'hôtel* unbent. The orange was with the compliments of the management: there would be no charge. Blurting thanks, clutching the fruit as if it was a golden nugget, Tersilla backed from the dining-room. Curious eyes watched her go; a small proud figure in rusty black, only a white crocheted shawl to shield her against the night air.

Back at the hospital, she squeezed the orange, segment by segment, dribbling the juice between Oscar's cracked dry lips. Presently, to her alarm, he began to shake all over, as if with cold, the sweat sliding down his face and chest like water from a shower. Tersilla bent, stripping off her shawl, spreading it over his back and shoulders. Once more Oscar spoke: his back was in agony, and the doctors could find no way to relieve it.

How long she stayed there, Tersilla did not know – although afterwards she discovered that it had been more than thirty hours. At times, she realised, she had dozed off, so that momentarily she was no longer here at all, but in other places, at other times ... always with Oscar, there had never been any man for her but Oscar. The orchard that the Vicenzotto and Nardini families had owned at Udine, where somehow young Tersilla and Oscar had found it necessary to water the vegetable patches at least four times a day ... the outer stone staircase of the two-family house, the night when Oscar proposed to her, looking up at the sky and telling her: 'God will bless us, and the stars too.'

It was once more night when she awoke. In the darkness, the barrage seemed very loud; a nun was shaking her by the shoulder but at first she could not distinguish the words. 'We should take him to the shelter, under cover,' the nun was saying. Tersilla looked at her husband's face; he was barely conscious. Feral instinct told her that her vigil would not be long. 'No,' she objected. 'Let him stay here now.'

Eleven p.m. ... midnight ... one a.m. Somewhere a long way off the guns still grumbled. Turning, she saw that Oscar was looking directly beyond her, his eyes unasking yet afraid. He said, and she was never to forget, nor fully comprehend, his words: 'Now the train is coming and I'll go under it.' Briefly his left hand was lifted from the blanket, three fingers extended, and this time she knew what he meant without need of words: Antonietta, 4, Angelica, 2, and Dora, 1.

Then Oscar came upwards from the mattress, all in one movement, and into her arms, and died.

CHAPTER FIVE

'Four Quinine Tablets and a Heap of Hay to Die on'

13 October—21 October 1918

Mrs Cornelia Goedhart could scarcely believe her ears. Normally, the Goedharts' family physician, Dr Gerrit Broekma, was the soul of courtesy, almost one of the family. Times without number, he had taken coffee and cakes or a glass of Bols gin in the Goedharts' comfortable first-floor apartment in the little Netherlands town of Oosterbeek. But this Sunday morning, having stabbed the doorbell he was bawling unceremoniously from the hallway like a street vendor: 'Have any of you got the flu?'

Startled, Mrs Goedhart answered no. But instead of ascending the stairs, Broekma only followed up with a string of shouted injunctions: 'Then don't go in trams, don't visit anyone, don't receive people. If you feel weak, take a strong drink.' Then, before Cornelia Goedhart could even gather breath, he was gone, the street door slammed behind him – one of the swiftest prophylaxes in medical history.

It was only to have been expected. By dawn on this troubled Sunday, doctors everywhere were fighting a losing battle against the pandemic – and time, as never before, was of the essence.

Thousands, like Dr Charles Hickey, of Bennington, Nebraska, somehow kept going twenty-four hours a day; for long weeks, Hickey's bed was the front seat of his buggy, his faithful horse steering him home as he slept, in time for the next sick call. In Enid, Oklahoma, Dr David Harris ate with whatever family he dropped in on at mealtimes – but on his feet, right hand taking the patient's pulse, left hand grasping a chicken drumstick snatched from the pot, the broth drip-dripping on to the coverlet. And in Roanoke, Virginia, Dr Waller Jameson later recalled, his only sleep in three consecutive days was a two-hour nap sprawled forward on little Jean Gray's bed – the boy, cautioned by his mother, lying as still as a mouse for fear of waking him.

Every doctor could tell the same story. Each morning, after an all-night round, Dr Willem van der Harst, of Goes, Holland, slumped against the bathroom mirror, as drugged as a man in shock, fast asleep in the act of shaving. From the fashionable Bois de Boulogne to the garrets of Montmartre, Parisian doctors calculated that 200 visits in a twelve-hour day worked out at exactly three minutes per patient. Dr Gordon Walker, in Queenstown, Tasmania, almost regretted his offer to stand in for a sick colleague: a routine surgery now involved 250 sufferers. More disturbing still, at the local hospital, Walker was signing death certificates solely on the Night Sister's say-so. He was now confined to bed, too ill to examine the corpses, and so were the coroner and most of the police.

It was, thought Dr Clement Bryce Gunn, the strangest irony. Thirty-three years back, after setting up his brass plate in the little market-town of Peebles, Scotland, he had waited six vain weeks for his first patient; though she had been the town prostitute he had borne her in triumph all along the High Street to his surgery. Now, even in tiny (pop. 5216) Peebles, he was called out seventy times a day.

In vain, the men at the top did their best to lighten the load. On 1 October, the United States Congress had approved a one million dollar flu fund for the Public Health Service, bent on securing more physicians for the battle line; Boston alone was pressing for 500 extra doctors. As Surgeon General Rupert Blue saw it, the pandemic could not only impede the mobilisation of troops but imperil every industry on which the war effort depended: mining, munitions, ship-building. (5000 miners were down with flu in West Virginia.) Now Blue had both funds and authority to recruit another 1085 doctors and 703 nurses – but where to find them? Forced at last to scrape the barrel, Blue sent out a call from the Butler Building to old folks' homes and institutions for the debilitated all over America.

One volunteer was 85, another was handicapped by a wooden leg, yet a third had an addiction problem, but all of them, 1000 strong, had one thing in common: the right to add the magic letters 'M.D.' to their names, so they could be of service somehow. And gamely, dusting off their battered Gladstone bags, they started out.

Almost everywhere, doctors were suddenly as rare as frost in August. For every 200 Viennese, there was no more than one practitioner. In Rome, the one way to contact your physician was to leave a note in his pigeonhole at the nearest pharmacy – and hope. Afterwards Quebec's city fathers opined that at at least 10,000 victims received no medical attention at all, and it was as bad all over Canada. So scarce were doctors in Otterville, Ontario, that desperate farmers even offered the deeds of a homestead as fee for one consultation.

Even in the fighting forces, men fared little better. Lieutenant Ivo Cobb, of the Royal Army Medical Corps, reporting to a field ambulance near Amiens, was disconcerted when the no. 2 burst out to the C.O.: 'By God, sir, we've got a real doctor at last.' On enquiry, Cobb, a fashionable London consultant, found two of his colleagues were subalterns a month out of medical school, and the Major, after years of farming, had forgotten which end of a stethoscope was which. 'For God's sake don't you get it, or we *shall* be in the cart,' they implored him, but in vain. Four days later Cobb was as sick as any of his patients.

At Blandford Royal Air Force Camp, Dorset, Flight-Lieutenant Halliday Sutherland, ordered to inspect 2000 airmen in two hours flat, fell back on a classic military manoeuvre: as the men formed a square of two ranks, six paces apart, in the tradition of Omdurman and Tel-el-Kebir, Sutherland passed briskly along front and rear ranks, taking the pulse-rate of any man who stepped forward. Halfway through, the inspection took an unexpected turn; without warning Sutherland's feet shot from under him and he fell flat on his back in the sticky brown mud.

The situation was saved by a sergeant-major of the old school, whose stentorian voice called the men to order : 'Silence in the ranks! Not a flicker! Not the flicker of an eyelid!'

Almost any man who could read a thermometer was at a premium now. Egypt fell back on the medieval tradition of the barber surgeon, and in New Orleans, 175 dentists, cancelling all further appointments, stepped in to help. In Reykjavik, Iceland, the world's most northerly capital, veterinary surgeons now gave the sheep second priority in a battle to save humanity.

As fortunate as any were the people of Kirksville, Missouri, by chance the seat of the American School of Osteopathy. As doctors all over town began to feel the pressure, 500 students put aside their anatomy text-books to help out. Often five minutes skilled manipulation, elevating the rib-cage and loosening up the pleural cavity, was enough to bring precious relief, although once, in the case of a faulty heart-beat, students worked in relays for thirty-six hours to stimulate the vagus nerve, which accelerates the heart action.

Above all, it was no time for niceties. Hungary's Dr Ferenc Kukarik, rural medical officer, was facing a military tribunal on a charge of supplying soldiers with fake leave passes for hard cash, when a surprise defence witness burst into court – the Commissioner of Police for Kukarik's district, Cinkota. Guilty or no, he urged, Kukarik was needed back home to treat the sick. Without demur, the tribunal dropped all charges.

In Dublin, the Lord Mayor and Corporation spoke up with equal success for Dr Kathleen Lynn. A noted Sinn Fein leader she had been jailed six days back and was awaiting deportation, but now she was needed to tend the stricken in the rookeries of Baggot Street.

Some doctors, in any case, found it hard even to reach their patients – automobiles were still a rarity and petrol hard to come by. One of Rupert Blue's Health Officers, assigned to visit patients for fifty miles along the North Carolina coast, had the boon of a naval hydroplane, with his own pilot and mechanic: possibly history's first flying doctor. But rarely were they so privileged; most made do with bicycles or travelled by horse and buggy, swaddled, on these raw autumn nights, in fur robes, with a heated soapstone or a charcoal foot-warmer in the bottom of the cutter.

Few rated such low priority as the doctors of Budapest; their sole concession was to use the elevators, forbidden to tenants to conserve electricity, in apartment houses. For many oldsters, those high crumbling city tenements were a hazard in themselves, but in Milan, eighty-year-old Dr Lorenzini, with his white spade beard and broad-brimmed hat, solved the problem neatly. When his legs gave out, a strapping washerwoman, Ida Carlini, carried him piggyback from floor to floor.

Some showed infinite ingenuity. The doctors summoned from Emerald to Comet, Queensland, finding all existing roads choked with prickly pear, covered the twenty miles by ganger's trolley. At Green Point Rapids, British Columbia, a medical team caring for sick lumberjacks, working as far as Port McNeil, eighty-five miles north, would never have made it without a 'one-lunger', a 40-footer with a heavy duty one-cylinder engine, built wide to take rough water. Battling nausea, buffeted by racing twenty-foot tides, they somehow struggled on until the following spring.

Yet once at the patient's bedside, few doctors had any concept of the deadly disease they were fighting. Aboard the troopship *City of Marseilles*, bound for Murmansk, the ship's doctor diagnosed every case as one of yellow fever. Not all were so positive; in Wairoa, New Zealand, Post Office messenger Bernard Teague was one of many needing a sick leave certificate, but the puzzled Dr W. R. Aitchison could ascribe no other cause than 'general debility'. When the pandemic struck down every child in Bloomington, Indiana, 'as though the

Pied Piper of Hamelin had strolled his second stroll', one baffled doctor asked a young victim. 'Have you been eating green walnuts?' In Central, Arkansas, housewife Lillie Ladd still recalls how a visiting practitioner cried out to her husband, Melvin: 'This is my twenty-fifth case and I've lost the first twenty-four.'

There were almost as many theories as there were doctors – but too many at first placed reliance on heavy overdosage of drugs. Philadelphia's Dr J. M. Anders and New York's Dr Simon Baruch joined forces to condemn the indiscriminate use of phenacetin, a coal tar product that could induce nephritis, and Baruch's neighbour, Dr Henry Berg, found that it acted as a heart depressant, too. Columbia University's Dr Walter Bastedo came out against expectorants 'which doped the patients with paregoric'. Some were loud in their praise of phenol, but to Washington's Dr Noble Barnes this could result only in lasting renal damage.

Did morphine reduce the respiratory rate? Often, claimed Major Walter Brem, U.S. Army Medical Corps. Not so, chimed in Dr Herman Bryan, from Fort McKinley, in the Philippines, it dried up the secretions of the lungs. From Greece and Austria came lavish praise of mercury perchloride injections – which could only harm the gastric functions, charged Dr Frank Fitchett, in Dunedin, New Zealand.

Was tobacco the 'germicide' that British factory doctors believed? On their recommendation, smoking was now permitted for the first time in many war-plants – and in Australia, some pathologists conducted their autopsies through a thick blue smoke-screen of pipe-tobacco. Yet when chain-store grocer Johan Zijlstra, on his doctor's advice, made cigar-smoking compulsory for his staff in Zwolle, Holland, the one man who refused on religious grounds alone escaped the flu.

Yet if British doctors approved tobacco, they condemned liquor as heartily. The Royal College of Physicians went on record: 'Alcohol invites disaster,' and the Danish Government, in full accord, banned liquor even when prescribed by a doctor. But others were strongly in favour – the patients no less than the doctors. In Louisiana, still a 'wet' state, Scotch whisky soared to the unheard-of price of $20 a quart. When alcohol became available on prescription in Canada, queues of 500 at a time formed, stretching four deep for more than a city block – sometimes with varying results. After Vancouver's Dr Henry Milburn tried to break a city fire chief's fever with a massive dose of brandy, he called next morning to see if the man had passed a restful night. The fireman's wife was frosty: he hadn't slept and nor had anyone else. Her husband had passed the whole night singing.

There were many bizarre situations. Didio Brazão, a young clerk in Rio Maior, Portugal, had brandy prescribed as a preventative, but all through the pandemic, to mollify a tee-total employer suspicious of the smell, he claimed to be wearing an alcohol poultice on a sprained knee. In Danzig, following an authorisation of cut-price medicinal brandy, the tally of alleged sufferers doubled overnight. One city, Wellington, New Zealand, doled out all liquor from the Mayor's parlour – and it was His Worship himself, J. P. Luke, who acted as the bartender.

Both quinine and strychnine had their staunch defenders, but Dr (later Sir) Adolphe Abrahams, at Aldershot's Connaught Hospital, found the first 'useless', the second prone to increase a patient's delirium. From Delhi the veteran Dr Nanjunda Rao complained that the smart young doctors in Bombay and Madras were recklessly misusing the new wonder-drug, aspirin, fatally weakening the heart and bringing on pneumonia. But one Harley Street, London, old-timer, Dr Edward Turner, disagreed hotly: a patient should be 'drenched' with aspirin, twenty grains an hour for twelve hours non-stop, every two hours thereafter.

It was small wonder that Dr James B. Herrick of Chicago's Presbyterian Hospital, fulminated: 'This is poly-pharmacy run riot.'

And not only poly-pharmacy, but hydrotherapy, too. Dr Bernard Reams of Richmond, Virginia, swore by wash-tubs of scalding water; the patient's feet and legs were plunged in, a blanket draped round to retain the heat, and more water added, often for hours at a time, until the sufferer was as red as a beet. Sweden's Dr Karl Gronstedt, against all advice, packed his charges in icy sheets, then set four attendants to rubbing the chest and shoulders 'until their hands were about to catch fire', Blanket baths, camphor injections and soap-and-water enemas completed this high-pressure treatment, and to the astonishment of his colleagues at least twenty patients survived.

Not many were as unremitting as Dr Roland 'Kill or Cure' Burkitt, a blunt vigorous G.P. who was a byword among the settlers of Nairobi. As staunch a believer in cold packs as Dr Gronstedt, Burkitt had every one of his patients bedded down in wet sheets on their verandahs, relays of African servants standing by to douse them with watering-cans like so many flagging plants.

It was a bold man or woman who abandoned this soggy therapy for a comfortable bed. Normally Burkitt's old Ford was chugging up the drive as early as 5 a.m. to check that his orders were obeyed to the letter.

To Dr Juan Zamora, in Malanquilla, there were no such infallible standbys. From the first, the young Spaniard was certain of but one thing: as this disease spread like a brushfire, almost every patient in the little town was exhibiting contrary symptoms. The only sure treatments would be symptomatic, according to individual needs – though often rest, warmth and a liquid diet proved as efficacious as many more pretentious cure-alls.

Minutes after Don Mosen Buenaventura had hurried off towards the church, where a group of citizens clad in the grey blankets of the mountain folk stood guard over a pile of coffins, Zamora had his second intimation of the magnitude of the disaster. Across the street, what looked like a bundle of black rags was piled untidily in a doorway. Moving closer, he realised it was a man. He must have died at the moment of leaving the house – perhaps to seek a pharmacist's aid for the woman and two children whom Zamora found helpless in an upstairs room.

In truth, Zamora never knew, for all of them had been beyond his help, too far gone even to reveal whether this had been their father. Within seconds, death had reduced the man to a cipher.

Now, as for thousands of doctors all over the world, time, for Zamora, became a blur: a cycle of alarms by day and by night, of calloused hands tugging like beggars at his sleeve, of steep flights of spattered stone stairways, admonitions, advice, and soon, more and more often, death certificates.

In Bijuesca and Verdejo and Torrelapaja and Clares de Ribota, the pattern was the same. For classic bronchial congestion, syrup with sodium benzoate, sometimes with an infusion of crushed foxglove leaves, for the digitalis that would strengthen the heart. At other times, an expectorant with a pine resin base. For an inflamed thorax, a wet towel sprinkled with mustard powder.

Hasty meals at the pharmacist's house where doctors, by custom, were always invited to dine: roast kid, smoked cheese, a light mountain wine. More visits, more prescriptions. For retention of urine a diuretic made from maize. For serious debility, injections of Kola Robert, a tonic based on iron hypophosphite. On and on, hour after hour, until midnight had come and gone, and the only sound in the cold clear mountain silence was the hoofbeats of his Arab picking its way homeward under the stars.

It had to come to an end, Zamora knew. Day after day, the pandemic struck at the youngest and healthiest like a scythe through ripe corn, and day after day the young doctor felt his own resistance growing less. One night, towards the second week in October, he retired early to bed, hoping to stave off the inevitable, but within what seemed like minutes, Doña Paca, the schoolmaster's mother, was knocking at his door. Another townsman was sick and needed help.

An hour later, when he returned, Juan Zamora knew he had reached breaking-point. He lay in bed, swathed in blankets,

but the shivering would not stop. Though his head was burning his whole mind, even now, remained strangely calm and
lucid. This is the end, he thought, the Spanish Lady has found
me, too, and he noted, with almost clinical approval, that he
was not afraid of death. To the last he was abiding by his own
rigorous standards: a doctor must preserve his detachment.

Suddenly, to his surprise, strange vibrant chords burst from
the four brass knobs of the bedstead – almost as if an orchestra
was tuning up. By degrees the music grew louder and faster, as
turbulent and full-blooded as a *flamenco*, and his heart was
beating wildly in rhythm. With his last conscious thought,
Zamora fumbled for a thermometer, and held it between his
lips until he was sure the temperature would have registered.

Even now, he didn't bother to switch on the bedside light.
Coolly, he had reached his decision: if he were spared throughout the night, daylight, when it breached the shutters, would
reveal the gravity of his fever.

As the strain reached breaking-point, more and more doctors
followed Juan Zamora's example. Try as they might, they
just could not keep going.

Some were philosophical. At St Bartholomew's Hospital,
London, house physician Geoffrey Bourne kept a clinical eye
on both his temperature and his delirium; a Chinese pagoda
had suddenly become a fixture in an angle near the door. When
Sir Thomas (later Lord) Horder, the hospital's Assistant
Physician, strode in, enquiring briskly, 'What's all this non-
sense about a Chinese temple?' Bourne was professional
enough to correct him: 'Excuse me, sir, it's a pagoda, not a
temple.'

On the other side of London at no. 10 Harley Street, Dr
Alfred Schofield crawled painfully to bed with a sobering
reflection: if he did die, his insurance company's estimate of
life expectation would be right after all. (In fact, he recovered
in two days.) At Chaumont, France, Dr Harvey Cushing, a
senior consultant on Pershing's staff, was careful to note in his
diary: 'I wobble like a tabetic ... spells of diplopia' – in lay

language, a man with a wasting disease, afflicted by double vision. Then a cheering thought struck him: 'If it really hit the German Army thus hard, we may ... thank it for helping us win the war.'

Some gave up reluctantly. On the fringe of the New Forest, at Christchurch, Hampshire, Dr Sidney Snell fought off all sensations of diplopia; jumping into his car, he set off to visit a patient. Meeting two donkeys side by side, he endeavoured to steer between them – knocking down the only one there was. Returning home, Snell knew that he *must* give in – once he had steered his car between three gateposts.

Others, struggling to carry on, recalled the words of Jesus in the synagogue at Nazareth, 'Physician, heal thyself' – though often with varying results. At Sliema, Malta, Dr Joe Galizia, striving to bring down his fever, sprang blithely into a cold bath – then expired after eleven days in a coma. Surprisingly, Dr Victor Henrikson was luckier in Växjö, Sweden; no sooner had the fever struck him on his hospital rounds than the heroic Henrikson gorged himself with a huge meal, followed up with a monster dose of calomel, topping off with a bottle of port. Then, fully dressed, he slept until the calomel unceremoniously awoke him – relieved to find his temperature now normal.

Most country doctors had no chance to give in; like it or not, their patients pursued them to the bitter end. Gales lashed the Shetland island of Yell, and the one doctor, Harry Pearson Taylor, was down with a temperature of 102°F – but it was to his bedroom that a woman hit by a car was brought one night for primitive medication, and it was on the floor beside his bed that she died in the small hours of the next morning. It was the same with Dr Ronald French in the quiet Surrey hamlet of Burgh Heath. Like all country doctors, French was his own dispenser – so automatically his counterpane became the dispensary where, under the anxious eye of his wife, Dorothy, he mixed up potions and powders.

And to make the doctors' lot harder yet, hospitals everywhere were crammed to suffocation, unable to carry on.

Now a hospital ward had become the easiest place in the world in which to die.

Reporter Gison Thonfält was horrified. A seasoned veteran of the Stockholm daily, *Folkets Dagblad Politiken*, Thonfält had had the share of tragedy that is any newsman's lot: fire, bloody slayings, street accidents. But never had he seen sights to equal those which he now witnessed at Västmanland Regimental Headquarters.

Not only the hospital but the gymnasium, the chapel, the canteen, were crammed with sick and dying men. Even the corridors were littered with stretchers placed head to toe – men whose end was fast approaching, cleared from the main wards to make room for new patients. Distraught relatives were everywhere; a Russian woman who knew no word of Swedish bent over her dying husband, beckoning pitifully to passers-by, frantic to communicate. Not far away, a young wife had fainted over her husband, who lay dead in a pool of blood. A father who had kept the final vigil over his son was hunched in a dark corner, sobbing like a child.

Then, as Thonfält watched, two orderlies gingerly approached a man who had died only a few minutes earlier. A letter had just arrived from his home – and after a muttered colloquy they agreed it must be opened. Drawing close, Thonfält read an anxious mother's last message: 'We've heard the Spanish flu is about down there. You do take good care of yourself, don't you, and wrap up well when you go out?'

Beside himself, one orderly burst out, 'This is murder.' Somehow nobody, not even the doctors near at hand, could bring themselves to answer him, let alone disagree.

Such shameful conditions were due in part to Sweden's coalition government of ineffectual liberals – dubbed by newsmen 'the too-late government' – to all intents subservient to the stiff-necked militarist clique dominating the court of King Gustav V, and reluctant to abandon conscription. Now the Radical-Socialist Party, spurred on by delegates like Edvin Malmsjö, launched a dramatic two-week probe of military hospitals all over Sweden – to spotlight cases of sick soldiers bedded down on straw in stables, moribund men shaken rudely awake and accused of malingering, convalescents forced to exercise horses in defiance of regulations.

Faced with the threat of a Socialist-inspired General Strike, the government now climbed down and cancelled all military manoeuvres.

Yet by 15 October, such sights were commonplace in every hospital in the world. 'It is best not to move the patient to hospital,' warned Dr Victor Scheel, head of the Special Influenza Unit at Denmark's Bispebjerg Hospital, 'The contagion is so strong that official measures are purely illusory.' The French Academy of Medicine agreed. Galling though it was to admit it, the risk of death was far greater than in a private home.

In Boston, the hospital death-rate had now reached an all-time high of fifty per cent – even with the beds screened off by draw-sheets, the chances of nursing twenty patients to a room and avoiding secondary infections were impossible. Even in asceptic Switzerland, one-third of all those admitted to Zurich's hospitals contracted pneumonia – and many Swiss hospitals, like those in Britain, were now so overcrowded they refused all further admissions.

It was worse still in the camps of the United States Army. Despite the protests of the Army's Surgeon-General, William Gorgas, sixty-four-year-old victor of the battle against yellow fever in Panama, many doughboys shivered all through winter in summer uniforms – often in jam-packed camps lacking both hospitals and steam heat. A man's average floor space was 21 square feet, as against the 60 recommended by Gorgas. Never once was Gorgas consulted on the selection of cantonment sites or hospitals – and the nursing orderlies who staffed them, ex-farmers and clerks, were woefully lacking in experience.

As thousands daily fell victim, more and more unlikely buildings were pressed into hospital service. At Charlesville, Queensland, it was the church hall, with sheepshearers weighing in to boil up billies of soup ... at Enderline, Nebraska, a run-down railway hotel called the Hilton House, with fifteen teenagers on round-the-clock duty as orderlies. For Montreal's Department of Health Director, Dr Seraphin Boucher, the city yielded up a curling rink and the Grenadier Guards Armoury; Copenhagen made do with an Oddfellows' Lodge. In Richmond, Virginia, it was the John Marshall High School, with its daunting sign: 'Castor Oil To Be Given Immediately To Incoming Patients.'

At St John's, Arizona, it was the abandoned county jail ... a railway waiting-room in Harwich, England ... a Masonic Temple in Waterbury, Connecticut. At Montego Bay, Jamaica, the deserted offices of the 'Northern News' ... a dance hall in Wellington, New Zealand, with the men's rest room standing in as a morgue ... an Ursuline convent in Parma, Italy ... a newly-built oil plant in Vastmänland, Sweden ... the Post Office at Windhoek, South Africa, where postmaster Robert Nisbet had his patients tucked up in mail-bags.

Of all these unconventional hospitals, the shining example was Sing Sing Prison, twenty-five miles up the Hudson River from New York. Despite the damp low-lying buildings, Warden William Moyer and prison physician Amos Squire lost not one man among the 106 convicts who went down – fourteen of them with severe pneumonia. Clamping down a rigid quarantine – which ruled out the five visits a month by prisoners' relatives – Moyer and Squire next established an isolation ward to which every suspicious case was promptly banished. Absolute quiet and rest, rooms at outside air temperature, and a diet of milk, whisky and four raw eggs daily saw every man on the road to recovery.

But untold millions knew no such comforts. In Riga, Latvia, isolation was an unheard-of luxury; flu patients were packed alongside others mortally sick from typhus and cholera. One nurse recalled Drumheller Hospital, Alberta, as 'an inferno of sick and suffering', but that same description would have fitted hundreds of others – like Gothenburg's Sahlgrenska Hospital, where the bereaved had literally to grapple among mounds of naked bodies in the mortuary to seek out their dead for shrouding. At Hong Kong's Tung Wah Hospital, patients lay not only in the beds but between them and under them as well. Even in the Exhibition Building Emergency Hospital at Adelaide, South Australia, inmates were packed two in a bed and depended on family food parcels to survive.

At the Bumper Hall Hospital, Kingston, Jamaica, patients sometimes waited twenty-four hours before getting even a cup of milk – and facilities were as bad everywhere. Many of New Zealand's rural emergency hospitals had only dairy thermometers used for testing the cream when making butter – one foot long, as thick as a finger, with mysterious legends such as 'Scalding' and 'Boiling'. The top floor wards at Melbourne's Wirth's Park Rest Home, reached only by outside stairways, had no plumbing facilities whatsoever; all water had to be carried up and all refuse carried down. The roof was of galvanised iron, too, so that the sick sweltered all day in a temperature of 105°F.

Few but the most modern city hospitals had such essentials as oxygen cylinders, inhalers or intravenous feeding apparatus; oxygen tents were then unknown. Often rusty tins did duty as spittoons, and standards of hygiene were unspeakable.

At Christchurch General Hospital, a distraught Sister hastened up to Senior Nurse Winifred Pollard: 'Have you any sputum cups?' But Nurse Pollard shook a weary head.

'None? Then what are your patients doing?'

'Spitting on the floor.'

The Sister knew when she was beaten. 'Then mine will have to spit on the floor, too.'

It wasn't surprising that many now shunned a hospital as they would a lazaret. Every Brazilian in his senses gave a wide berth to Rio's Santa Casa Hospital; to make room for newcomers, it was said, the hopelessly sick were given a lethal brew called 'midnight tea'. The fear was more logical in Budapest, for a new ban on hospital visitors – who alone provided food – meant virtual starvation. Thousands would have endorsed Venetian Tito Spagnol's bitter epitome of hospitalisation: 'Four quinine tablets and a heap of hay to die on.'

Private Frederick Frewer, of the London Scottish Regiment, owed his life to his widowed mother, Constance, a woman whose determination proved a match for any Army non-com. Booked for leave and sensing that he was coming down with a 105°F fever, Frewer headed not for the M.O. at Wisbech Camp, near Cambridge, but for his mother's house at 44 Malden Road, New Malden, Surrey. As a matter of form, having put her son to bed and called the doctor, Mrs Frewer informed the local military authority.

But when an Army ambulance called to collect him next morning, Mrs Frewer refused the sergeant all access to her house – arguing spiritedly that a mother's care rated far above any crowded military hospital. She resisted so forcibly that the ambulance men, pressed for time, finally gave in – and later Frewer learned that one friend from the next street hadn't even survived the draughty journey to the hospital.

There were men who showed bitter determination. Near Foggia, on the Adriatic, Leonardo Martella stood guard over his sister with an axe for two days and nights until she recovered, determined to behead any man who tried to take her to hospital. Aboard the barque *Lange de Fécamp*, en route to France after eight months on the Grand Banks, Seaman Joseph Chevalier had one fixed resolve: no hospital would ever claim *him*. The flu had been sweeping Newfoundland when they left, and now, at every watch, Chevalier looked death in the face anew: two, three or more comrades whom he couldn't shake into wakefulness. When the barque reached Cherbourg, he knew, every man would be booked for inspection at the Military Hospital.

Once in port, the wily Chevalier soon saw the way out; the hard-pressed duty doctor contented himself with a cursory inspection of each man's tongue. Retiring to the head with a toothbrush, Chevalier scrubbed away until his tongue glowed a rosy pink – and was the one man among the crew to gain a coveted leave permit.

Back in Cherbourg after an eight-day bout in his hometown, Chevalier found himself the *Lange de Fécamp*'s sole survivor. Every other man had entered that hospital; none had left it alive.

Over by Belvedere, the fog bell was tolling. Like a veil of yellow-white gauze, the sea-mist, heavy with the salt of the Pacific, came drifting through the Golden Gate. Soon it would blanket all San Francisco, from Fisherman's Wharf to Nob Hill and the Mint end of Market Street. But down by the Embarcadero, aboard the s.s. *Newport*, the fog bell was only dimly audible above the strident cries of 'All ashore' that echoed in the corridors, the long blast of the whistle sending a tremor through the ship. Fog or no, the *Newport* was sailing on the night tide – bound for Panama and Corinto, Nicaragua.

In a panelled stateroom on the saloon deck, Emilio Alvarez Lejarza was alone. Reflected in the mirror before which he stood were reminders that a gay farewell party had just concluded: long-stemmed Baccarat roses, empty champagne glasses, ashtrays piled high. But Lejarza had no eye for these tokens of old friends just departed and a pleasant voyage to come. With curiosity and wonder and a lurking sense of shame, he was studying his own face.

Even now, the thirty-two-year-old Lejarza could scarcely believe that he had been capable of such an action. He, an official delegate of the Nicaraguan Government, soon to be first secretary of Washington's Nicaraguan Embassy, had shamefully deceived the country that had been his host and had even made a blatant attempt to bribe a ship's officer.

Yet the whole trip had promised so well. As the forthcoming first secretary, Lejarza had been sent on a good-will tour of every Nicaraguan Consulate in the United States, and on the spur of the moment had made it a honeymoon voyage, bringing with him his bride, Juanita. Then, ten days earlier in Chicago, a sudden dizzy spell, a stabbing pain in the small of his back, had told him the worst. The virus of the dreaded Spanish flu had somehow entered his body.

Lejarza knew real fear – not so much of the disease itself but of dying in hospital in a strange land, 3000 miles from

Nicaragua. Somehow, he determined, he must deceive the health authorities until he and Juanita were safely aboard the *Newport*.

It was no easy task. In San Francisco, Lejarza was feeling worse still; he wondered if he could ever keep going. Moreover, doctors were stationed at the Customs House to examine all arrivals and departures, with uniformed police standing by to remove suspect cases to hospital.

Then, at the eleventh hour, desperation drove Lejarza to do what he had to do. A brief enquiry at the shipping company's office revealed that the ship's surgeon was Dr A. E. Dilley. At a Market Street jeweller's, Lejarza invested in an ornate gold pocket watch – asking the craftsman to do a rush job of engraving the initials 'A.E.D.' If he passed the health authorities and Dilley was still suspicious, this should help to put him in a trusting frame of mind. But first there were the port doctors to be reckoned with. Half an hour before settling the bill at the Hotel St Francis, Lejarza, borrowing Juanita's rouge, locked himself in their private bathroom.

Now, as the *Newport* inched away from the pier, he stared with growing disgust at the face he had thus transformed – painted like a Mission District street-walker's, yet healthy enough to pass muster in the garish half-light of the Embarcadero. He had even sought out Dr Dilley and the surgeon, although surprised, even curious, had accepted the watch gratefully.

So he was safe. Once they were well past the Gate, he would summon the doctor and confess his deception. It would be too late then for the ship to be put back. It was strange, he thought, that the ambitions of a newly-married man, a shining diplomatic career ahead of him, should scale down to one final intention: to die 3000 miles away in Managua.

She had prayed for a sign. Night after night, lying wakeful in the darkness after one more fruitless argument with Marius, Else Dahl had prayed that God should in some way signify his need of her. And now, in the night, it came.

Even at 1.30 a.m. she was wide awake, for her conscience had troubled her badly, ever since the epidemic had reached Ejstrup, so that when the rapping came at the window she was out of bed in an instant and past Marius' bed, running towards the sound. 'Mrs Dahl,' a man's voice was calling, 'Mrs Dahl!'

'Who is it?' she called, her voice pitched low, in the hope that Marius would not awake.

'Nils Hanson, Mrs Dahl. Please, will you come to my wife? I think she's dying.'

So this was proof enough that God wanted her, as she had always believed. 'I'll come,' she answered, without hesitation.

Swiftly, for the first time since her marriage, Else donned her crisp white nurse's uniform, checking that her thermometer was securely in the pocket. She would have need of that, she knew, in the days to come; almost no one in Ejstrup, let alone on the farms, owned a thermometer, and if anyone suspected they were coming down with flu they would be bound to send for her, if only to check their temperature.

If medicine was needed, then she would have to send to Dr Thorup at Kolding, ten miles away, for Penisetyl tablets that would reduce the fever. But Thorup himself was too overburdened with work to pay calls in Ejstrup, so that unless a patient developed pneumonia and she had to beg the doctor for an ambulance, the whole weight of the epidemic in Ejstrup and district would rest squarely on the shoulders of Nurse Else Dahl, who had only her bicycle to carry her wherever she might be needed.

Passing to the bathroom, she first collected soap and a nailbrush for her personal use, then on to the linen cupboard for clean rags; she would surely need these to sponge her patients. Finally, to the kitchen for soda-water. She had learned the value of that in her nurse's training, back in Copenhagen; half a cup of boiling milk topped up with soda-water was a powerful aid in clearing the chest of phlegm.

Moving through the silent house, she looked with an emotion akin to love at the everyday symbols of her life with Marius: the solid oak and mahogany furniture, the beige-coloured lounge carpet they had chosen so carefully, the white curtains offset by blue plush-covered chairs. It had been a good marriage, all four years of it, never marred by quarrels until now, but strengthened by their love for Kirsten, and with a faint twinge of shame she wondered how Marius would feel when he awoke in the morning to realise she had defied him. Would he ever understand her innate belief that she, a lone professional, must see this through?

But only fleetingly. Briefly, Else paused in the bedroom doorway, and in this moment she saw that Marius was awake. In the half-light, their eyes met, and though neither spoke a word she realised that he was aware of her decision and accepted it – perhaps even, from the expression on his face, with a perverse sensation of pride.

She slipped quietly from the room.

At times like these every veteran nurse could feel, with Else Dahl, a professional's lonely pride. Whatever the challenge, years of tough training and practical experience had armoured her to meet it.

Duties which once would have left her aghast were suddenly commonplace. Attached to a French ambulance train on the Italian front, Red Cross Nurse Henrietta Tayler now viewed thirty-six hours of continuous duty as just a way of life. Nurses like New York's Permelia Doty worked on uncomplaining when twenty-bed wards were stretched to fifty, and cots and wheel-chairs did duty for beds – yet the total nursing staff remained the same.

At Toronto General Hospital, Nurse Gladys Brandt spent hours each day escorting bodies to the morgue – in an elevator so cramped she had to lean on the corpse to manipulate the switch. The long nightwatches, when the delirious fought their nightmares and the wards grew stale with the approach of death, were part of it, too; then the nurse tiptoed from bed to bed, torchlight playing briefly on each tormented face and rumpled blanket. To keep herself wakeful through nights like these, when the red cotton screens were drawn round bed after bed, Nurse Marguerite Pugnaire, at no. 53 Military Hospital, Marseilles, crocheted nineteen bed-covers.

If doctors were hard to come by, nurses, it seemed, were scarcer still. Some nurses from New York's Henry Street Settlement were even locked in houses or kidnapped by desperate relatives – and one, with only two months training, was offered $100 dollars a week to tend a wealthy New Yorker and his wife. (The standard pay for a trained nurse was $50 a month.) And as nurses, too, fell sick, those still on their feet were truly beyond price: at Cape Town's Summit Hospital, sixty-eight of them went down in one day. At Masterton Public Hospital, New Zealand, things were so desperate that the 'Sister-in-Charge' was a three-month probationer and her no. 2, christened 'The Bedpan Queen', a typist in a garage, promoted from kitchen-maid.

It was hardly surprising that in Cleveland, Mississippi, when Peggy, her six-month-old baby was stricken, Mrs Sylvia Wiggins gratefully accepted a nurse not ordinarily welcome: a girl-friend of her husband before marriage.

Faced with unimaginable horror, it was only human that some felt like giving up. At Brunswick City Hospital, Germany, Nurse Erna Wäsche, brushing the hair of a mortally sick girl, was suddenly filled with revulsion. 'You are going to die,' she thought, then, as she took in the serried rows of faces, 'and you, and you, and you!' But soon, as thousands of others were doing, she took a grip on her emotions and worked on.

At Edmonton, Alberta, the Victorian Order of Nurses found, with dismay, that their charter prohibited the nursing of epidemic cases – then, to a woman, voted to disregard it. At Chicago's Augustana Nursing School, the nurses kept going with unpalatable if prophylactic doses of beer spiked with castor-oil. Rank was no barrier; at Bellevue Hospital, New York, with 144 nurses down, fifty-year-old Superintendent Carrie Brink, twenty-five years a Bellevue veteran, herself took over a ward nurse's duties ... opening a round-the-clock snack bar for her charges ... working on to care for 3000 cases, although her feet and ankles swelled so painfully she was forced

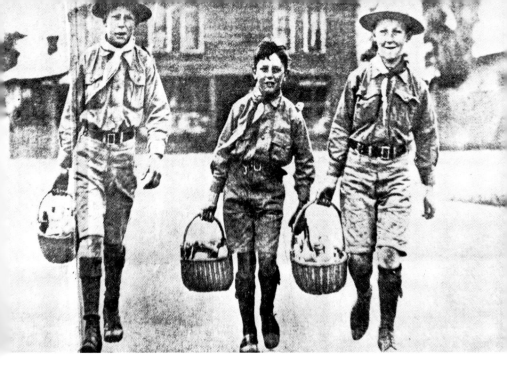

Above : Boy Scouts in twenty-seven countries carried soup and bland diets to flu-stricken households. *Below* : Hastily-converted transportation, from Model Ts to delivery vans, stood in as ambulances in Wellington, New Zealand.

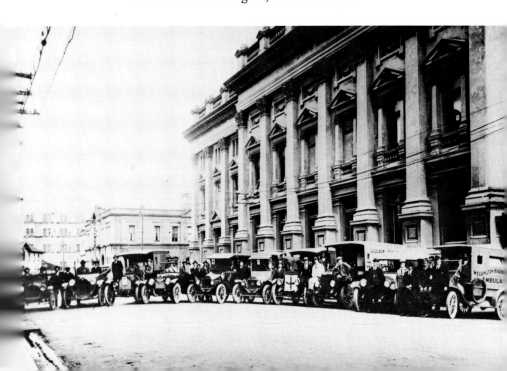

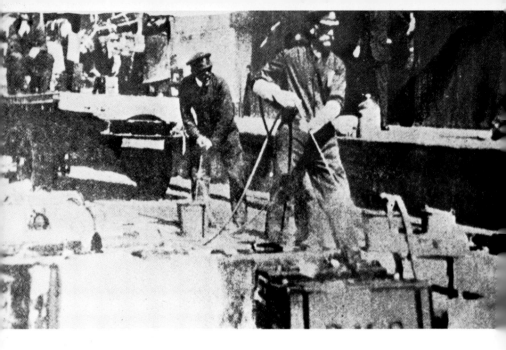

Above: Futile emergency precautions abounded across five continents. Here zealous Harbour Board officials in Durban fumigate travellers' baggage. *Below*: For many, like these policemen in Seattle, Washington, medicated masks became compulsory.

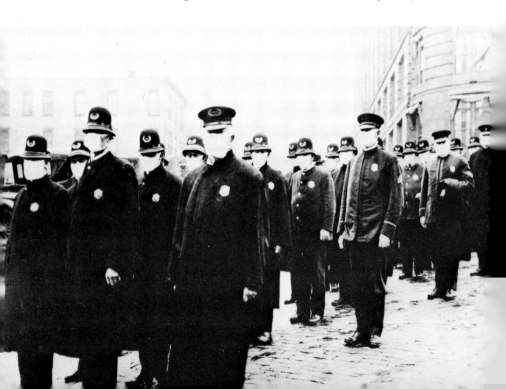

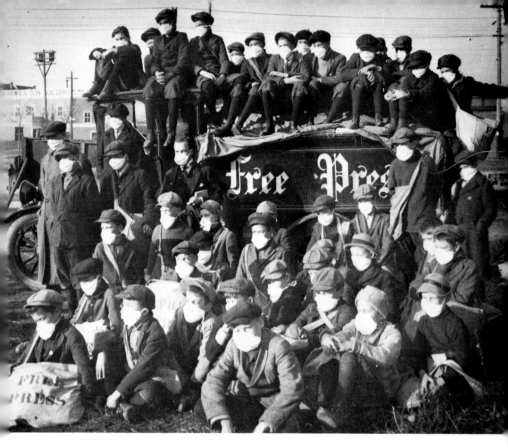

Above: Business as usual for newsboys in Winnipeg, Manitoba.

Below: Bank-tellers in Sydney, New South Wales.

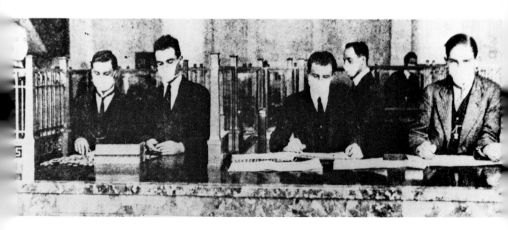

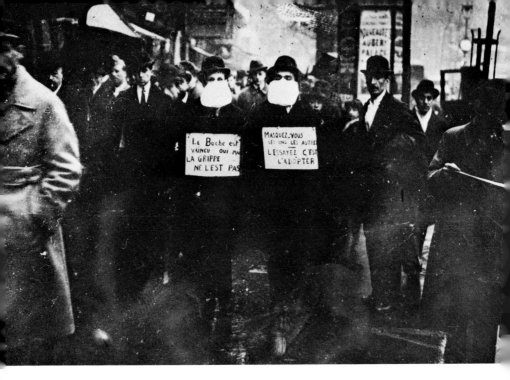

Above: Placard worn by Parisian boulevardiers reads: "THE GERMANS ARE BEATEN BUT NOT THE FLU". *Below*: For 10,000 Australian travellers, border checks, long sojourns in cramped quarantine stations, became routine.

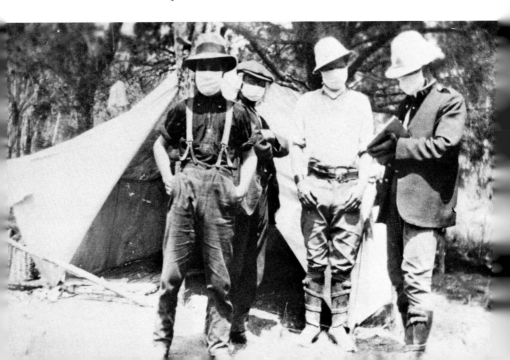

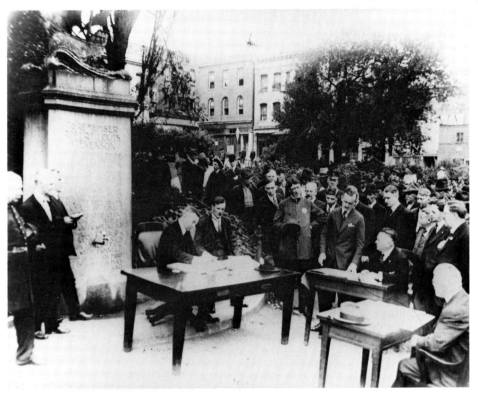

Above: Some law-courts, as in San Francisco, transferred to the open-air. *Below*: In Copenhagen's *Politiken*, the Angel of Peace laments: 'They won't have anything to do with me, but that detestable Spanish woman can go anywhere'.

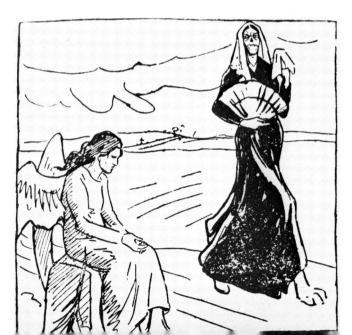

METROPOLITAN MOVIES.

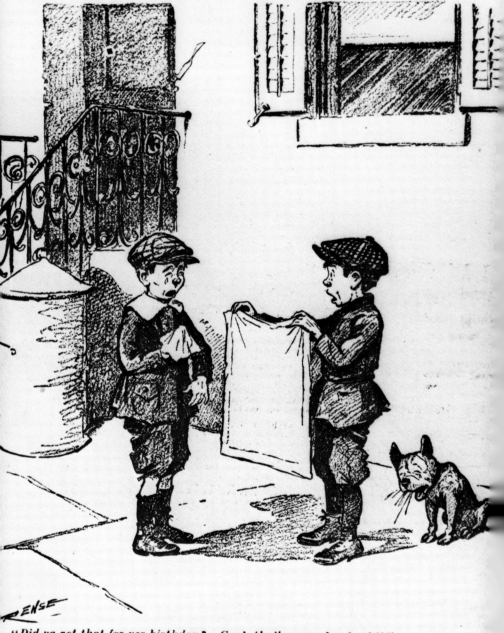

"*Did ya get that fer yer birthday? Gee! that's some hankachif.*"
"*Yeh, me mother made it fer me. It's good fer a hundred sneezes.*"

For newspaper cartoonists, the pandemic was a field-day: street arabs pictured in Joseph Pulitzer's *New York World*.

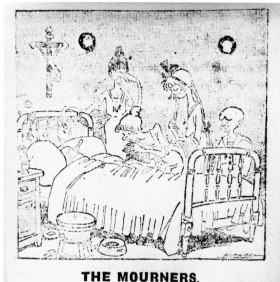

THE MOURNERS.

"That's just like papa. He goes and dies just as the new Chaplin film visits our village."—"Esquella," Barcelona.

Above: Unfilial daughters as seen by Barcelona's *Esquella*. *Below*: Milan's *Avantix* saw the killer virus as the new Napoleon, undisputed conqueror of Europe.

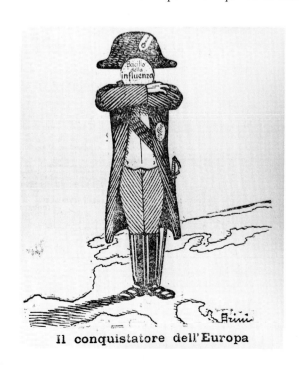

Il conquistatore dell'Europa

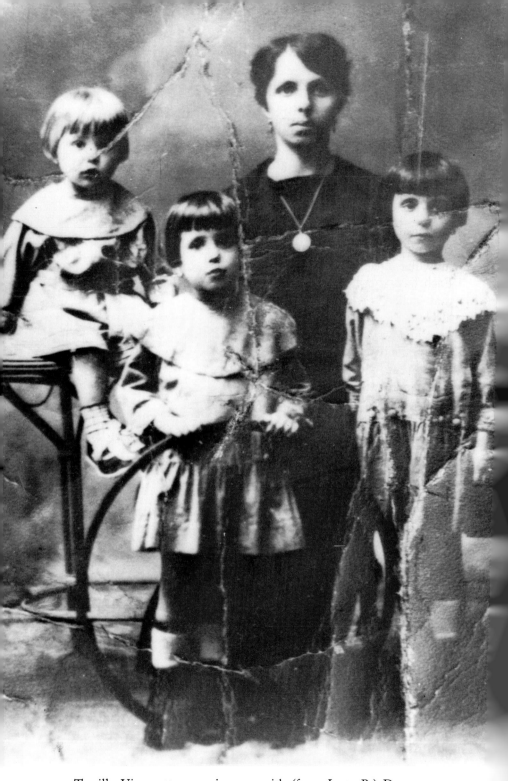

Tersilla Vicenzotto, seen in 1919 with (from L. to R.) Dora, one, Angelica, two, and Antonietta, four.

to wear cloth-covered canvas shoes over plaster casts.

The more hopeless the case, the greater the challenge. In a tent hospital at Hirson, France, Nurse Germaine Girod, caring for a pain-racked soldier, called in a doctor who had only one verdict: *'Il est foutu.'* (He's done for.) But somehow Germaine couldn't accept it; the man's lips were violet and he could no longer speak, but she vowed: 'Come what may – I shall bleed him.'

Each day she cut harder and deeper into his back and chest, eight incisions at a time, following up the cupping with intramuscular injections of camphorated oil to strengthen the heart. Each day, she noted, as she sponged the incisions, the blood that welled forth grew less black, and the blanket baths in alcohol, the hot drinks, helped, too. They were the two most gruelling weeks of her life, but at the end she knew a sense of infinite triumph, for the soldier walked confidently out of the tent, bound for convalescent leave, a young unknown Frenchman with all life before him. She had brought back a human soul from beyond the grave.

Often an itinerant nurse had the scantiest equipment; her overnight bag held little more than a thermometer, a nailbrush, alcohol, creosol, green soap, feeding cups and drinking tubes, gauze, rubber sheeting and formaldehyde. Yet they achieved therapeutic miracles; one Public Health Nurse, at Muscle Shoals, Alabama, cared for 139 patients for three days and lost only one.

They were nothing if not resourceful. New Orleans nurse Grete Judis, unable to obtain quick transit from call to call, solved the problem by commandeering a hearse. In Udine, which had fallen to the Austrians a year earlier, the Ospedale Dante's Sister Serena knew her flu patients needed nourishing broth – but ingredients just weren't to be had. So one dark October night, retiring soft-spoken Sister Serena stole past the sleepy Austrian sentries to the cattle pound and as quietly led back a bullock to the slaughter.

It was harder, by far, for the volunteers. By Tuesday, 15 October, the scale of the pandemic was so unprecedented that no previous standards held good. By local consensus, one of Surgeon-General Blue's Public Health Officers had now assumed command in every one of the forty-eight States. This day alone saw 1722 deaths in Berlin – and two days later 1900 died in Paris. Simultaneously, the sickness had reached its peak in Liverpool, Baltimore and Vienna – where the red-and-white city flag streamed from the *Rathaus* flagstaff edged with black ribbon.

Anyone willing to sponge down a patient, fill a water bag or even make a bed now had a part to play – yet to some harassed professionals, it seemed, would-be helpers had never been more obtuse. At Christchurch General Hospital, New Zealand veteran nurse Sybella Maude was beside herself with vexation: a volunteer given a thermometer to take temperatures hastened back ten minutes later with the mercury parted. Near to tears, she confessed: 'I just put it in the soup to see if it was hot.' In Vancouver, B.C., Dr Henry Milburn would have sympathised – after posting an untrained volunteer by a sick bed overnight to administer castor oil 'when necessary'. Next morning, the patient enquired of Milburn weakly: for how many hours, on the hour, must he go on taking castor oil?

Luckily, only a handful were as short on know-how as those ministering to a troop of Sea Scouts, hospitalised in the National Stadium on Rome's Via Flaminia. Their sole contribution was a few cans of preserved meat – without benefit of a tin-opener.

But many a volunteer – and medical man, too – found their patients equally obtuse. One Yorkshire doctor, who absent-mindedly left his thermometer beneath a farmer's armpit, returned next day to find it still in position – though the man complained it had cost a night's sleep to keep it there. A Cape Town victim, given a scarce egg for nourishment, promptly fried it and clapped it as a poultice on his stomach. Another, in Sydney, New South Wales, hastened back to his doctor for a booster injection of vaccine; the first, he claimed, had cured his corns. And at Christchurch Hospital, New Zealand, one irate house-surgeon, sounding a woman patient, found it near impossible to detach his stethoscope; as an interim precaution she had anointed her chest with treacle.

Few were as literal as the Vancouver patient who greeted his doctor tucked snugly up in bed fully clothed in overalls and boots. He explained that he had merely followed Board of Health instructions: go straight to bed if seized with sudden pains.

Sometimes sheer snobbery was a volunteer's sole motivation; if one helped the less fortunate, one must still adhere to certain standards. One Society woman declined not only a motor-cycle and sidecar but the first automobile offered her, which was 'only a Ford'; it took a five-seater to coax her on a mercy errand. The one woman arriving at Napier Technical College, New Zealand, wearing a serviceable gingham apron was given immediate charge of the steamed custard; by week's end she had taken over the mutton broth and the beef tea as well. The others, all wearing modish dresses, had come to 'organise'.

But many more were moved by a warm and simple desire to help their fellow-man – as Dr Doris Gordon recalled later: 'The drama of the Priest, the Levite and the Samaritan came alive again in 1918.' One hundred women volunteers in Toronto, known as the 'Sisters of Service', had only two lectures and a hasty perusal of a nursing booklet, but they started out the same evening in masks and cotton overall aprons and in three weeks cared for 1000 families. Those 400 altruists staffing Copenhagen's Doctors' Bureau, which co-ordinated calls for help, worked on night after night until past 3.30 a.m. And not all even knew the stimulus of working as one of a team. Armed with no more than ether bottles of linctus and a 20-lb. bag of linseed, Mrs Alice Ransom nursed the Australian outback town of Byrock single-handed, for out of twenty-seven families, twenty-three were down. A trained nurse, Mrs Ransom was also the railway's level-crossing keeper, but there was nothing for it but to double up the jobs.

Times without number, the Salvation Army proved themselves, as General Bramwell Booth had styled them, the

'Servants of All' – and nowhere more so than in Nasaker, Sweden. When sickness brought the town to a standstill, Captain Ester Pettersson took over the entire community, not only nursing the sick but checking the farmer's grain, running the bread bureau, doling out clothing cards. As she worked, desk-bound, far into each night, her Lieutenant trudged from farm to farm, feeding the cattle and poultry.

All of them needed a willingness to face grim scenes. One Philadelphia nurse found a house in which a lone woman had lain dead and putrefying for a week. Another found a husband dead in the same room where his wife lay with two new-born babies: a home where the quick and the dead were ranged side by side. But most had more than their share of what one admiring city official called 'six penn'orth of pluck'. Wasn't she scared, one teenage girl volunteer was asked, in Richmond, Virginia, to traverse that dark road from hospital to street-car? 'If anyone speaks to me,' she replied scornfully, 'I'll just COUGH.'

They needed stamina, too – the women no less than the men. At Ferrara's Casa Pia, whose concern was unmarried mothers and their children, the Mother Superior, the gynae-cologist, Professor Merletti, and Emma Libretti, an eighteen-year-old foundling, were the only three hale enough to carry on. But fortified with steaks and cognac – and a strong Tuscan cigar apiece when they bore the dead to the mortuary – they stuck it out.

Nothing was too much trouble. At Whakatane, on New Zealand's Bay of Plenty, volunteers manhandled milk churns of soup to homes as much as five miles distant along rough bush track. Few sought for reward, but one man, Government Inspector F. G. Wayne, did receive an unexpected tribute. After weeks of providing the Maori settlements with food and medicine, he dropped in one day on a christening party. To his astonishment he learned that the newborn had been bap-tised 'Aspirin Wayne'.

For one moment in time, class barriers were put aside: the haves and have-nots worked together as one. In her father's luxurious apartment in Owensboro, Kentucky, Clementina Wolf, a wealthy merchant's daughter, spent long secret hours with needle and thread, leaving each morning with a half-hidden bundle beneath her arm. Only when the flu had taken Clementina's life, did her family discover she possessed hardly one stitch of clothing: all her stylish dresses and lingerie had been made over to clothe the sick.

In a public ward at San Francisco Hospital, call-girl 'Billie' Gibson was dying, too. Now, for the first time, Red Cross workers realised that the girl who for weeks had worked with them under an assumed name in the slums of the Mission District was once the darling of the scandal-sheets: the delin-quent whose reluctant testimony had earned Barbary Coast politician Jimmy Lawlor a two-year stretch for transporting her for immoral purposes across the State Line, in flagrant violation of the Mann Act. Forswearing her old life, for months disguised as a man to ensure anonymity, 'Billie' had chosen this way to redeem herself. She had no fine clothes or lingerie to give to the sick: only her life.

Hastening up to William Wallace of Auckland's Hospital Board, an excited crony thought to impart startling news: a man they both knew well had sat up all night with a dying woman. Smiling patiently, Wallace explained: 'But it's hap-pening hundreds of times every night.' Death, if it came, would find all of them ready – like the woman volunteer who arrived at Chicago's State Council of Defence outfitted from head to foot in gold: gold tinsel dress, gold bonnet, gold muff, gold slippers. It was, she said, her resurrection dress; eager to serve, she was also ready for heaven at a moment's notice.

Sometimes these newcomers gave the old-timers fresh per-spective. At the John Marshall High School Emergency Hospi-tal, Richmond, Virginia, one blackboard notice loomed larger than any: infants in the Baby Ward were *not* to be picked up and petted. The signatory, Dr McGuire Newton, a leading pediatrician, had firm views on the subject: babies must be allowed to 'cry it out'. Hence, Newton's anger, arriving one night, to find a teenager unrepentantly fondling a lone infant.

'Can't you all read?' he demanded, his pointer stabbing the blackboard. But the girl was undaunted. 'We can read,' she retorted, 'but this baby isn't ill. He's been brought here because everyone at his house is down with flu. He's lonesome and frightened and he needs love, and that's what I'm doing.' Without a word, Newton walked to the blackboard and scrubbed out what he had written.

Many no more than children themselves played their parts to the full. From the first, Sir Robert Baden-Powell's Boy Scouts, then ten years young, blueprinted the traditions later generations would follow. Dutch Scouts acted as guides for locum doctors, unfamiliar with the terrain; Lisbon Scouts rushed hot meals to night hospital workers. All over, they stood in as tram conductors and postmen – or chopped wood and tended furnaces. One Wellington, New Zealand, Scout worked twenty-one hours non-stop – then, following three hours' sleep, was back on the job again.

For most, at first, it was just a glorious game. Lads like ten-year-old Hilbert Mathiesen, in Townsville, Queensland, had never felt so important: he alone was responsible for four streets in the suburb of Hermit Park, briefed to report back instantly a telltale Red Cross, signalling help, appeared in any window. Fiercely proud of his place in the battle-line, he even slept in a medicated face mask. Everywhere Scouts delivered billies of junket and gruel to hard-hit households – and learned that a squirt of boiling soup was the surest defence against a truculent house dog.

For some volunteers, like Lydia Phillips, in Johannesburg, their days of service were like a slow coming of age. After that first morning at Twist Street School Emergency Hospital, when the chafing of the vagrant's feet had brought her to the point of nausea, she had believed that she could never return the following day. Yet long wakeful hours in the silence of that night had convinced her that she must. How could she renege after one day and still face her mother, or her fellow typists at Heymann & Gordon? If rubbing a man's feet was to be her contribution, then Lydia would rub.

At 8 a.m. next day, without even checking first, she returned to the cramped little room. Abruptly she stopped short. The bed was empty – remade with freshly laundered sheets and stacked pillows. She sought out the Staff Nurse.

'Oh,' the woman replied abstractedly, busily checking linen, 'he died in the night.'

Lydia was inexpressibly shocked. Despite everything she had done to save him, the man had died. She was torn between compassion for a human being who had passed on unfriended and a feeling, almost, of affront. A blow had been struck at her professional pride.

That was the beginning of it. From this moment on, Lydia Phillips resolved that come what might, she would not betray the profession she had sought to embrace. Whatever the days ahead had to offer, they would find her ready.

It was easier to resolve than to achieve. Daily the chores went on – sordid, unglamorous, unavoidable. Lockers to be scrubbed and bottles to be emptied. Temperatures to take, medicines to administer. Faces and hands to wash, fingers and toe-nails to pare, pyjamas and bed-linen to change – and always a niagara of stained stinking linen and pyjamas to be carted away.

And who would have thought so many sick men could raise so many petty objections? If the Staff Nurse told her to pare toe-nails, then Lydia must pare them – but most patients protested vigorously. 'Get away,' one grouchy old man shrilled at her, 'I'm not having no chit of a girl mess around with me.'

A shy, gently-born girl, Lydia Phillips, by the standards of later generations, had lived a sheltered life until now. Her English childhood, in a village on the fringe of Epping Forest, had been almost a rural idyll: rowing on Highams Park Lake, with her brothers and sisters ... early morning cycle rides to Chingford Old Church, said to have been built by William the Conqueror, to roam among the ruins and read the old inscriptions on the tombstones ... musical evenings ... elocution lessons.

Now, in Johannesburg, she was rapidly making new friends

of her own at the Parkview Golf Club – but never, except for brief glimpses from the windows of a tramcar, had she seen the seamy side of life as the patients at Twist Street School lived it.

Each hour brought fresh horrors, fresh humiliations. Later that second day a nurse explained how to clean a bedpan: press it firmly against a high pressure faucet. Awkward and again giddy with nausea, Lydia grasped the pan – but not firmly enough. The sudden gush of water spurted the contents clean into her face.

Soon after, a senior nurse asked her to help turn a man over in bed. Gladly, Lydia obliged – wholly unprepared for the sick-sweet gangrenous stench that rose like a miasma from the mattress. Despite her vow, she turned away, her stomach heaving frantically. The nurse, whoever she was, did not lack compassion. 'Poor child,' she sighed, 'you'll soon get used to this sort of thing.'

Not all were so understanding. One afternoon Lydia was crossing another ward on the far side of the building with a message for the sister-in-charge. It was the most crowded ward that she had ever seen, the beds so jammed together there was barely room for lockers. At first Lydia could see no one in charge, but there was a door at the far end which seemed to lead to another ward.

She was halfway towards it when she noticed a patient trying to attract her attention. Approaching, Lydia could see at a glance that he was very ill. His whole body, from the crown of his head to his finger-tips, was a bright unnatural red and the sweat was running down his face and arms.

Though he could scarcely speak, Lydia saw what was troubling him. Immediately behind his bed was an old-fashioned sash window, raised about eight inches from the sill. Outside, a high hot wind boomed through the city streets; the man was in dire discomfort. Lydia hesitated. She had no business to interfere, but the stark fear in the man's eyes tore at her heart. Suddenly, making a supreme effort, the man choked out: 'Pneumonia ... die ...'

As Lydia stepped forward, a woman's voice from behind her cut like a whip: 'Don't you dare touch that window!'

Startled, Lydia swung round. It was the sister-in-charge, who had suddenly appeared from nowhere, her manner as stiff and unbending as her starched white coif. Again Lydia hesitated. It was so draughty for the patient ... didn't Sister think ...?

Outraged, the sister snapped back: 'It's the only bit of air we've got in the ward.' To herself, Lydia had to admit that this was true: the long room was as fetid as a zoo. Sick at heart, she delivered her message and departed.

Now she knew she would have to go on, day after day, to work until she dropped. If only to wipe out the memory of fear in a man's eyes.

CHAPTER SIX

'The Only One Who Knows is God'

22 October—26 October 1918

Faces haggard with fatigue, the two scientists wearily surveyed the laboratory's serried benches. Ranged about them between the sterile white-washed walls was the apparatus that had played a vital and determinant part in the three-month quest now ended: test-tubes, retorts, binocular microscopes, slides magenta-coloured with Giemsa stain, shallow glass Petri dishes, porcelain Berkefeld filters. Now they must render their report.

Outside, it was a bleak morning. The *hamsein*, the swirling desert wind, lashed the date palms; curtains of drifting sand obscured the blue-grey waters of El Bahira. To a layman, it was a scene as remote from the plague ravaging the world as any place on earth – yet here, in the laboratory of the Pasteur Institute, Tunis, Doctors Charles Nicolle and Charles Lebailly had, on 15 October, scored a notable if disturbing victory in the war against the Spanish Lady.

In the wire cages of the annexe, beyond the main laboratory, was the first tangible proof of a new unsuspected virus which had thus far baffled bacteriologists in a score of countries: two shivering disconsolate monkeys, a Chinese bonnet and a macaque, who had somehow survived the full impact of the dread disease. Within the four walls of the Pasteur Institute, the virus was now trapped: a killer at bay, awaiting only positive identification by the sleuths Nicolle and Lebailly.

The assignment had been handed them only three months back by Dr Emile Roux, the Institute's Paris chief. For the first time since the epidemic's spring wave, grave doubts were assailing the world's scientists. Was a new and deadly agent, hitherto unknown to science, insidiously at work across the globe?

Until that moment, flu fighters everywhere had assumed their common foe to be the haemophilic (blood-nourished) *Bacillus Influenzae* – known also as Pfeiffer's Bacillus, after the German bacteriologist, Richard Pfeiffer, who had isolated it two years after the pandemic of 1890. Yet in the weeks past, this 'delicate and fastidious organism', as the German styled it, had time and again eluded cultural recovery. Measuring no more than one-hundred millionth of a millimetre – one-sixteenth of a red blood corpuscle – the bacillus was a will-o'-the-wisp that had foxed even such eminent pathologists as Britain's Dr Bernard Spilsbury.

Since September, so many Londoners had died mysteriously that Spilsbury had carried out a score of autopsies at the behest of local Coroners – yet almost never had he succeeded in tracing the bacillus that bore Pfeiffer's name. At the moment of death, Spilsbury reported, the organism seemed to vanish clean away.

All over the world, laboratory reports had been as bewildering – and as contradictory. From Camp Devens, Massachusetts, true fountainhead of the pandemic that hit the U.S. Army camps, the Medical Corps' Major Lesley Spooner reported Pfeiffer almost daily – in the naso-pharynx, in pleural fluids, in the sputum of pneumonia cases during life, from the heart's blood and lungs in almost every post-mortem case. It was the same, doctors reported, with troops laid up at no. 3 Scottish General Hospital, Glasgow – and with every patient treated by the Rockefeller Medical School, Peking.

But in Germany, Pfeiffer's fellow scientists – whose findings were eagerly studied abroad through medical journals culled from neutral Switzerland – afforded no such confirmation. At Königsberg, Dr Selter examined thirty-one patients and failed to find the bacillus in any one case. And from Kiel, Frankfurt, Dresden, Berlin and Metz came reports that were as negative.

It wasn't always for want of trying. Many scientists, understandably reluctant to abandon a thesis that had held good for twenty-six years, spent fruitless hours at their microscopes – or blamed younger up-and-coming bacteriologists for failing to recognise the bacillus when they saw it. To some, it seemed the Pfeiffer legend was a hard one to kill. At the New York Microscopical Society's autumn exhibition, the bacillus was still the prize exhibit, vying with a snail's tongue. And at Camp Sherman, Chillicothe, Ohio, the harassed pathologist, Major Carey McCord, unable to pinpoint the organism, was even threatened with court-martial by an irate superior.

Nicolle and Lebailly had thus been faced with one challenge above all. If Pfeiffer's bacillus was discredited as the culprit, why were untold millions contracting influenza – and why did virulent broncho-pneumonia so often supervene to result in death?

Three distinct stages had marked the Frenchmen's experiments. First, using an emulsion of unfiltered human sputum, taken from a feverish three-day-old influenza case, they inoculated the monkeys – both with swabs in the nostrils, to simulate the ordinary method of 'snuffing up a cold', and in the conjunctival sacs. Nor were they disappointed. By the fifth day the macaque was sick and moping, at times resting its head on its arms. Refusing all food, its coat was dull and matted, its eyes suffused. The fever had reached a critical 103°F. One day later, the bonnet was stricken too.

Within a week, both monkeys were on the mend – yet for Nicolle and Lebailly, the violence of the attacks was proof enough of the toxic nature of the secretions. Next, this time using filtered sputum diluted with salt solution, the scientists infected two volunteers from the local Army base. Both came down with classic Spanish flu – headache, backache, 102°F fever. It was twelve days before both were groggily convalescent.

For the French scientists this was a critical juncture. Both men knew well enough what other scientists had posited in the weeks just past: that the luckless millions were being attacked, in their flu-weakened state, by common bugs that often live without harm in a man's throat – for just so long as he is well. Not only Dr Pfeiffer's blood-loving bacillus, but the pneumococcus, or the streptococcus, whose colonies, under the microscope, resemble short chains of beads. Among the latter, some doctors had recently reported more than half as haemolytic – possessed of toxins that would dissolve the blood corpuscles as surely as snake venom.

Often, in the later stages of the infection, bugs like these completely swamped out Pfeiffer's, but even these organisms, many doctors suspected, played a secondary role: there was no master strain. Nor was any one organism present in every case. From New York's Department of Health, the Director of Laboratories, Dr William Park, reported a family of six stricken with influenza – with every member afflicted by different bacteria.

But suspicion was no substitute for scientific proof. In the second week of October, the third and most vital stage of their experiments still confronted Nicolle and Lebailly.

This time, calling for fresh Army volunteers, they injected the filtrate intravenously – along with three c.c. of the blood of the infected bonnet monkey. Next, the blood of an influenza patient in the second day of the attack. Each time, the results were as negative as the conclusion was plain. The virus did not exist in the blood of men or of monkeys.

But now, on the morning of 15 October, as the weary scientists prepared their report for Dr Roux, another factor, too, was frighteningly evident. When the two men had injected the monkeys, the bronchial secretions were unfiltered – but at Stage Two, with human volunteers involved, the diluted sputum had been filtered under pressure.

Pfeiffer's bacillus, pneumococci, streptococci, all had been effectively blocked off by the filter – yet still the volunteers had contracted the disease.

What scientists had for some weeks dreaded, Nicolle and

Lebailly knew now to be truth. Somewhere within the walls of this laboratory were micro-organisms so small as to be invisible through the lens of a pre-electronic microscope, then the most powerful in existence. Small enough, even, to traverse with impunity, the fine-grained walls of a laboratory filter. The true killer, the secondary invader, was there, maddeningly, tantalisingly close at hand — but imperceptible to any human eye.

Within seven days it would strike down the man on whom the eyes of all the world were focussed, who held within his grasp the whole outcome of the World War.

The attack came quite suddenly, as it had with all the others. One moment he was the distinguished public figure whom millions of Germans were hailing as a saviour or reviling as a traitor: a tall slim fifty-one-year-old, his ascetic features sharply etched with fatigue after that day's traumatic events, now making ready for a frugal dinner in a royal suite of Berlin's Hotel Adlon. Within minutes, he was a gasping pitiable figure, bent double with pain, tugging at the bell-rope to summon Friedrich von Prittwitz, his adjutant.

In the most critical hour of his life, the disease, with cruel impartiality, had struck at Crown Prince Max of Baden, Imperial Chancellor of Germany. It was shortly before 8 p.m. on Tuesday, 22 October.

In the twenty days just past, Max had lived a waking nightmare. Before him, as newly-appointed Chancellor, had lain a bitter and unenviable task: somehow, with a beaten army and country behind him, to negotiate an honourable peace with President Woodrow Wilson. Yet his every request for a breathing-space — to his cousin, Kaiser Wilhelm, at Supreme Command Headquarters in Spa, to Field-Marshal Paul von Hindenburg, even to General Erich von Ludendorff — had met with pointblank refusals.

'The Army needs a rest,' the frosty punctilious Ludendorff had insisted. 'The Armistice offer must go out at once. I must save my Army.'

None knew better than the fifty-three-year-old General how

closely that army faced annihilation – from an enemy encamped within his lines as securely as a Trojan horse. 'It was a grievous business,' he recalled later, 'having to listen each morning to the Chiefs of Staffs' recital of the number of influenza cases.' Later Prince Max was to complain that Ludendorff had clutched at the news of the pandemic hitting France 'like a drowning man at a straw' – but Ludendorff was painfully aware how little resistance his troops could offer to British soldiers who remained miraculously free from flu. In one German division now, a man's average weight was estimated at eight stone – and quartermasters had to assure the troops that worms in the rations, if unpalatable, would not impair a fighting man's health.

This grim reality embraced not only the Army but all Germany besides. Cold, hungry and ragged, the people had lost all heart for war. Meatless weeks were commonplace; the bread ration had been cut, and potatoes, too. In Germany's industrial heartland, the Ruhr, the silent smokeless chimneys told their own story. And six days earlier, on 16 October, when the German Armies had begun their great retreat from Belgium, 1000 workers had thronged the streets outside the Reichstag, clamouring for peace.

Max, too, knew that peace was inevitable – but still, intent on a peace with honour, he had pressed for time. Again, on 9 October, in Berlin's Chancellery, he had begged Ludendorff for some measure of military support. But the General, weighed down by the presence of the pandemic, was as stubborn as before: 'We need rest.'

If the German front contracted further, Ludendorff knew, he must fight on without Rumanian oil, Ukrainian wheat, Serbian copper or Belgian coal. Soon Turkey would sue for an armistice, the Austro-Hungarians would crumble before the Italian onslaught at Vittorio Veneto – and always, in the background, was the looming ever-present shadow of the Spanish Lady.

Prince Max was in anguish. Despite his 3 October note to Wilson, penned at the Kaiser's insistence, he must somehow avoid the shame of total capitulation. To the Reichstag he would deliver a fighting speech: a critical analysis, stage by stage, of the Fourteen Points that were Wilson's blueprint for a League of Nations. But Chancellery experts begged him to desist. Wilson was a proud and sensitive man, easily offended. His Fourteen Points were 'the conditions of peace', not 'the basis for a negotiation'.

That morning, 22 October, the panelled chamber of the Reichstag was packed to suffocation. All Berlin had avidly awaited the programme that the Chancellor would outline, the measures he would propose for the safety of his country. Then, as Crown Prince Max mounted the tribune, a stifled murmur arose from the close-packed benches. Max, some onlookers noted, looked 'as pale as death', but it was another more ominous factor that drew comment. In place of the Chancellor's resplendent uniform, the Crown Prince wore morning dress.

Speaking in a low toneless monotone, Max began. 'The nation has today the right to ask the question,' he said, 'if a peace on the basis of Wilson's conditions should not come about, what does it signify for our lives and our future?' Yet he could not agree with critics who charged that the acceptance of those conditions 'would mean subjection to a tribunal hostile to Germany'. For Germans, the standards must no longer be 'what we ourselves regard as right but only what would be recognised as right in open discussion with our enemies'.

All over the Chamber now, the delegates exchanged incredulous glances. What strange double game was the new Chancellor playing? It was as if the German, lacking all will to fight, had tamely accepted the services of Woodrow Wilson's speech-writer.

Doggedly, Prince Max went on. The kernel of Wilson's programme was the League of Nations, which required the surrender by nations of part of their sovereignty if justice for all were to be realised. Calmly, he put it to the assembled delegates: 'If today in this dark hour for our people I commend the idea of a League of Nations as a source of comfort and renewed strength, I will not for a moment try to conceal the tremendous obstacles yet to be overcome.'

So softly did he speak that to many, at times, his words were unintelligible. So low did he bend over his typewritten draft, as if he hung his head in shame, that only those seated close at hand could glimpse his face. Yet to old-guard Germans the import was brutally plain. To Frau Margarethe Ludendorff, seated in the Royal Box, 'it was the moment that the Hohenzollern dynasty received its death-blow'.

Now, nine hours later, after discharging his duty as he saw it, Prince Max was out of the fight. The plague that had sapped the Kaiser's Army had cut down the Imperial Chancellor to the size of any Hindenburg Line rookie: a sickbed greasy with sweat, pain crushing and grinding, a heaving kaleidoscope of walls advancing and receding.

Within days, as an earnest of good faith, Germany's Social Democrats would adamantly demand the Kaiser's abdication – a move which only the ailing Crown Prince Max had any power to enforce.

Prince Max of Baden was luckier than he knew. Despite the raging 103°F fever that pinned him to his sick-bed, he was still in good enough physical shape to follow the daily reports of Chancellery advisers. For scores of men and women as renowned as the German Chancellor, death was the one way out.

There never had been a casualty list like it. The Dowager Queen of the Tongan Islands ... General Louis Botha, first Premier of the South African Union ... playwright Edmond Rostand, author of *Cyrano de Bergerac*, whose revival of *L'Aiglon* was just then due in Paris ... Lu Kuang, would-be Emperor of China whose bid for power had been foiled one year earlier ... silent screen-star Harold Lockwood ... the Maharajah of Jodhpur, patriot and turf patron ... Harry Elionsky, America's strongest swimmer, who had once swum ninety miles non-stop.

Some died in settings befitting their status. Guillaume Apollinaire looked his last on a rose-coloured room on Paris's Left

Bank: white chrysanthemums glowed like pale moons in the dusk and a log fire guttered on the hearth – an apt backdrop for the *avant-garde* poet who had celebrated the aeroplane and the phonograph, the art critic who had helped launch Picasso, Chagall and Dufy.

Prince Erik of Sweden died within the white walls of Drottningholm Castle, the flag at half-mast, a chill wind ruffling the waters of Lake Mälar. Duke Leopoldo Torlonia, one of Italy's first families, lay in his Frascati villa, under a gold-fringed damask pall; later his gold-studded sarcophagus would be followed to the grave by footmen of the Senate, who bore aloft blazing torches as symbols of his glory. A few would even merit the nine-gun salute that marked the end of the Sultan of Perak.

Some died full of years and honour. Sir Hubert Parry, composer of King George V's Coronation music and the stirring *Jerusalem*, was seventy when the end came at Rustington, Sussex. Actor-knight Sir Charles Wyndham, founder of the London theatre that bore his name, had reached the ripe age of eighty-two; his actress wife, Mary Moore, watched over him until the last. Others had known the bright lights and the fanfare, but death, in the end, found them in obscurity ... 'Admiral Dot', one of Phineas T. Barnum's first midgets ... Irma Cody Garlow, daughter of Buffalo Bill.

Some had cheated death once, but he was a pitiless adversary. Captain William Leefe Robinson, V.C., first airman to bring down a zeppelin over Britain, survived two years of combat, but not the flu at Stanmore, Middlesex. Canada's youngest-ever Victoria Cross winner, nineteen-year-old Alan McLeod had jousted with death at 10,000 feet; only seven months back, after a dog-fight with Richthofen's Air Circus, his Armstrong-Whitworth became a blazing fiery torch above St Omer, but McLeod had scrambled on to the wing, flying the plane from that position, until he crash-landed, badly burned, near the British lines. He took his leave of death near St Omer; it caught up with him during a hero's home-coming to Stonewall, Manitoba.

For other illustrious names, there were happier endings. Assistant Secretary of the Navy Franklin D. Roosevelt collapsed aboard the battleship *Leviathan* – but family friends weren't surprised to hear that despite his thirteen-year-old marriage to his cousin, Anna Eleanor, it was at his mother's home on New York's East 56th Street that he was recovering. By now Sara Delano Roosevelt's meddlesome interference had reduced the union to an in-name-only charade. In Chicago, a sixteen-year-old Red Cross ambulance driver, who had faked his age in the hope of getting to France, was lying sick in a camp near the Edelweiss Gardens, when a compassionate stretcher-bearer decided: 'We'll take you home – you'll have a better chance there.'

Sped to his parents' home nearby, the youngster, Walter Elias Disney, was delirious for a week – but recovered to delight untold generations with his immortal bestiary.

From the first, the disease was no respecter of persons. The richest woman in the world, Mary Pickford, grossing £138,000 a year, was seriously ill in Beverley Hills – but so too, was Queen Alexandrine of Denmark ... Wencelas Braz, President of Brazil ... the Sultan-Caliph Mohammed VI of Turkey ... Prince Yamagata of Japan ... and Madame Réjane, darling of London and New York, creator of Sardou's *Madame Sans-Gêne*. It was impervious to frontiers, and even front lines ... Marshal Joseph 'Papa' Joffre, victor of the Marne, had cancelled all appointments in Paris – and now General John Pershing and Kaiser Wilhelm came down with it, too.

The most disgruntled of all the invalids was the British premier David Lloyd George, laid up in Manchester in a week of teeming rain. The flu had been depressing, the 'Welsh Wizard' complained, but more distasteful by far had been to watch from his hotel window, the rivulets running down the statue of a man whose politics he revered: the Radical statesman, John Bright.

For some doctors, the mounting toll of disaster was a challenge – among them Captain George T. Palmer, of the U.S.

Sanitary Corps. In Washington, D.C., Palmer had spent some days pondering the sober conclusion of his chief, Major Victor Vaughan: that simple contact from man to man might infect a million souls a week. Now he decided on an experiment.

How many chances would the average man have to acquire infection in the course of a single day? Palmer set out to discover.

Even morning ablutions, he noted with surprise, involved seven distinct contacts – from the toilet flush-handle to the bathroom door-knob. And once in the street, *en route* to breakfast at the Officers' Club, they began to multiply – the *Washington Post* from a newsboy, the trolley-car handle. Hastily Palmer put on his gloves.

Breakfast proved an undreamed-of hazard. The back of the chair, the coffee-cup, the toast, the shredded wheat – all told, the Captain had clocked up an alarming twenty-two hand-to-mouth contacts by the time he paid his check. It was lucky that office routine was marginally less risky. Shaking hands with visitors, blowing his nose, again using the toilet, accounted for only fifteen.

There were further dangers ahead. At lunch, a minimal nine. Yet visiting the Post Office he had no option but to lick the stamp the clerk had handed out. Next, a visit to the bank: to hold a pen used by the general public, to receive used bills from the teller. Back to the office now – the contacts spiralling with every move he made. And dinner was still to come.

Late that night, as he retired to bed, Palmer made his final tally. It was dismal reading. Only one man had laughed in close proximity to him, none had coughed or sneezed, and he had assuredly kissed nobody at all. Yet all told, through touching what others had recently touched, he had totted up no less than 118 opportunities for direct contact infection.

Almost Palmer wished he had never carried out his survey. One last despondent thought had come to him as he switched off the light: contact 119. The way it looked now, the only safe course a man could pursue was to stay in bed.

*   *   *

Tall and resolute, another American doctor was facing an unique audience. A thousand strong, they stood reluctantly to attention before him on the asphalt parade-ground of Deer Island's Naval Prison, Boston Harbour – the most unlikely assembly, thought prison doctor Robert Parsons, to call on for any supreme self-sacrifice. Most had landed on Deer Island for the very crimes of putting self before country: outright desertion, overstaying furlough, slugging a non-com.

But the speaker, Dr Joseph Goldberger, a lanky hawk-faced veteran of the U.S. Public Health Service, seemed undeterred. Moments earlier, arriving in company with Harvard's Dr Milton Rosenau, he had laconically announced his mission: fifty prisoners were needed as volunteers for 'certain influenza experiments'.

Shrugging, the prison officials had passed the buck back to Goldberger. He could take his pick – if he managed to realise even three volunteers from the delinquents ranged before him.

Privately, Dr Parsons acknowledged, he could blame no man for resisting Goldberger's plea. The average prisoner's age was twenty-five – and almost every man's sentence was short. Within months, most could look forward to release. Though liberty was restricted, the chow was tolerable and gripes were few. The promise that each volunteer would be pardoned and returned to Navy duty was small inducement to face such risks as Goldberger now spelt out.

Powerful hands fiddling with his gold watch chain, brown eyes sweeping the ranks, the P.H.S man did not seek to minimise those risks. All volunteers would be isolated on Gallops Island, quarantine station for the port of Boston. Their first duty would be to snuff a culture of pure influenza bacillus into their nostrils. If this failed to take, they would be injected with other strains, some taken from the lungs of the dead at the time of necropsy. Later, secretions from patients in the Chelsea Naval Hospital would be sprayed into their nostrils, eyes and throats.

Then, as a final attempt to chart the course of infection, Goldberger would take selected volunteers to the hospital itself.

Each man would be assigned a patient – to sit beside his bed and chat for five minutes. Then, his face barely two inches distant, the sick man would breathe hard at his visitor – while the 'guinea-pig' breathed in. Finally the patient would cough five times – straight into the volunteer's face.

For Dr Robert Parsons, and many listening, it was more truly a moment to hold one's breath. Not for one moment was he, or any of the audience, fooled by Goldberger's quiet unemotional delivery. That others, as yet unaffected, might live, Surgeon-General Blue's man was quite literally asking for fifty men to die.

What followed was a revelation. As Goldberger finished speaking, a hush fell over the parade-ground. Abruptly, the command rang out: 'Volunteers – one pace forward.' Without hesitation, not three but close to three hundred now stepped from the ranks – so swiftly, Parsons noted, it more resembled a stampede than a drill-ground manoeuvre.

Within the hour, after winnowing out the fittest of the contenders, Goldberger, his aides, and three truck-loads of human guinea-pigs were pulling out from the Naval Prison. In the steps of Doctors Nicolle and Lebailly in Tunis, and Captain George Palmer in Washington, 100 men, seeking the secrets of the plague, had chosen a rendezvous with death on Gallops Island.

Hand raised urgently above his head, like a pupil seeking the teacher's attention, the delegate bobbed from his seat. From the rostrum of the Council Chamber in Montreal's City Hall, Mayor Médéric Martin nodded acceptance of the question – one of sheer economic survival. As spokesman for 2000 theatrical employees, the delegate wanted urgently to know: when could Montreal's cinemas and theatres reopen their doors?

For answer, Mayor Martin regretfully shook his head. 'We will be happy to let you go on as soon as we get rid of the epidemic,' he promised, 'but the only one who knows is God.'

It was a mortifying if understandable reply. As early as 8 October, Montreal's Health Board had closed down all schools, theatres, dance-halls, movies and concert halls, throwing hundreds out of work – and all over the world, municipalities were reaching identical decisions. Some British showmen carried on, though compelled to ban children under fourteen and reduce showing times – one Liverpool cinema installing a camphor block under each one of its 647 seats – but few were so lucky. Theatre-owners in Winnipeg and Sydney, N.S.W., were forced to urge a moratorium, for everywhere the lights and the big names were winking out on the marquees: Theda Bara in *Camille* and Mary Pickford in *Amaryllis of Clothes Line Alley*, Charles Ray in *The Hired Man*, Douglas Fairbanks in *Bound in Morocco* and William S. Hart in *Riddle Gawne*.

Already many theatres whose attendances had slumped sharply had closed down of their own accord, and scores of touring companies, stranded without hope of work, were now literally destitute.

Typical was the plight of Princess Oyapela's company, a maidenly trio marooned on a six-month tour of Nebraska and South Dakota. The Princess – whose real name was Eloita Stidham, of Eufaula, Oklahoma – claimed to be one-eighth Creek Indian, and her dances and recitals from Indian folklore, backed up by violinist Fannie Weinstock and pianist Corinne Shroeder, were normally a sell-out through the prairie states. Often the girls collected their wages in gleaming silver dollars.

Now, though public meetings were banned, the company's contract still compelled them to visit every town on the circuit or forfeit their fees – though most towns, Fannie Weinstock recalls, refused point-blank to pay up.

The low point of their lives came one October night in the whistle-stop of Elwood, Nebraska. Arriving late at the tiny railway station they found the whole town cloaked in darkness. Trudging the streets in search of a night's lodging, they spotted the main hotel with its lights burning bright – but a sign on the door warned all comers: 'We Have the Flu.'

Near at hand was a smaller hotel – main door standing open, coal stove burning, but not a soul in sight. Resigned to taking pot luck, the Princess bedded down for the night on the reception counter, while the others made do with three chairs and a desk. At intervals they shovelled coal on the stove with the only means available – a small tumbler.

At 6 a.m. next day, without having seen one living soul, Princess Oyapela's company took the first train out of Elwood. And though they carried doggedly on for five more months through 151 towns they gave not one concert.

But far more than theatres were affected. Cities as distant as Brandon, Manitoba, and Berne, Switzerland, clamped down a total ban on all public gatherings; not even the department store's Santa Claus was exempt in Hamilton, Ontario. Lodge meetings, poolrooms, concerts and racetracks now belonged to the peaceful past. In Montreal and elsewhere, all stores must close by 4 p.m., and motor-cycle cops sputtered through the streets on a daily spot-check. For some, old habits died hard. In Charleston, South Carolina, the merchants dutifully closed down at this same hour – then loitered uneasily outside their shuttered premises until going-home time, 8 p.m.

Many cities now advocated walking to work, to avoid over-crowding on street-cars, but New York was the first metropolis to go further still, compulsorily staggering both hours of work and opening and closing times. Promptly, in Washington and Philadelphia, Health Commissioners Louis Brownlow and B. Franklin Royer followed suit – but in some quarters, graft proved too strong. In Kansas City, Missouri, 'Boss' Tom Prendergast, mindful of the payola, successfully blocked every move by the Health Board to close down movie theatres and saloons – and the city's ultimate death roll topped 1800.

Often, even in law-abiding communities, such measures prompted bitter opposition, for though theatres and saloons were closed, war plants, of necessity, were operating seven days a week round the clock. Did the flu bug, scornful opponents asked, go by the book as rigorously as a Board of Health official – infecting cases in street-cars but not in food queues, and never visiting a store until after 4 p.m.

Was nowhere in the world immune? Only, it seemed, where authority declared and enforced a rigid quarantine – rarely practicable in a world at war. St Helena, in the South Atlantic, famed as the scene of Napoleon's six-year exile, escaped altogether – as did Yerba Buena Island in San Francisco Bay. Here the Captain of the United States Naval Training Station clamped down a nine-week quarantine on 4000 souls – forbidding all liberty, sterilising drinking fountains hourly with blow torches, compelling new trainees to exist twenty feet apart from one another. Another community, Coromandel, New Zealand, cut itself off from the outer world through a roster of vigilantes armed with shotguns – and their system worked. Yet Liberia, which imposed a three-month quarantine from 4 October on, was stricken nonetheless.

Others just did the best they could. To some townships, three was now a crowd, and even little (popn. 906) Johnstown, Ohio, had guards patrolling the streets to disperse gossiping groups. In Cork, Ireland, young Jean Flanders had an identical precaution enjoined by her mother: if approaching more than two people she must hold her breath until safely past. Soon enough Jean became an adept – once Mrs Flanders had conducted private dress-rehearsals with a stop-watch.

In Milan, one man nourished an obsession all his own: a man who so disliked human contact that twenty years later, as the dictator, Il Duce, he would forbid all Italians to shake hands under penalty of imprisonment. Debar every Italian from the filthy custom of hand-shaking, he trumpeted in his rabble-rousing newspaper, *Il Popolo d'Italia*, and the pandemic would vanish overnight. But sadly for Benito Mussolini, only one town in the world – Prescott, Arizona – put this ordinance into effect.

Overnight, as the restrictions mounted, the lives of millions underwent an abrupt sea-change. For avid readers, it was a barren time, since most public libraries shut down – or piled the chairs on the library tables to discourage casual browsing. It was an anxious time for those with sick relatives; many hospitals forbade outsiders or allowed only ten-minute visits. Often it was hard to place even an emergency call; in many cities the telephone-booths, a likely source of infection, were padlocked. It was hard, too, for indigent Maltese: the authorities had closed the pawnshops.

As always, the people were swift to adapt. When 800 Melbourne hotels and bars closed down, sandwich lunches for office workers were suddenly all the rage. In New Zealand, where barbers' shops were closed, the sale of safety-razors boomed. So many victims were losing their hair – for the high fever caused the follicles to cease production – that Parisian wig-makers did a land-office business, and restaurateurs noted with glee that the after-dinner cognac, esteemed as a 'preventive' was now mandatory. In Rio Maior, Portugal, Didio Brazão noted a less auspicious change of habit: so commonplace were funerals, a man no longer raised his hat to the dead.

Scores of advertisers found a way to cash in. Every electric sign in Madrid's Puerta del Sol blazed out some sure-fire flu remedy. One Danish newspaper carried no less than 117 plugs for different brands of mouthwash. Druggists in Argentina even invited the nervous to have their sputum analysed at a bargain price of eight pesos.

For those confined at home, the Paragon Shorthand Institute of New Orleans suggested their new simplified correspondence course for budding stenographers. At least 20,000 house-bound Swedes had already devoured Dr Henrik Berg's 'The Spanish Flu and How to Cure It', now in its fourth edition. Few struck a note so glum as the Simon Art Studio in Johannesburg: 'Keep the Memory of Dear Ones Alive with an Enlargement of Their Photograph.'

In thousands of cities, the queue was now a way of life: for food cards, for scarce milk and vegetables, for medicines, even at the cemetery gates, and the Paris daily L'Oeuvre grumbled: 'Having queued to live, now we must queue to be buried.' Yet in a time of grief, there was patience and compassion, too. When an Athens dairyman closed down to mourn his dead, his customers queued uncomplainingly outside his shop for the entire weekend.

Inevitably, some found the pandemic the best reason ever

to please themselves. To the London *Daily Express*, it was 'the new excuse that has ousted the dying grandmother', and in Buenos Aires, suspicious employers noted the onrush of fresh cases every Thursday morning – six hours before the horses came under starters' orders at Palermo racetrack. But none exceeded the ingenuity of four young clerks in Patras, Greece, who stretched a fictitious convalescence into a three week non-stop poker session.

It was a slow-witted malefactor who couldn't profit by it somehow. In St Marylebone Police Court, West London, one man, arraigned for stealing a £20 car, promptly produced a doctor's certificate: the after-effects of flu had 'clouded his moral sense'. Two Chicago Chinese, caught smoking opium by a narcotics inspector, protested indignantly that it was a flu preventive: 'One puff – flu gone'. And only weeks after the men concerned had dropped from sight did startled Isolation Hospital nurses in Adelaide, South Australia, discover that the two most conscientious orderlies had been sneak-thieves on the run – hiding up in the one bolthole the police were understandably reluctant to enter.

The palm for ingenuity went to Chief Petty Officer Arthur Nathro of the United States Navy. When private detectives, along with irate husband Walter Larsen, burst into Nathro's room in Chicago's Plymouth Hotel, they found the sailor in a compromising position with none other than Mrs Larsen. Unsuccessfully, Nathro sought to put their minds at rest: 'I'm recovering from Spanish flu and she's measuring me for a sweater.'

Youngsters, albeit in harmless ways, were profiting by the epidemic, too. Needy students in Turin soon found that the priests paid a lira per funeral to those who would carry the Cross – and often there were fifty funerals a day. Thirteen-year-old Albert Baumgardt, in Malmesbury, South Africa, spent all his spare time on the veld gathering wild garlic; currently the greengrocers were paying him a penny a bulb – and reselling at six times that figure. In Richmond, Virginia, another teenager, Walter Browning did a brisk weekly trade with the Greek Orthodox Church, whose funeral ceremonies involved the release of a flight of white doves. Since Walter's 'doves' were homing pigeons, come Monday he could sell them back all over again.

No man benefited so unexpectedly as Dr James Ayson Marshall, of Auckland, New Zealand. At the time the s.s. *Niagara* brought the pandemic to his native city, Marshall was embarking on his honeymoon – a leisurely car-trip to enjoy the scenic beauties of the South Island's Pacific coast. But in the 450 miles between Blenheim and Invercargill, every hotel where he and his bride stopped off had its quota of flu victims.

Condemned, willy-nilly, to a busman's honeymoon, Marshall always recalled in wonderment that aside from gasoline bills the entire trip cost him precisely nothing. Without exception, not one grateful hotel proprietor would present any bill at all.

The churches, too, were under fire. In many cities – Winnipeg, Budapest, Dunedin, New Zealand – they closed down for the first time in history. Others indulged in Christian compromise – limiting services to thirty minutes, or congregations to ten, with the preacher sited twelve feet away from his flock. Milan's Archbishop Cardinal Andrea Ferrari, laid down as many hygienic do's and don'ts as a sanitary inspector: always scrub out the confessional, change the Holy Water daily, disinfect robes after the last rites. By common consensus, the communion goblet was retired – but few churches took such stringent precautions as in Zurich, where a ban on singing and oral responses decreed a city-wide congregation of deaf mutes until 1919.

A few had reservations. One Hamilton, Ontario, minister argued that closing down the churches would affect the people's health; with no need to look spruce and put on their Sunday best, none of his congregation would take a bath. But the most poignant heart-cry came from Rhodesia's Archdeacon Etheridge, when the church at Gatooma remained closed for the fourth Sunday in succession.

The loss of four collections in a row, he confessed, had put the diocese in a dilemma; there were simply no funds left to pay the parish priest. So would all churchgoers please come to the rescue – and send in without delay at least as much as they would have put on the collection plate?

Coughing and choking, her eyes red and streaming, Annie Petrie moved blindly in circles. For the moment she had lost all sense of direction. Smoke from the shovel of hot embers and formalin disinfectant that she held before her billowed like a fog, blotting out even the walls of the little pitch-pine classroom, in Sandstone Rural School, five miles from Riversdale, New Zealand.

More by luck than judgement, she found the door at last and staggered gasping into the sunlight. But at least, a dutiful schoolteacher, she had discharged her final duty, just as the Education Board's letter had directed. She had dismissed her pupils, fumigated the school and formally closed it down. Now there was nowhere to go but home, more than 100 miles away in Dunedin.

It was almost a symbolic gesture. Afterwards, looking back to that autumn, the survivors held fast to one memory above all: the deserted asphalt playground of the neighbourhood school, its silence unbroken by the faraway cry of children's voices. Countless thousands of schools had closed down for the duration of the epidemic, and when they would open again was now any man's guess.

At times, many citizens benefited indirectly; the services of 2000 public school teachers in Buffalo, New York, enabled Health Commissioner Franklin Gram to conduct a house-to-house canvass of every family in the city. Yet the problem – to close or not to close the schools – was one to tax medical officers and education boards everywhere. Often there was little choice; in the cotton kingdom of Manchester, the Medical Officer of Health, Dr James Niven, always recalled the horror of one school inspection, the children collapsing as he watched 'like poisoned flowers' across their desks. Soon the rows of empty desks in Manchester and a thousand other cities told their own story. And one Dublin magistrate, Patrick Lupton of the Northern Police Court, proved to be the friend of whom every schoolboy dreams – refusing to enforce any summons against a child playing hooky for as long as the epidemic lasted.

Elsewhere, the authorities wavered, undecided – though none were as forthright as Amsterdam's Dr H. G. Ringeling, who refused to close schools lest the children indulge in an orgy of pilfering. But few could agree on a common course of action: if schools were closed in Athens, Melbourne and Winnipeg, they stayed open until the end in Stockholm, Paris and Cairo. For those teachers still at their blackboards, some special problems arose. In Ferrara, Italy, Giuseppina Galli, on her first-ever assignment, had pupils of all ages ranged on the hardwood benches – not only children sobbing with fright but sobbing parents who had stayed to comfort them.

Some schools which kept open devised unique methods of keeping the flu at bay. At Christ's Hospital (the Bluecoat School), Horsham, Sussex, where the pupils still wore the long blue coats, yellow stockings and white neckbands of the sixteenth century, medical officer Gerald Friend devised a solemn twice-daily drill: on a monitor's word of command, 800 boys blew their noses in unison six times both when rising and retiring. At least one group of schools whose pupils were dispersed, in Modesto, California, even hit on a hotly-resented plan to ensure that the curriculum didn't suffer. By arrangement with the morning *Herald* and the evening *News*, assignments were published twice daily – and the fuming pupils sent in written answers by mail.

One man resolutely refused to close down New York's schools – and though a storm of criticism burst about his head, there is no doubting he was right. To Dr Royal Copeland, the Health Commissioner, it had at first seemed the natural thing to do – but with barely six months in the job, Copeland was still feeling his way. An amiable prosy fifty-year-old, whose long-winded orations in the U.S. Senate later earned him the nickname of 'General Exodus', the Commissioner was no Public Health man but a noted eye-specialist, who had jumped at the chance of the political career offered him by Mayor John 'Red Mike' Hylan.

Midway through October, Copeland summoned Dr Sara Baker to his office in the Health Department's tumbledown headquarters on 55th Street. Ten years Chief of the Bureau of Child Hygiene, Sara Baker was renowned as a cool outspoken feminist who sported elegant man-tailored suits and four-in-hand ties.

All public schools, Copeland told her flatly, were to close down as of now.

Dr Baker saw her chance. 'If you could have,' she asked Copeland, 'a system where you could examine one-fifth of the population of the city every morning, and control every person who showed any symptom of influenza, what would it be worth to you?'

'Well, that would be almost priceless,' Copeland agreed impatiently, 'but we haven't got anything of the sort and why talk about it?'

Fervently Sara Baker disagreed. Out of her years as a health worker in the squalid tenements of Hell's Kitchen, on the city's west side, had been born the pioneer experiment which her department represented – for until 1908, preventive medicine in New York had been almost unknown. Now, for ten years, that department had done its share of reducing the toll of contagious diseases among the city's children – measles, scarlet fever, whooping cough.

Now, she stressed to Copeland, the control system she had outlined was already in being. Her staff of inspectors and nurses were uniquely equipped to keep the six to fifteen-year age group – 800,000 children in all – free from all danger of Spanish flu.

Let the schools, she urged, be kept open at all costs. Children would go straight to their classrooms on arrival, and each morning bureau doctors would visit the schools to check out every pupil. No class would come in contact with any other.

As soon as school broke up, each child would go directly home.

'Won't you let me try out the idea for a week or so?' Sara Baker begged. 'I don't know that I can do it, but I would awfully like to have a chance.'

For a long moment Copeland pondered, but finally he decided: 'All right, I'll give you that chance. But remember – the responsibility is on your head.'

It was a masterly decision. Though business giants like department store tycoon John Wanamaker and newspaper magnate William Randolph Hearst took Copeland severely to task, cases of influenza among New York's children, thanks to this lynx-eyed daily scrutiny, were almost non-existent from the first, and significantly, the teachers kept well, too. Soon enough, other health top brass, like Chicago's Dr John Dill Robertson and New Orleans' Dr William Hasler, recognising the schools as 'positive agencies for preventing disease' had followed Copeland's example.

The outcome was still in grave doubt – yet where teenagers in many American cities were concerned, there was scant evidence that the visitation even existed.

Even now many officials were unwilling to believe the worst – as a man hesitates to open the telegram that may spell out unthinkable news. All were acting independently, yet every pronunciamento might have been penned by the same hand: an ill-advised attempt to stem panic by playing the epidemic down.

Most were as complacent as the Chief Health Officer of Christchurch, New Zealand, Dr Herbert Chesson; even a month after the s.s. *Niagara* scandal, with the epidemic at its height, Chesson refused all offers from nursing volunteers, having had no official orders from Wellington. 'Tell your readers not to get upset,' was the beaming counsel of Dr Alfred Gascuel, President of the Seine Medical Association, when the Paris daily *L'Oeuvre* sought practical advice, and Rome's Chief Sanitation Officer pooh-poohed it in the same terms, 'a transitory minuscule phenomenon compared to the war'. From Poland's Public Health Commission and Rhodesia's Medical Director came this identical bromide: 'There is no cause for alarm.'

Few bodies were as rapacious as the municipal council of Kandy, Ceylon, which levied a minimum three-rupee tax on burials for even the poorest coolie – yet donated only three hundred rupees (about £20) to the town's disaster fund. The majority, like the Town Council of Salisbury, Rhodesia, voted 'to drop discussion' of the matter – though six days later one doctor was treating 400 cases single-handed.

What followed, in scores of instances, was as sorry a chapter as any in colonial history. In Georgetown, British Guiana, the Governor, Sir Wilfred Collett, stubbornly brushed aside his Surgeon-General's advice to clamp down a quarantine; it would be an expensive luxury and upset the business community. Then, ignoring all warnings on the dangers of congregation, Sir Wilfred, a keen music lover, invited the port's leading citizens to a Government House oratorio, following up with a party for 400 children. Anyone who ignored the surgeon's warnings in the local press, he avowed, was 'to be congratulated on his good sense'.

In Bermuda, the refusal of the Governor, General Sir James Willcocks, to impose a quarantine laid low 4000 islanders, cost 200 lives.

And despite all pleas from his Board of Health, Jamaica's Governor, Sir Leslie Probyn, adopted the same short-sighted policy. Urged to close down schools and churches and to permit the erection of emergency hospitals, Sir Leslie was inflexible: 'The danger is grossly exaggerated.' Later the *Jamaica Gleaner*, comparing him to Nero, charged that the deaths of more than 7000 Jamaicans 'will be laid down to his refusal to comply'.

At times, sheer defeatism lay behind the authorities' refusal to act. 'We are demonstrably powerless,' shrugged Budapest hospital chief Zsigmond Gerlóczy. Milan's Chief Medical Officer, Professor Bordoni Uffredduzzi, was as despondent: 'It isn't humanly possible to arrest the course of such an epidemic.' Accepting that every susceptible human would catch it anyway, Oslo's Sanitary Commission advised: 'Better catch it now, while the weather is warmer.' Promptly the angry citizens demanded: 'Are they Muslim fatalists?'

When well-wishers urged that the Pacific island of Fiji impose a quarantine, confining all shipping to the chief seaport, Suva, both the Governor, Sir Cecil Hunter Rodwell and his Chief Medical Officer, Dr George Lynch, offered only a counsel of despair. If the flu reached Germany and the United States, how could one hope to stop it reaching Fiji? Thus, on 9 October, when the *Niagara* docked at Suva, *en route* for New Zealand, no man made a move to impede her passengers from going ashore.

Soon, across Fiji's 100 inhabited isles, more than 8000 corpses were 'piled like copra' by the roadside – yet on Taveuni two resolute planters, imposing their own quarantine, kept the southern half of the island free and saved 600 lives.

There were a resolute few who held events in their grip from the first. On Western Samoa, the American Governor J. M. Poyer, imposed a five-day quarantine which kept the area around Pago-Pago free from all infection. In Lyons, France, Mayor Edouard Herriot functioned as a kind of one-man sanitary squad, to keep deaths to the minimum ... organising rapid burials ... forbidding funeral processions ... closing all theatres and schools and personally supervising the disinfection of the buses, cafés, banks and post-offices ... installing the first underground toilets with free washing facilities. And Australia's Director of Quarantine, Dr John Howard Cumpston, by isolating 10,000 travellers for a week at a time over a three-month period, effectively kept deaths to a minimal 13,000 in a population of five million.

Some authorities enforced precautionary measures that were as futile as could be. Self-appointed pundits, like the Mayor of Santiago, Chile, even forbade the eating of uncooked vegetables – and in cities like Dublin and Nottingham, mobile water carts sluiced the gutters with hundreds of gallons of useless disinfectant. Ludicrous ordinances multiplied. Athens abolished the sale of shaving brushes, apparently mistaking the virus for anthrax, and in Christchurch, New Zealand, with memories of bubonic plague, sanitary inspectors launched a city-wide rat hunt.

It was forbidden to throw flowers to Swiss soldiers on the march, or confetti at French weddings. Some townships enforced the fumigation of everything from newspapers and mail to tram tickets. Even the employees in Washington's State, War and Navy Building were solemnly marched from their desks into the open several times a day, aired for twenty minutes and then marched back again.

At Camp Sherman, Ohio, when one eager company captain sought guidance on how to protect his men, Major Alfred Friedlander, Chief of Medical Service, thought he knew: soluble quinine salt would kill off any pneumococci, presumed cause of fatal pneumonia, in the throats of men who gargled with it. Promptly, the captain came up with an offer: if the hospital furnished the quinine, his company's 258 officers and enlisted men would gargle as often each day as Friedlander advised.

This was a major prophylactic exercise, for Friedlander opined gargling would be necessary twice a day at least – so that first medical corpsmen were assigned to weigh-out and wrap 3612 packages. And the captain was as good as his word. For the next seven days, the company gargled so wholeheartedly that the local *Gazette* even assigned a photographer to record them in action. But by week's end, the despairing Friedlander recorded one more failure: the company's pneumonia mortality rate was higher than any other in the stricken camp.

Paramount among all the panacea favoured was the emergency inhalation chamber – hastily-rigged booths of wood and hessian, where up to twenty at a time inhaled a fine cloud of formalin or sulphate of zinc at a jetting 80-lb. air pressure. One indignant Spaniard, Tomás Aguirre, would always recall that before he and his friends could sunbathe on the beach at Bilbao, dim-witted officials penned them all in a windowless hut, to inhale burning sulphur for twelve suffocating seconds.

Whatever the location it was a fruitless precaution from the first. At Venice, California, where health officers fumigated both animals and performers of the Al G. Barnes Circus with coal tar and formaldehyde, the only casualties were the performing fleas and the 'Albino Girl', whose silvery hue abruptly gave place to dusky Filipino. But often the effects were more damaging. For Colonel Charles Averill, R.A.M.C., it was plain that British soldiers who passed through spraying chambers came down with flu more readily than any others: the chemical, irritating the mucous membranes of the throat, devitalised the surface cells.

It was a verdict wholeheartedly shared by railway worker Rupert Mattson in Blenheim, New Zealand. Put in charge of the inhalation chamber at Blenheim Station, he spent the entire day before inauguration giving himself sample treatments – only to come down with the first case recorded in the city.

Yet even now, only two American cities – New York and Chicago – and seven countries – Australia, Brazil, British Honduras, New Zealand, Poland and South Africa – saw fit to classify influenza as a notifiable disease.

Now, almost everywhere in the world, the people were hedged in by restrictions and precautionary measures – and assailed with slogans, too. Never had the population been so exhorted and cajoled – 'treated by placard', as one cynical doctor put it. To be sure, some were sensible enough and meticulously far-reaching; all through the villages of Ceylon, tom-toms proclaimed, for the benefit of those who couldn't read, that it was unwise to visit the sick except in dire emergency. 'Avoid Overcrowding', the posters urged – or 'Keep Your Feet Dry and Warm'. And almost every city in the world had stickers advising: 'Go To Bed At Once if You Feel Unwell'.

But some advice was plainly contradictory. 'Go to bed between warm blankets,' advised the Wellington, New Zealand, Health Department – in disconcerting contrast to an Auckland doctor's: 'Go to bed between wet sheets.' 'Get nine hours sleep non-stop,' counselled Chicago's Health Commissioner Robertson – no easy task when a Cape Town doctor insisted: 'Take fluid nourishment every two hours.' Other precepts had a ring of Alice in Wonderland. Rhodesians were pressured to remove their artificial teeth at bedtime, Paris doctor Louis St Maurice urged all to wear a nightcap, and Vancouver City's Health Officer, Dr Underhill, cautioned youngsters: 'Boys! Don't lick your marbles' ...

Mirroring the total confusion prevailing at every level as October drew to a close was the solemn advice tendered by no less an authority than the Greek Ministry of the Interior: 'Convalescents should be particularly careful not to have a relapse – this is always more dangerous.'

Across 197 million square miles of the earth's surface, the world was grinding to a standstill. Down India's Ganges Valley, fields ripe for the sickle remained unreaped: in Poland, the potato harvest grew brown and pulpy in the furrows. One-third of Guatemala's coffee crop was lost, too, and many Malayan rubber estates, their tappers sick and dying, closed down.

For many industries, large and small, it was like a death-blow. Peru's copper mines had shut down, like those of Union Minière, in the Belgian Congo, with 500,000 black workers mortally sick. On the Rand, goldfield production was to suffer a staggering £256,000 drop in output. New South Wales, like Manitoba, declared a moratorium, for 50,000 Australians were jobless, and the Government had guaranteed half rent and board to all those out of work. Often there was bitter resentment. When the Hon. John Bowser, Victoria's Minister of Public Health, suggested that all unemployed theatricals enlist as medical corpsmen, the renowned actor Frank Harvey flashed back: if Bowser deservedly lost his post at the next elections, he was welcome to a job as Harvey's dresser.

At the National Phonograph Records headquarters on New York's East 40th Street, bankrupted by the disaster, the employees enacted a solemn closing-down ceremony: smashing several thousand gramophone records on the tiled basement floor.

To the insurance companies, it was a nightmare they would never forget. In South Africa alone, companies were faced with claims of £1 million, the sums ranging from £100 to £20,000. Many Swedish and German benefit societies just suspended payments altogether, for even the giants were hard put to meet their obligations. The three weeks ending 19 October saw the Prudential Insurance Company's headquarters in Newark, New Jersey, paying out $1 million; in one day alone, they disbursed $506,000, then the largest total ever paid out in a twenty-four hour period.

'Pay out all claims within the day,' was now the golden rule – often, as in Philadelphia, to a line of claimants stretching all the way round the block. Daily, accounts were overdrawn, though the banks continued to honour the Pru's cheques until new deposits were made. All over the world, insurance offices stayed open far into the night, the volunteers working fifteen hours a day, including Sundays, to keep pace. Routine methods went by the board; in place of written memos and the regular reference of claims came the 'Floor-Walker Claims Adviser' – a specialist who made the rounds of the staff, giving snap judgements on specific problems.

Those who still had jobs to cling to struggled on somehow. In Rio de Janeiro, bank clerk Gino Dazzi and his colleagues knew just how grave the crisis was; the bank was even footing the lunch bills of all those still on their feet, to keep them close to the office, and turned a blind eye to the swigs of *cachaca* (sugar-cane rum) from which the tellers sought Dutch courage. But soon Brazil's banks, like those of New Zealand, closed down for a whole week; lacking staff, many vital services now ceased to function. With thirty-four M.P.'s on the sick list, New Zealand's Parliament closed down. For the first time in history, all the coastguard stations on America's eastern seaboard were out of commission for sixteen days.

Slowly each country, each capital, grew more isolated, thrown back on its own resources. No trains now ran from

Berlin to Sweden, or from Spain to Portugal; the Dutch frontier was closed to refugees. In South Africa, with 15,000 railway workers down, the lines between the Union and Rhodesia shimmered for miles under the sunlight, empty of traffic. Even families were split up for fear of infection, and in Budapest the newspapers' agony columns were each day crammed with announcements, anonymous, cryptic, pathetic: 'Arnold. Dear Mother completely recovered. Papa' ... 'Gáborka. Am hovering between life and death. God be with you, little sweetheart.'

Telephones could have eased the stress, but few families were subscribers then, and many towns had to lay down draconian rules on who could call whom – and when. Switzerland allowed no calls passing through more than three main exchanges; in Hamburg, with 650 telephonists down, the switchboards were unmanned after 7 p.m. Some exchanges, like Lillehammer, Norway, closed down altogether, and those that kept going, like Auckland, New Zealand, working double shifts for more than a month, gave top priority to emergencies: the red discs on the switchboard that bespoke doctors, hospitals and clergy, the black that meant undertakers and police. So frantically did calls pile up, on one memorable night in Washington, D.C., that it was fifty minutes before the Relief Centre's phone could be replaced on its hook.

Everywhere in these desperate weeks, the mind recorded small vivid cameos, which even half a century would not erase. It was the deafening cry of ambulance sirens screaming through the streets ... florists' girls in Rome, hurrying by with wreaths of mop-headed chrysanthemums ... the blinds down in every house along the streets leading to Paris' Pantin Cemetery. It was doctors' coupés with lighted green crosses gliding through the night in Shreveport, Louisiana ... the clop of horses' hooves through an Aberdeen dawn ... crepes on doorway after doorway, black for the men, grey for the women.

It was an Irish setter in Oslo, Norway, howling for seven nights beneath his master's deathbed ... or knots of people, anywhere on earth, clustered uneasily at street corners, asking, 'Who's got it? Have you had it yet?' It was, for Nurse Eunice Saunders, in Milwaukee, Wisconsin, 'the year men cried'.

For teenager Irene Corbett, in Cape Town, it was grass sprouting in the streets outside a once-thriving fruiterer's, its display window, 'just a sheet of green mould', the marble slab beyond a black sticky sea of rotted fruit. To Annie Everitt, an engineer's wife, more than 6000 miles away in Björneborg, Sweden, it was the silence each day as darkness fell that oppressed her: no flicker of flame from the smelting works in the Björneborg's Bruk iron foundry, 'only darkness and silence and the sound of somebody coughing – a doctor passing in a hurry'.

The world was dying.

CHAPTER SEVEN

'Doctor! Doctor! Do Something!'
26 October—30 October 1918

The Right Reverend Bertram Lasbrey caught his breath. Until this moment, his anguished progress in the motor-cycle's side-car had occupied all his attention. Skilfully as his African missionary, Mr Onyeabo, was steering, the Lord Bishop On The Niger found the rutted roads a torment, choked with brown billowing dust, thronged with Ibos and their goats, bound for the little Nigerian town of Ata on market day.

But what drove all thoughts of discomfort from the Bishop's mind was the sight of the first field outside the mud-walled town: a succulent green plantation of yams, with their gaudy yellow-white flowers, twining through a thicket of stakes. And fringing them like some nightmare palisade was a whole line of polished glistening skulls, grinning emptily beneath the tropical sun.

As the motor-cycle ground to a halt, the Bishop posed a shuddering query, but Mr Onyeabo sheepishly craved his people's pardon. In times like these, despite Christian teaching, the old pagan beliefs were wont to resurrect themselves. What the Lord Bishop saw demonstrated here was the landowner's belief that the skulls of flu victims formed a powerful *ju-ju* – so that neither rural thief nor evil spirit would dare with impunity to steal his yams.

All over the world, in this last week of October, the same

criterion held good. The spiralling death-rates, the breakdown of the hospital system, the supine inertia of many authorities – all these had conspired, in both east and west, to lend powerful impulse to age-old superstitions.

To millions, the flu was a deadly if unseen killer, hovering like a sword of Damocles above *their* community – and the one thing that made sense was somehow to propitiate or deceive him. In scores of Japanese villages, a guileless placard outside every dwelling announced: 'No one at home' – and by common consent the citizens of Meng Feng, China, staged an unofficial New Year's Day, hoping to divert the flu spirit with red paper mottoes and a shower of firecrackers.

Strange beliefs multiplied. In Yatung, Tibet, the lamas haunted the sick night and day, pounding drums and clashing cymbals; if a sick man slept too much, more devils would enter his body. Touring the Maori settlements around Auckland, New Zealand, Nurse Alice Whittaker found the inhabitants would accept nothing but brown medicine – in harmony with their own skins. And even prosperous Indian villages now looked as derelict as could be, with old baskets, dustpans and rags festooning every tree. If Kaliathal, spirit of the goddess of death, saw such poverty, she would hardly think the village worth visiting.

For doctors like Richard Van Geuns, such outlandish beliefs were a constant thorn in the flesh. Following his wearisome horse-and-trap journey from Cape Town to the German mission station at Uamre, the missionary had tolled the church bell, assuring the villagers that a doctor had arrived 'to drive away the evil spirit' – but one glimpse of Van Geuns' hypodermic sent the people stampeding for the bush.

Yet things were as bad in the west. To maintain contact with the dead, ouija boards and automatic writing were suddenly all the rage. In New Orleans, citizens of both sexes and all ages flocked to Canal Street to purchase voodoo charms – anything from a white chicken's feather to an ace of diamonds for the left shoe – or paid fifty cents for an incantation to be repeated three times a day when rubbing vinegar over the face and palms:

> Sour, sour, vinegar-V
> Keep the sickness off'n me.

Whatever the nation, there was a superstition to fit. On the rocky promontory of Gibraltar, the British were fearful for the first time in more than a century; the Barbary apes were down with flu, and an old wives' tale had it that if the apes left the rock, so, too, would the British. In a village churchyard near Sogn, Norway, painter Lars Prinz had not long set up his easel when he beheld a sight from another age: a group of mountain farmers, approaching a freshly dug grave, solemnly laid on it a plump salmon trout, along with a bowl of porridge and a mug of home-brewed beer. An old Viking tradition of generosity towards the dead had been upheld.

At Cracow, Poland, another graveyard witnessed a ceremony as bizarre. In an effort to save all mankind from the epidemic, two young orphans, surrounded by hundreds of faithful Hebrews, united for a 'sacrificial wedding' in the Jewish cemetery – swayed by a dowry of 20,000 crowns and a fully-furnished flat. Facing the Rabbi beside the grave of the latest flu victim, they pledged their vows in a desperate attempt to exorcise the plague, watched by scores of weeping widows and a troop of armed soldiers who had come to maintain order.

In Yingshang, China, a one-time soldier in the army of the Emperor Kwang-su came to perhaps the most appalling decision which the epidemic was to prompt. Weeks earlier, bowed before the idol in the temple of Cheng Huang, the god of the city, he had sworn a lonely oath: if the god would spare the life of his mother, now stricken with flu, he would willingly make the supreme sacrifice. Now the doctor had pronounced his mother out of danger. It was time to honour his vow.

That day, Yingshang City was crowded; there was a festival in Cheng Huang's honour, and the temple was packed with worshippers. A blue fog of perfumed incense hung before the altar, and in the press of people no one noticed the ex-soldier furtively elbowing his way towards the front of the crowd, his one-year-old son cradled in his arms.

Suddenly an indescribable scream shivered the air. Realising the awful import of that sound, a score of people now leapt forward, grappling with the man. It was too late. In an insane attempt to pay homage to Cheng Huang's victory over the flu demon, the soldier had kept faith: in one apocalyptic moment thrusting his only son far into the red hot cauldron of incense.

The porch door swung noiselessly on its hinges. As intangible as a shadow, Tersilla Vicenzotto stood again within the Basilica of San Antonio of Padua.

The white crocheted shawl was once more drawn tightly about her shoulders, but not because the morning was raw. It had been draped round Oscar when he died, and blindly, irrationally, she hoped that in some mysterious way he had transmitted his sickness to the soft woven material. Thus, she, too, would find release in death.

But first she had a mission to perform; a mission so urgent that this morning her right hand didn't even stray towards the stoup of holy water. As swiftly as before she crossed the nave, deserted now, three hours after Angelus.

This time she did not genuflect before San Antonio's altar. She stood, her eyes strained upwards in the gloom, her face a mask of hate, as far from the love of God as any pagan. It was a terrible accusation, not a prayer, that burst now from her lips: 'San Antonio, you didn't *hear* my appeal.'

Then she spat savagely upwards into the sightless golden face of San Antonio.

Two hundred and forty miles east of Padua, in Turin, the death rate, in this week, topped 400 a day. In Rome, 240 miles south, the casualties were as grave. But no matter how closely an Italian examined each morning's edition of *La Stampa* or *Il Messaggero*, such grim statistics were denied him. In an ill-advised attempt to consign unpleasant reality to limbo,

Liberal Premier Vittorio Emanuele Orlando had clamped down a censorship as totalitarian as any that dictator Benito Mussolini would later impose upon his people.

Though Italy's death rate was higher than any European country except Russia, every outward display of grief was now forbidden by law. No bells tolled. Funeral processions, mourners, wreaths, the familiar black-edged obituary notices pasted on city walls, were banned. Prohibited, too, was the time-honoured closing of the *portone* – the main door of a building – as a sign of mourning.

Only one lone Deputy, the Honourable Luigi Petravalle, himself a doctor, vainly urged Orlando's government to publish the true facts about the nation's health, 'to quash the rumours undermining the moral resistance of a working community at war'.

But not only Italy was at fault. The bells were silent, too, in France, Spain and Holland; in Zurich the Director of Public Health personally rang every city editor to beg them: 'Please don't mention influenza in your obituary notices.' And in New Zealand, until the Government at length refused to issue any statistics at all, many hospitals laboriously scissored all pandemic items from the newspapers before the patients saw them – what the *Dunedin Evening Star* called 'a well-intended effort to allay panic creating panic in another form'.

For the most part, such furtive evasions bred only scepticism and distrust. When Paris newspapers admitted that the capital was suffering 1000 deaths a week, seventeen-year-old Jean Prévost and his school-fellows at the Lycée Henri IV exchanged knowing glances. If the papers admitted to 1000, you could safely multiply that by five.

Some newspapers made a bold attempt to winnow out the hard facts, but ran into a stone wall of bureaucratic silence – and increasingly, as the pandemic swept on, most were reduced to a few pages of agency syndicate stories.

In Clearfield, Pennsylvania, the first-ever Sunday issue of the *Progress* was hammered out by just two men, the managing and city editors, but they were luckier than most. Everywhere, as their staffs went down, papers like the Hampton, Virginia, *Monitor* folded altogether, or, like the Beaufort, Cape Province, *Courier*, bade a long farewell to their readers: 'Don't expect the next *Courier* till you see it'.

Soon there would be no way to check the rumours.

On a misty autumn morning at Camp Hancock, near Highlands, New Jersey, a white-faced assembly of Medical Corps officers and nurses stood erect and blindfolded before a firing squad. All had been convicted, as German spies, of spreading flu among the troops by hypodermic shots. Now, as a volley rang out, these guilty men and women toppled dead.

Simultaneously, squads of street-cleaners in blue overalls set out from municipal depots all over Italy. Overtly armed with canisters of disinfectant to sweeten the streets, they were, in fact, under orders to broadcast flu germs among the crowds – an undercover plan of Premier Orlando's government to keep down the population.

Around this time, in Old Willesden Cemetery, North London, another truck-load of flu victims arrived for burial. Not for one instant, though, did this cover-story fool grave-digger Francis King and his mates. Since the rich began hoarding all the food, the poor were dying of starvation – and the Government had invented 'Spanish flu' to account for the soaring death-toll.

Bumping over a grassy strip outside Cape Town, a Voisin biplane began a slow climb towards 7000 feet. Strapped to the fuselage like some outsize bomb was the skinned carcase of a sheep. Abruptly, at a point where the troposphere teemed with germs, the carcase turned black.

A fanciful scenario? Not entirely. So radically had the pandemic changed the lives of the people that these were four rumours currently circulated and widely believed as October drew to a close – though often the details changed radically according to locality. Almost every U.S. Army Camp, as well as Hancock, had witnessed that mass execution – and other South African cities, in place of an aeroplane and a sheep turning black, had a curious schoolboy flying a piece of liver – which turned green – on his kite.

In vain, authorities like the Army's Acting Surgeon General, Brigadier General Charles Richard, fulminated: 'There have been no medical officers or nurses or anyone else executed at camps in the United States.' Still the rumours persisted – so insidiously that South Africa invoked the Public Welfare and Moratorium Act of 1914 to prosecute anyone circulating rumours about Spanish flu. In Waterbury, Connecticut, the Scovill Manufacturing Company, who organised the city's volunteer aid, adopted a recognisably modern technique: hiring a public relations man to counter each rumour.

It wasn't surprising that such legends died hard. As the pandemic gained ground, and authorities everywhere were less than frank, fear swept the world like a hurricane – as schoolgirl Georgina Cragg remembered it in Gerald, Saskatchewan, 'fear so thick that even a child could feel it'.

Sometimes a man had good reason. In Bangalore, India, Private Jim Wasding of the Ox and Bucks Light Infantry, was down with a mild attack, but try as he might he just couldn't follow the hospital orderly's advice and get a really good sweat on. Soon Fate came to his aid; when the man on his right died and then the man on his left, Wasding found sweating all too easy.

But all too often blind panic lay behind it. Twelve-year-old Geerling Klos, perched on a gate in Enschede, Holland, queueing for the family milk coupons, felt suddenly dizzy and toppled to the ground. At once, fifty people scattered as if someone had lobbed a bomb: 'Take care, he's got flu!' And a housewife who entered a store in St George's, Bermuda, was outraged when one clerk blew a cloud of cigarette smoke at her, while the other, swallowing a pill, retreated to the rear. As she followed up, convinced the man was ill, he shouted hysterically: 'To tell you the God's truth, I'm afraid of you – keep away from me!'

Even lawmen weren't immune. In Grafton, New South Wales, where suspect cases had to report to the police station, one panicky policeman was responsible for sending scores of fit men to the isolation hospital. Unwilling to allow any man nearer than ten yards he placed a thermometer for their use on a post outside the station then retreated – oblivious that it was the broiling Australian sun which sent the mercury to fever-pitch.

In Superior Judge E. P. Morgan's courtroom in San Francisco, the judge himself was the one man remaining impassive when stevedore William Doyle, defendant in a divorce suit, announced he had quit his sickbed to appear. Within minutes, bailiffs, cops, spectators and even attorneys had stampeded from sight – leaving the court to Judge Morgan and the Doyles.

For at least two hungry men, the public's jittery state proved a short-cut to an ample dinner. In the Federal Hill district of Providence, Rhode Island, where Italian immigrants congregated, twenty-year-old Peter Morsilli had a dinner-date with his brother-in-law, Saverio Iafrate, at their favourite restaurant, Marconi's. But the *maître d'hôtel* shook an implacable head. The two were welcome to repair to the bar – but it would be a two-hour wait for a table. At once, Iafrate winked covertly at his brother-in-law. 'You head for the bar,' he muttered, 'I'll catch up with you.'

Minutes later, he reappeared – overcoat collar turned up, hat pulled low over his eyes, coughing strainedly. Catching on, Morsilli demanded loudly: 'What's the matter with you?' As if over a loud-hailer, Iafrate replied: 'Gosh, I don't know – this morning I woke up with a headache, fever, pains in my chest' – then doubled up, coughing convulsively.

To their unfeigned delight, the ruse worked. Within ten minutes the bar had almost emptied, tables fell vacant as at the touch of a wand, and the wily brothers-in-law, napkins tucked in their necks, were impressing on the waiter that their *pasta*, above all, must be cooked al dente.

Yet, tragically, even family ties were affected. One Rome householder, Ida Mengarini was so fearful of the neighbours' hostility when her sister died from flu that she arranged for male nurses to smuggle the dead woman out at night on a stretcher. It was an ugly phenomenon that troubled ambulance operator Ben Buck in Portland, Oregon: all too often, his drivers found the patient alone. After putting through an emergency call, the family had fled.

Even the most innocent sights could prompt mass terror. At Mazatlan, Mexico, passengers from a Panama-bound liner, trooping ashore to buy take-home goods, were appalled by the sultry silence of the streets: the whole port must be in the grip of plague. Running and stumbling, casting fearful glances behind, they hastened back to the ship's gangway where a sleepy peon disillusioned them. Nobody in town had Spanish flu; the people were taking their accustomed siesta.

For thousands in unfamiliar surroundings, fear was now as insidious as the germ itself: not for nothing did one New Zealand physician counsel his patients with advice from Solomon: 'Keep thy heart above all that thou keepest.' In New York's Municipal Lodging House, now an emergency hospital, twenty-five Chinese patients, taken direct from a liner, were convinced that the white-coated doctors and nurses were brigands who had kidnapped them. Refusing to eat, undress or even allow an interpreter near them, seventeen of them died as much of fear and hunger as of flu.

More sinister still was the panic that swept 1500 black recruits at Camp Wheeler, Macon, Georgia. No sooner had their train arrived at the railhead than they scrambled terrified for cover – certain that the platform reception committee of masked medical orderlies were Ku Klux Klansmen.

At least one doctor experienced such terror at first hand: Dr John Hogan, Assistant Commissioner for Health in Baltimore, Maryland. Never, in fifteen years of practice, had he known fear such as assailed him one October night, as he made to enter an apartment in the downtown Clifton Park district.

Suddenly, from the gloom of the hallway, there came a stampede of wild-eyed women, streaking towards him, drawn, as if spellbound, by his black calfskin bag. In one primeval moment, Dr Hogan saw himself as he appeared to these desperate harpies: a magic Aesculapian symbol of health, the key to life itself, possessed of powers akin to witchcraft.

Frantically, they clawed at his lapels and tore at his sleeves, their breath hot and nauseous in his face. 'Doctor!' they screamed, 'Doctor! Do something, give us something, doctor!'

Now Hogan himself knew fear; jungle instinct drove out all sense of professional etiquette. Clutching his bag beneath his arm he lowered his head and plunged violently through the screaming mob into the street.

Through the murmuring shadows of Clifton Park he ran like a man possessed, seized by a nameless inexplicable dread, not daring to look back.

The night was a time for listening. On her verandah at Stratford, in the lush dairy farming country of Taranaki, New Zealand, Dr Doris Gordon had a new yardstick on these October nights: she listened for the crack of a whip. Within days, she had come to gauge the gravity of each case approaching her nine-bed hospital by the frenzy of those whip cracks. If the 'cow cocky', the dairy farmer, was plying his whip furiously, urging the horses that hauled the old milk-waggon ambulance to even greater speed, then she knew that pneumonia threatened.

In the Moravian mission house at Hopedale, Labrador, the Reverend Walter Perrett was listening too. Above all, he longed to hear the joyous whistle of the mission barque *Harmony*, for the ship was days overdue from Jamaica with a cargo of molasses, and Perrett was worried. For some time, too, the Eskimos had been calling his attention to the small signs that all was not well. Not a hare or a partridge had been seen all that winter – and always, when trouble threatened in Labrador, the hares seemed to sense it and lope silently and intently away from the scene of the disaster.

Worse, on his last visit, the *Harmony*'s Master, Captain Jackson, had brought the first word of the pandemic, and Perrett was now more concerned than he liked to admit. 'One rather quakes when one thinks of what might happen if that made its appearance among us,' he wrote carefully in the mission journal. 'May the Preserver of men protect our little nation from that disease.'

But though he listened intently, he was listening only to the absolute silence of the Labrador night, broken at intervals by a soft persistent scratching and scuffling: some huskies had clambered up a snowdrift to the slippery roof of a house, seeking the greater warmth of the chimney. Still not entirely at ease, Perrett returned to his journal.

In a sparsely-furnished subaltern's room at Bramshott Camp, England, Lieutenant Arthur Lapointe was listening to his own despondent thoughts. Thus far, Lapointe had steered clear of Spanish flu, though the damp English countryside had brought on a sharp attack of rheumatism and he was troubled by violent headaches – the effects of the gas he had inhaled at Neuville Vitasse, the M.O. assured him. But every day more and more men at Bramshott were reporting sick, a constant reminder of what this pandemic could do, and still no word had come from home.

'Oh, why don't they write to me?' Lapointe scribbled frantically in his diary, for now the triumph of his commission, his desire to have the family bask in his new-found glory, had all but faded. More than anything he yearned for reassurance and peace of mind, but each week's mail-call left him restless and uneasy, a prey to thoughts he somehow dared not voice.

In the beach-hut at Taunoa, Tahiti, the night winds brought only familiar sounds to the ears of Hector MacQuarrie: the tireless hush of the surf off Moorea, where the pin-point lights of the fishermen's boats sparkled like diamonds on dark velvet. Yet the New Zealander, too, was uneasy, for though Tahiti had no newspapers and relied solely on the daily bulletins of Governor Gustave-Henri-Jacques Julien, news had come of the casualties in Paris and the French in Papeete were gravely concerned.

It hadn't then struck MacQuarrie that this could threaten Tahiti, too; somehow the languorous life of the Society Islands made such a grim reality unthinkable. But he thought of good friends back in New Zealand and the United States, and how they must be faring, and for the first time since reaching Taunoa he felt a dim stirring of conscience. Now he was once more restored to health, he could surely be of service elsewhere in the world at such a time. The thought was to trouble him, unresolved, for many days yet.

On another verandah, eighty miles north-east of Nairobi, the Reverend Handley Hooper, of the Church Missionary Society, watched moonlight bathe the crater of Mount Kenya, towering 17,000 feet above the skyline. But Hooper, at the same time was listening, too: to the monotonous beat of the tom-toms sounding through the night from the Kikuyu Hills. From the villages, the people were calling to the Creator-god, who dwelt within the mists of the mountain, to free them of the scourge about to destroy 155,000 of their number.

As the missionary listened, a cry rent the darkness. Unwittingly, he gasped. It was a cry expressing the Kikuyu's pain and bewilderment in the face of an unseen enemy, yet more prophetic than any man among them could have realised. It was a sentiment which millions in the weeks ahead would come painfully to accept: 'Ni uhoro wa Ngai.' (It is God's affair now.)

One man was afraid for the first time – yet for him, ironically, the pandemic was over.

Through the high wooden gates of Lager E, Josefstadt, Bohemia, came an old and frail man, fur-hatted, walking with a stick, escorted by armed sentries. Beneath one arm he supported two wicker cages. As he drew closer, Lieutenant Enrico Bedeschi, the camp doctor, saw that one contained a rat, the other a dormouse.

Now Bedeschi, whose German was spotty, grew puzzled. Though the old man was fluent, he could understand nothing except that this was a doctor who wanted to inoculate the animals with the blood of patients convalescing from *Spanischer Krankheit* (the Spanish sickness).

What was that, Bedeschi asked, mystified. In his mind he

was sure the old man meant the 'Celtic disease', as the Italians called syphilis. Not for a moment did he call to mind the appalling death rate among the Russian prisoners that autumn, with the cyanosis and the mysterious abscesses – which Bedeschi had always ascribed to malnutrition. In any case, the deaths had ceased weeks ago, as abruptly as they had begun.

Frustrated, the old doctor grappled to bridge the communication gap, then suddenly it struck him: as a doctor, Bedeschi must surely understand Latin. When the Italian nodded, the old man announced very loudly and distinctly: *'Novus morbus'* (a new disease).

Then, as Bedeschi watched, the other grasped his walking-stick. With the ferrule, he began to draw, and little by little, in the dust of the compound, the Italian saw that it was a map of Europe which was taking shape: Spain, France, Germany, the outline growing inch by inch, until it spanned Russia and the near east.

It had swept all these countries and more besides, the old man explained in precise school-book Latin: unearthly, unidentified, unchecked.

Now for the first time Bedeschi realised the magnitude of the scourge that had befallen Lager E, and there in the warm autumn sunlight he shivered and knew fear.

With the *Newport* two days out from San Francisco, Doña Juanita Lejarza knew an anguish all her own. Despite Emilio's trick with her rouge-pot, which had gained him safe passage aboard the ship, there was no disguising the gravity of his condition. Fiddling selfconsciously with his new gold watch, Dr Dilley, the ship's surgeon, made no bones about it: both her husband's lungs were badly affected. It was only a matter of days.

Emilio was sleeping deeply, almost in a coma, on the morning that Juanita rummaged stealthily through her jewel-case, then with an anxious glance at her husband, stole from the stateroom. It was the first time, day or night, that she had left his side since the onset of the illness, but now she had business to do.

On deck, the slim dark girl sought out two of Emilio's closest friends: Don Adolfo Benard and Don Dolores Morales, both influential Nicaraguan politicians. Juanita came at once to the point. Emilio had wanted to die in Nicaragua, but his race was almost run. Would Don Adolfo act as her intermediary with the Master, Captain Yardley, to ensure her husband was at least spared a burial at sea?

Now she produced her jewel case. There would be enough, she said, to defray the Pacific Steamship Company's expenses in making a diversion to some Mexican port like Progreso. There the funeral could take place.

Both men were appalled. All of them, Don Adolfo reminded Juanita, had paid $4000 American for the return trip. There was no question of Emilio being buried at sea, or even in Mexico. 'Keep your jewels,' he concluded with brusque kindness. 'Emilio is our friend.'

Touched, yet strangely reassured, Juanita returned to the state room. Emilio might not live to know it, but at least in death he would fulfil not only his own but, perhaps, every man's last conscious wish: finally to go home.

The fears that now beset the world barely registered with Lieutenant Charles Clapp, Jr, American Army Air Corps. He was drunk.

Ever since that spur-of-the-moment lunch date at Sherry's, with Margaret Macdonald, Clapp had continued his steady binge – sometimes discreetly, in Margaret's company, at others on marathon weekend jags with his buddies. But now, posted overnight to Paine Field, West Point, Mississippi, the young aviator was at the lowest point of his twenty years.

Despite a confident belief that his previous bout of flu – plus the generous shots of White Rock that had cured it – would immunise him, Clapp had come down with it yet again. To be sure, he had suffered a mild enough bout, like most of his fellows, but coupled with the depression that followed it was the bleak knowledge that so far as overseas flying was concerned, Paine Field spelt zero. Some numskull in a swivel-chair had finally once for all decided that there were aviators enough in France.

For days on end, rain had curtained the airfield, the planes were in worse shape than the aviators, and a strict flu quarantine, which decreed lights out by ten, made liquor hard to come by and life intolerable. But in this last week of October, Clapp had discovered one place in the camp where a light, of necessity, burned dimly all night: the officers' latrine.

Now, locked away in foul-smelling privacy, a writing-board on his knees and a pint of hard-won rye conveniently at hand, he was thinking of Margaret. Already, in such squalid surroundings, his judgement warped both by flu and by rye, he had begun to invest her with a wholly unreal glamour.

Their theatre dates, those suppers at the Plaza Grill, the dances – to Clapp's fancy, Irene Castle had never glided through a dance more smoothly. And though Margaret loved a good time, she was cultured and refined, her personality as subtle as her perfume – a far cry from the over-scented broads the bell hops laid on during those weekend benders.

Never after being with Margaret had Clapp the strange guilty feeling that women like that prompted in him. Instead he felt elated, exalted, as when the day's first drink began its work, and suddenly the thought struck him: Wouldn't it be wonderful to go through life with someone like that at your side? She might laugh if he asked her – but hadn't some fellow said, 'Faint heart never won fair lady'?

Emboldened, he took another swig of rye. He settled the writing-board more firmly on his knees. Abruptly conscious of the stench and squalor of the latrine, he thought disgustedly, what a God-awful place for romance. Yet even so, his mind racing with guilty excitement, he was already planning the courtship that was to involve both of them in seventeen years of alcoholism and debt, of shabby affairs and broken promises.

First, a telegraphed order for fifty dollars worth of American Beauty roses. By careful calculation, they would arrive on the same day as the letter which he now began, to be sent special delivery. They were words which had been penned many times before, though rarely in a stranger setting: 'I wonder what you would say if I asked you to marry me ... ?'

Painfully, Private John Lewis Barkley tugged at the laces. Inch by inch, the sodden mud-caked thread yielded: with his last remaining ounce of strength, he pulled off his shoes and sank back in the straw of the barn. All told, he thought, it was twenty-one days since he had last removed those boots.

Looking back, it seemed to the stuttering slightly-built doughboy that those three weeks had somehow symbolised his whole war: the traumatic fear, then the numb resignation, the muddy squelching monotony of survival, then the fear again, coiling like a fist in the stomach.

It had been a fear like this that had engulfed him on that autumn afternoon at Cunel: the ringing in his ears as the shell from the 77 burst above the tank he had hijacked, in the woods facing Hill 253, the nasal haemorrhage he believed was Spanish flu, the blackness.

Then, within seconds, as he thrust blindly from the turret, gulping at cool air, he realised what had happened. That last shell had torn loose the caterpillar chain of the tank, so that it whiplashed upwards to strike the barrel of his Maxim machine-gun. It was the Maxim's stock which had recoiled with such agonising force and caused that nose-bleed.

Then, as conscious thought returned, all Barkley's hatred of the war had concentrated on that 77. Momentarily he had forgotten that as of then he was stalling the entire German advance. He was going to get the gun that had thrown a scare into him if it was the last thing he did.

Hastily he thrust a new belt into the Maxim. Some 600 yards off he could see several gunners clustered round the 77. Pushing the muzzle out, using battle sights because of the long range, he gave the 77 a whole frenzied burst – under it, over it, to the right and left, finally straight at it. An aching silence followed, and by degrees he realised that the 77 would trouble him no more.

But Barkley himself was not out of trouble. Once more the

Germans had realised his tank was still in business. Now one deadly sound again became apparent: the clamour of machine-gun bullets against the Renault's steel sides. And in this moment, too, the Maxim began to give out – jamming after every four shots. Within minutes it became a single action. Barkley was having to pull the operating crank for each shot.

He had held the advance for as long as he could. Now the scout realised the one way out of this was through the driver's compartment, in the end backing on to the woods. He must crawl into this, wait for a slackening of fire, then run for it.

At that moment a grenade hit the Renault's turret like a thunderbolt. A German patrol had stolen so silently and skilfully up on him that Barkley hadn't even heard them.

As if by reflex, he lunged for the Maxim. This time it worked, and as the patrolmen dived headlong for cover he saw one man had left a satchel of grenades abandoned in plain view. Swinging the barrel, he fired. With a roar like a six-inch shell the bag blew up, a concussion so intense the tank shook all over, and everywhere across the hillside men were falling.

Then, as suddenly as it had begun, Barkley's stand inside the tank was over. For a long time he had waited for the gun to cool, before sneaking a look through the port to take aim. Then he gasped. All across Hill 253, the Germans were doubling for the woods. And behind them the khaki-clad lines of the U.S. 7th Division were sweeping down over the top of the hill.

After that, to Barkley, all of it had seemed anticlimax. There had been his link-up with a 7th Division patrol, who just couldn't credit that one man had stalled an entire German advance. There had been the jubilant reunion with 'Jesse' James and 'Nigger' Floyd – and the uproarious revelation that Jesse had been the lone sniper backstopping him all through that fearsome afternoon. Then there was a blind march by night, through rain, to Bois de Naulemont ... patrols ... hand-to-hand skirmishes. But somehow no one thought to mention his stand before Cunel.

Worst of all was the knowledge their partnership was fast

breaking up. Floyd's arm was growing steadily worse, from the bullet he had stopped all those weeks ago, before St Mihiel, and though they dressed it with iodine and clean gauze, soon Floyd was too sick to keep down food. That pact to stick together, no matter what, couldn't remain valid much longer. Then, on the night they were relieved from the line and started back towards Montfaucon, the medical orderlies had spotted Floyd's condition and hauled him before a doctor.

When the big Cherokee Indian reacted so violently the medic ordered him to be tied to the stretcher, Barkley and Jesse exchanged a long look. From now on, that pact concerned only the two of them. Floyd was booked to go down the line, and plainly they couldn't accompany him. Technically at least, they were still in fighting shape.

Until this night, in the last week of October, in the farmer's barn at Culey. Though John Lewis Barkley found strength to remove his shoes, for the first time in all the campaign he could not swallow food. Suddenly he slid sideways in the hay.

Minutes later, another Company K scout, Mike De Angelo, who spoke some French, was hammering on the farmer's doorway. To the comely girl who opened up, he gasped out: all the help they could muster was needed to save a soldier's life.

For hours on end, tossing and mumbling in an old-fashioned feather-bed, John Lewis Barkley fought his nightmares. But his was no lone example. It was a phenomenon that doctors everywhere, at October's end, viewed with increasing dread.

To every medical man, mild delirium, and above all, post-influenzal depression, was already a well-recognised condition. But the effects of this unknown and lethal virus upon the central nervous system was something that none of them had witnessed until now.

From St Mary's Hospital, London, Dr Wilfred Harris reported cases of influenza that had degenerated into cataleptic states, trances, and even spastic paraplegia. Often the illness involved such excruciating neuralgia of the trigeminal nerve – which controls the chewing muscles of the jaw – that many citizens mistakenly consulted their dentists. One rural mail-carrier, from Norristown, Pennsylvania, was found over 250 miles away in Marlboro, Massachusetts, suffering not only from flu but total amnesia, with no recollection of how he got there at all. And Dr William Jones of Minneapolis found that the disease had played such havoc with his patients' mental state that no less than three of them claimed to have started the war.

Many victims still recall delirium so unnerving that it more accurately resembled a hallucinatory drug attack. Across a hundred thousand bedroom walls and ceilings the patterns writhed and twisted in frightening arabesques ... monkeys grimacing from the lintels ... spiders scuttling from the cover-let ... cohorts of soldiers filled the room and firemen battled flames against a jet-black background. Somewhere behind the curtains a waterfall was tumbling, and the door dissolved into Braque-like cubes and circles. Huge snakes lay coiled in dark corners, and bats swooped and fluttered.

Strange delusions became stark reality to those who suffered them. At Edenton, North Carolina, eleven-year-old Sue Jordan found herself suddenly on the *Titanic*, struggling for a place in a lifeboat. The Kaiser was a fixture for days in the south bedroom window of Gertie Belle Damon's house in Dickens, Iowa. On a Wisconsin farm, fifteen-year-old Lina Davis thrilled every night at dusk when a quartet made up of her grandfather, her father and two strangers grouped round her sickbed to sing such heavenly music as she had never heard. But even when convalescing she never dared thank her father, for her grandfather, she now recalled, had died two years before.

Even beloved objects became sudden symbols of terror. In a bedroom facing the Vatican Gardens in Rome, five-year-old Gemma Olivetti was convinced that her favourite doll was turning black in the face, as if it, too, had developed the fatal cyanosis that had slain her father and mother.

Often such nightmare visions led to appalling violence. Along the corridors of Foxworth Hospital, Liverpool, alarmed medical orderlies fought a running pitched battle with delirious soldiers who had armed themselves with razor-blades strapped to broom handles. On Chicago's South Morgan Street, neighbours who heard labourer Peter Marrazo scream, 'I'll cure them my own way,' broke through the barricaded door too late to save his wife and four children from being slashed to death.

But most often the maddened victims wished no harm to anyone but themselves – and many hospital patients came to dread the nightly sound of running steps, the swish of a sister's full skirt, then the appalling crash of glass as a crazed victim leaped from a third-storey window. In Paris, with 200 policemen sick, appeals were made for volunteers to guard the Seine bridges, the tragic haunt of suicides – but even two who agreed to stand in leaped fatally from the Pont de la Concorde.

Few ended their lives for as strange a reason as Cape Town businessman Frederick Harris. Fearing that he, too, like his partner and several of his staff, would become a flu victim, he scrawled a farewell note in his own blood, then plunged off the esplanade into Table Bay.

Hundreds nourished the delusion that their lives were spared only by divine intervention. War correspondent Edgar Mowrer of the *Chicago Daily News*, delirious in an American Red Cross hospital at Padua, saw God as in a Renaissance painting, while below, like the Virgin in a Crucifixion, kneeling in profile against a background of dark pines, was Mowrer's wife, Lilian. Suddenly light suffused the whole scene and God announced: 'Because of her love you shall not die.'

Ex-soldier George Beardsmore, in Dunedin, New Zealand, fancied himself on the brink of a picture-book Hell, with the Devil and all his fork-tailed minions thrusting flu victims into swirling flames. Gamely as Beardsmore fought, the fiends were gaining ground until Jesus Christ placed a calm hand upon his shoulder and said: 'You are going to get well.'

Divine intervention or no, the strange case of Therese Göransson vividly recalled the warning of Moses: 'Be sure your sin will find you out.' Delirious with flu above the beerhouse she owned in Oskarshamn, Sweden, she raved in guilty remorse that she had taken a child's life. The unwitting confession triggered off a search until horrified neighbours, opening a trunk in an attic room, discovered a child's corpse.

Days later, when the fever abated, the wretched woman awoke to find police agents at the bedside, awaiting her statement. Unnerved, Therese Göransson confessed to not one but two cases of infanticide – in each case a child born out of wedlock, whose deaths were only now revealed through the strange agency of the Spanish Lady.

For Lydia Phillips, there was one moment in all her weeks at Twist Street School Emergency Hospital when she walked within the kingdom of fear. It was the turning-point, she afterwards recalled. From this time on she was a true professional – armoured against the worst that fear could do.

Although Lydia had done temporary duty in every ward at Twist Street, one-quarter of the rambling two-storey building had remained forbidden ground until now: the mortuary. Because of an imagined risk of infection, it was strictly off-limits to both nurses and volunteers.

Then, one afternoon, Lydia was chatting with a friendly orderly when the man revealed that only five minutes earlier he had taken a body there. Was it really true, Lydia asked diffidently, that the bodies turned black? For answer, the man gave her an appraising glance. 'If you really want to know,' he parried, 'now's your chance to see.'

Within herself, Lydia guessed the man was testing her nerve, but she did not demur. In a sense, all her life at Twist Street had been a test of courage: the chafing of the feet, the incident of the bed-pan, the eyes of the man who had begged for a closed window. All along she had subconsciously driven herself to see how much she could endure, venturing beyond established barriers, grateful that thus far she had not been found wanting.

Together, like conspirators, they crept along a passage, crossing a yard, finally into a rough shed littered with lumber and wood shavings. At the far end, on a rough heap of rags, a man was lying, unnaturally still.

Stooping gently, the orderly lifted the man's head, and

Lydia saw with a start that the nostrils, mouth and ears were tightly plugged with cotton wool. It was true, she thought with fascinated horror, discoloration was already marked, though the skin was by no means as black as rumour suggested. Kneeling beside the orderly she gazed with wonder and compassion at this unknown man, already beyond time.

Suddenly a wild scream turned Lydia's stomach to a block of ice. Galvanised, both she and the orderly swung round. A yard distant, a small girl of about eight years old, white-faced and trembling, was backing slowly away from them, her eyes mirroring her horrified disbelief.

'That's not my Daddy,' she cried out in passionate rejection. 'That's not my Daddy!'

Then before they could stop and comfort her she was gone – running from a memory that time might one day erase for her, but for Lydia Phillips, never.

In frowning silence, Dr Juan Zamora studied the list. Below this office where he now sat, in Madrid's Ministry of the Interior, traffic swirled past the building's baroque façade, through the autumn sunlight that flooded the Puerta del Sol. It was a scene as remote from the silent stricken mountains of Aragon that Zamora had but recently left as any on earth. Yet the typewritten list he perused made plain that the challenge to doctors was everywhere as great.

On that unforgettable night when the flu had riveted him to his bed in Bijuesca, Zamora's coolly lucid decision to postpone even checking his temperature until dawn had been wholly characteristic. He had been resigned to die – yet if Providence ordained it, and he was spared for new service in life, then he was ready.

At dawn, he had awoken blearily, clammy with sweat, and reached for the thermometer. Now he saw that at the onset of the fever his temperature had been almost 101°F. He shook the thermometer and tested it again. It was close to normal – so there was still work to be done.

Still weak and shaken, but knowing himself on the road to

recovery, Zamora had stayed on in bed for five more days – still prescribing for sick townsfolk according to the symptoms Doña Paca reported to him. By then, his colleague, Dr Martinez Solaz, had returned from tending his sick father. At once, Zamora set out to Madrid to volunteer for locum duties. All over Spain the situation was reported as near breaking-point.

And just how critical Zamora now saw, as he studied the long catalogue of place-names that the black-coated Ministry official had handed him. The choice was up to him. Already 200 Spanish doctors had died in the epidemic – and there was a crying need for stand-bys in places as far apart as Badajoz and Bilbao.

Though Zamora didn't then know it, the situation was as bad all over. In Coimbra, Portugal, the Medical School had brought the finals forward by three weeks, to rush through more qualified men – and the State Board of Medical Examiners in Sacramento, California, had catechised and passed ninety-seven candidates in one day. The Italian Supreme Command had put 800 Army doctors at the government's disposal. In Dunedin, fifth-year students, following a crash course in drugs, were already standing in as G.P.s.

And many veterans, following six weeks of unequal struggle, were finding it doubly hard to sustain their faith. In the words of one hard-pressed British Medical Officer of Health: 'The disease simply has its way. It comes like a thief in the night and steals treasure.' Hundreds had even begun to ask themselves the dangerous question posed by Dr Wilhelm Binnendijk of Amsterdam: 'Why did I become a doctor? I can do nothing to help, and soon there won't be any more people.'

But many more, like Juan Zamora, were only fired with a new determination by this seemingly insoluble challenge. If they had engaged in a losing battle, they would still be in there fighting to the end.

Now, like them, Zamora reached his decision. 'I'll take Algeciras and Gibraltar,' he told the gratified official. 'If my credentials can be made ready, I'll leave tonight.'

CHAPTER EIGHT

'I'll Take Orders from Dead Men'

31 October–4 November 1918

On a busy street in the Birmingham suburb of Ward End, a woman hastened up to a passer-by, drawn, as though by a magnet, to the black bag he carried. Was she right, she panted, in supposing he was a doctor?

Wearily, the man nodded assent. Then, the woman begged him, would he be kind enough to come to her kitchen right away? Her pet starling had just broken its leg, and the poor birdie so badly needed a splint.

Strangely heartened, Dr Alexander Mackie, works doctor to both Wolseley Motors and the Shell Petroleum Company, agreed readily. Though the woman could not suspect it, Mackie was so relieved to find any patient untouched by Spanish flu he would gladly have treated the bird for nothing.

On the morning of Thursday, 31 October, every doctor, nurse and pharmacist would have felt a kindred emotion. On this momentous day, the pandemic had spanned the entire globe, and nowhere was there any sight of a respite. In scores of countries, their daily routine bore eloquent testimony to the way the sickness had transformed all their lives.

Arriving home after an eighteen-hour day in Vancouver, British Columbia, Dr Henry Hall Milburn's first action was to yank the telephone off the hook. It was something he had never done in all his years as a practitioner, but somehow he must ensure himself six hours sleep. It was the same with Nurse Dorothy Deming of New York's Columbia Presbyterian Hospital. For her in these dedicated weeks, 'as truly under fire as though we were with our brothers in the Argonne', sleep was only possible if her eyes were masked with a black silk stocking and her ears plugged with cotton wool.

It was harder still for hospital residents. Dr Ernst Ottsen never stepped outside Berlin's 2400-bed Virchow Hospital for two whole months; though he could retire to his room to cat-nap, he and 120 other doctors were now on twenty-four hour call to check new admissions or certify deaths. And at Glasgow Infirmary, even Dr Agnes Bennett, a veteran of the Salonika front, carried on only through the compassionate blind eye turned by the night sisters and nurses. More often than not, at 10 p.m., when the Resident must go the rounds, they found Dr Agnes, exhausted and fully dressed, fast asleep at her desk.

The pharmacists, too, were rushed off their feet. Most, by government order, kept open at least until midnight, and at weekends, too, but when a local ukase made round-the-clock service compulsory, the situation became desperate. One such city was Paris, where cycle patrols, on all-night duty at police stations, rushed emergency prescriptions to chemists on the hour – so effectively that most ran out of supplies before dawn. One hundred grams of drugs was now sold out in exactly fifteen minutes.

In Oslo, a sympathetic government backstopped the pharma-cists' efforts by recruiting chemistry students and retired women dispensers – but elsewhere most had to shift for themselves. Fourteen-year-old Eric Parr, a second-year apprentice in Auck-land, New Zealand, kept the shop going, when the rest of the staff went down, for seventeen hours at a stretch – roping in three policemen to wash bottles and make up creosote capsules, keeping himself alert at intervals with three tonic drops of strychnine.

And most, in true Hippocratic tradition, carried on some-how – since their patients gave them little choice. At Stratford, New Zealand, importunate patients kept tabs on Dr Doris

Gordon's movements through bribing the telephone operator – or even pitched camp in her car drive until she returned.

Often their faith was touching. Trim little Dr Gasper Bioux, with his goatee beard, renowned through Charleroi, Pennsylvania as a state-licensed fringe practitioner who hadn't lost a flu patient, got an emergency call from Lawrence Frye, the town's leading undertaker. Smilingly, Dr Bioux teased him, 'Is it true you said I was the only doctor who never contributed to your business?' Tears starting to his eyes, the undertaker replied, 'Why else do you think I called you? Because I know you can save my daughter.'

At Fort Covington, on New York's Canadian border, Dr William Macartney steered his two-wheeled Concord buggy all through the night, often followed patiently by his big black Labrador dog, Mr Winkle. When sentimental ladies chided him that he would tire the poor dog's heart, Macartney had a sour rejoinder: Mr Winkle, at least, could quit when he was tired.

Age was no barrier in this unremitting battle. 'Working on borrowed time', as he himself put it, Toronto's Dr John Hall was well into his eighties, but on the day before he himself went down he visited ninety-four patients – and within weeks had recovered to fight on again.

Not all were so selfless. Some survivors still speak bitterly of far from professional conduct – most probably because the doctor concerned was strained beyond endurance. One doctor roundly reviled the first man to collapse outside one Indiana pharmacy 'for bringing this damned thing to Bloomington'. And when twelve-year-old Cecil Wilson – who survived to tell the tale – was stricken in Pueblo, Colorado, a doctor contemptuously brushed aside his grandmother's anxious query with, 'Get on the waiting list for a casket.'

There were cases of shameless rapacity. One doctor on the Rand charged an unheard-of £405 for nine visits, and in Medicine Hat, Alberta, another asked thirty-five dollars for disinfecting a seven-room house. Nor did his patients readily forget the Auckland, New Zealand, practitioner who demanded thirty shillings fee and transportation expenses before he would examine a patient. When the others in the house could muster only twenty-nine shillings and sixpence between them, the doctor waited, stony-faced, until someone had hurried out to borrow the missing sixpence.

More typical was the genuine distress of Dr Ashley Jago, country doctor for the Land's End area of Cornwall. As his son, Maurice, steered the gig through the narrow lanes, Jago confided earnestly: 'My boy, in the last seven weeks I've been making money – and if this is what's making money, I hope to God I never make any more.'

Many surprised even themselves with their resourcefulness. One Toronto doctor, working on a mass-production basis, wrote out batches of flu prescriptions in advance – handing them out immediately after walking in and touching the patient's forehead. In the old Hansa Viertel quarter of Berlin, Dr Hugo Freund, with one thousand potential patients, transgressed every medical canon by contacting all of them in advance: if they felt the slightest inkling of a cold, he had a quinine compound already made up.

Fewer than a dozen patients died – and Freund even escaped the censure of the German Medical Association by charging no one a fee.

Inevitably, some doctors had recourse to placebos. One Kirksville, Missouri, G.P. doled out pills in three different colours, white, yellow and pink, with appropriately mystic instructions: each was to be taken on the hour, the first with a glass of water, the second with two glasses of water, the third with three. Though none of them contained anything but sugar, the doctor claimed one hundred per cent success.

In the Croix Rousse quarter of Lyons, France, where the poor silk-weavers congregated and the air resounded day and night to the clacking of the looms, Nursing Orderly Ferréol Gavaudan was scratching his head. Seconded from the western front because of the shortage of doctors, Gavaudan had not even completed his medical training, yet now he was daily called upon to pose as a skilled physician and reach decisions on cases that defied all text-book definition.

Surveying the sick weaver in the bed before him, he thought the man was typical of many such cases he had seen in these cramped fusty apartment houses – sick, with a high fever and congestion, but almost certain to recover and in need, above all, of reassurance. As before, Gavaudan decided on a course of treatment he had rarely known fail in the past.

She must, he told the man's wife, procure a jug of red *vin ordinaire*, add sugar and then mull it like a punch. Then, leaning forward, he twirled the man's cloth cap from a hook behind the door and set it squarely on the knob at the foot of the bed.

'For you, *mon vieux*,' he announced confidently, 'I prescribe the "three hats" treatment. You drink the wine. You keep drinking until you see *two* of these, but don't worry – you're getting better.'

'And then?' the awe-stricken patient demanded.

'Keep drinking,' Gavaudan counselled, 'until you see *three* hats – and then, *voilà!* you'll be cured.'

The waiting-room door closed behind the day's last patient. Now an intense silence reigned, broken only by the raucous hissing of the gas-jets. In his dingy surgery at 113 North Street, Belfast, Dr Nathaniel Osborne M'Connell was alone.

Never in twenty years' practice had the tall greying Ulsterman been so truly thankful for a pandemic as he was now. On this forlorn Monday evening, 4 November, as a thin drizzle bathed Belfast's red-brick slums, the Spanish Lady, to Dr M'Connell, represented the one way out of the most desperate dilemma he had ever known. Without this sickness he might, within days, face not only being struck from the Medical Register but a charge of manslaughter, even murder.

To be sure, there had been risky moments in the past. In the city's poorer quarters, along Falls Road and Crumlin Road, M'Connell was known as a doctor who pronounced no moral judgements if a tearful girl visited his surgery and confessed shamefacedly that her fellow had got her in trouble. For a two-guinea fee M'Connell had terminated many an unwanted pregnancy, and no questions asked. As Ben Clarke, the Donegall Street druggist, well knew, the doctor had made use of twenty-four pounds of liquid ergot, used to contract the muscles of the uterus, in the past four months.

Then, on Friday, 1 November, everything had gone alarmingly wrong. That morning, M'Connell had reached his surgery at midday to find a message from his dispenser, David Thompson. A young girl, accompanied by an old woman, had been enquiring for the doctor. They had left the name of Reid, and the address, 817 Crumlin Road, dividing line between Belfast's strife-torn Protestant and Catholic areas.

He had been anxious to get them out of the surgery and back home, the dispenser added, for the girl was so ill she seemed on the point of collapse.

At first, Dr M'Connell had suspected Spanish flu – but it had needed only a cursory examination to determine that Mary Jane Reid, who lived with her mother and her brother David above the old lady's little shop, was pregnant.

M'Connell had used the blunt scraping instrument called a curette which he often employed in such cases, and it had seemed straightforward enough. But, as always with him, it was something that left a bitter after-taste. Early that afternoon, he had retired to the snug in John Muldoon's pub, farther up Crumlin Road. By 3.15, he recalled bitterly now, he had been drunk.

At Horseshoe Corner, he had boarded a tram-car for the city centre and launched into a rambling drunken conversation with the Reverend John Gailey, the Minister of Ballysillan Presbyterian Church. Though the Reverend Gailey didn't know the doctor, the medical man had recognised him, tapping him solemnly on the knee and announcing, 'You don't know me but I know you.' At this stage M'Connell was unaware that the Reverend Gailey, as Mary Reid's pastor, was a frequent visitor to the Crumlin Road shop.

Nor did he know that on the Saturday afternoon, with Mary's condition worsening hourly, David, her brother, had spent hours at her bedside. Why was she in such great pain, he had asked her, alarmed. Mary had hesitated, but finally she had told him: 'The doctor performed an operation ... they might get him for manslaughter.' Then she had added: 'David, will you pray for me?'

Early on the Sunday morning, a white and shaken David Reid had called at M'Connell's house. Was he the doctor who had attended Miss Reid of Crumlin Road? M'Connell had hesitated visibly before replying, yes. Young Reid begged him not to lose an instant. His sister was dangerously ill.

At 6 p.m. the same day, with the Reverend Gailey keeping watch beside her bed, Mary Jane Reid had died.

Now, on this rain-soaked Monday night, his first suspicions concerning the girl's illness came back to M'Connell as a sudden diabolical inspiration. Until now, Belfast had the smallest influenza death-rate of any town in the United Kingdom, yet even so the sick were numbered in thousands. Thus there was every chance in the world that this death would go unremarked and unsuspected.

In Column 6 of the Entry of Death form, under the heading 'Cause of Death', Dr Nathaniel M'Connell now unblushingly certified that on 3 November 1918, Mary Jane Reid, female, 26 years, cloth worker, had died of 'influenza and acute gastritis'.

One factor now conspired to help the doctors above all: the whole-hearted if belated backing of the health authorities. The closing-down of theatres and churches and all public gatherings had been the first stage. Now, accepting that only the hardest-hitting tactics could check the pandemic, many townships clamped down more stringent controls than ever before.

Many were aimed at the then widespread and insanitary habit of spitting – everywhere from tram-cars to sidewalks. In New York, Health Commissioner Royal Copeland, taking thought of the 'heatless Mondays' that conserved the nation's fuel, called for 'spitless Sundays' – a vain attempt to seek public co-operation, for soon enough State Commissioner of Health Herman Biggs had resorted to sterner measures. Any person who coughed, spat or sneezed in a public place without using a handkerchief would now be liable to the fullest rigours of the law.

Huge signs loomed on New York's streets – 'It is Unlawful to Cough and Sneeze' – and warned that violators were liable to a staggering $500 fine or a year in jail. Within days, more than 500 New Yorkers had been hauled before the courts, and other cities followed suit; Chicago's Health Commissioner Dr John Dill Robertson told the police department: 'Arrest thousands, if necessary, to stop sneezing in public.' Where churches remained open, ministers were asked to inveigh against spitting from the pulpit, and at least one township, Bergen, Norway, laid on spitting controllers for its street-cars.

Until this moment, health authorities everywhere had fought shy of inoculation. To introduce germs, either live, weakened or dead into the body had seemed pointless, even risky. To begin with, Dr Nicolle and Dr Lebailly had run into a stone wall: though they had confirmed the presence of an entirely new virus, no microscope could identify it. In preparing a vaccine to combat the disease, there could be no certainty that the organism at fault had even been included.

Thus the one hope was a 'shot-gun' vaccine – a hodge-podge of organisms found in the bodies of patients, some of which might have played a decisive part. As one Melbourne doctor put it: 'It may be a gamble – but it's the only rational gamble.'

At Camp Cody, New Mexico, on the theory that any immune serum might be better than none, Captain Frederick Lamb and Lieutenant Edward Brannin treated one batch of flu patients not only with diphtheria antitoxin but anti-tetanus and anti-meningitis serums as well. Their verdict: many cases which appeared malignant showed a marked improvement, and often recovered unexpectedly.

Then Dr Timothy Leary, of Boston, Massachusetts, took a hand. He, too, concentrated on patients at the Chelsea Naval Hospital – the same group of men from whom Dr Joseph

Goldberger's 'guinea-pigs', the tarnished heroes of Deer Island Naval Prison, were seeking to contract the infection. Both here and at the nearby Haynes Memorial Hospital, Leary and his co-workers made cultures enough to prepare 50,000 doses of vaccine – some from the pure Pfeiffer bacillus, others from mixed bacteria.

The results were startling. Between them, twenty-three Massachusetts physicians who received the vaccine inoculated 1483 patients. Of these, only twenty-one ever took the disease – and only two contracted pneumonia. But even in the flu-ridden Bay State, neither of these patients died.

Other doctors told a similar story. At the Chelsea Hospital, Lieutenant William Redden, U.S. Navy, treated 151 serious cases with a serum from the blood of convalescent pneumonia patients and successfully pulled through all but six. At Puget Sound Navy Yard, out of 4212 men inoculated, fifty-two later contracted the disease but none of them fatally.

Nor were these results confined to America alone. Across western Canada, 20,000 railway employees who received their shots stayed largely immune. From Newcastle West, Ireland, Dr John Cremin reported only two mild cases among fifty-two inoculated with a Pfeiffer-based serum. The Director-General of Pathology for Britain's War Office, Major-General Sir William Leishman, had even more conclusive evidence. Among 16,000 Tommies inoculated in the Home Command, there had been only two deaths.

The moral was plain: given determined leadership and prophylactic control, the disease, if not eliminated, could still be channelled and minimised.

Overnight, too, came the era of the mask. As far back as 23 October, Calgary, Alberta, as yet untouched by the pandemic, had ordered that all employees in contact with the public – in banks, buffets, candy stores, elevators, and barber shops – must don a medicated mask through working hours, like any hospital attendant. On this same day, 225 miles away in Edmonton, the ukase was extended to all passengers riding a street-car.

It was as vexed a measure as any the pandemic prompted. Medical men were divided, and some, like Britain's Dr Leonard Hill, condemned masks from the first: by raising the temperature and humidity of the air breathed, they struck at the respiratory membrane's natural defences. To thousands of citizens, it was a blow at their personal freedom and they reacted with bitter hostility – 'we look like so many muzzled dogs' one man wrote furiously.

But many communities cooperated from the first. Hooded bus conductors collected fares from masked riders. Australian bank tellers, as heavily disguised as Ned Kelly himself, passed out banknotes to long lines of anonymous eyes. At least 200 volunteers in Wellington, New Zealand, plumped for servicemen's gas-masks; in one Red Cross rally, in Cedar City, Utah, even the Goddess of Liberty was arrayed in a gauze-mask. And all later evidence suggests that when the public obeyed instructions to the letter these medicated gauze or cheese-cloth masks were a potent factor in reducing the deadly risk of droplet infection.

In San Francisco, the most mask-conscious of all American cities, it began, as early as 19 October, with a compulsory order on barbers. Then, three days later, on the advice of Dr Woods Hutchinson, a far-sighted emissary of Surgeon-General Rupert Blue, Mayor James Rolph urged every citizen to purchase a mask without delay.

Citing a slogan that the Italian Supreme Command had printed on every gas-mask – 'Who leaves this mask behind, dies' – Mayor Rolph warned his people that, maskless, San Francisco faced a possible 50,000 cases, with 1500 deaths.

With 15,000 masks snapped up at Red Cross headquarters, the day after his warning, Rolph at first saw no need for compulsion; even the plush Hotel St Francis had turned its entire staff of linen-workers over to mask-making for guests and employees. But by 24 October, with 1407 new cases and 82 deaths, city Health Officer William Hasler thought again. From 29 October on, masks made from four thicknesses of material, five inches wide and seven inches long, became compulsory for all San Franciscans.

Promptly, the *San Francisco Chronicle* ran a front-page photo spread to demonstrate how such prominent citizens as Dr Hassler and Postmaster Charles Fay had 'enhanced their beauty with influenza masks', but some were less enthusiastic. Within thirty-six hours, zealous cops had hauled in 161 'mask slackers', and on Market Street, Henry Miller, an over-zealous Health Department inspector, came near to provoking a shoot-out. When blacksmith James Wiser stubbornly refused to don a mask, Miller attempted to frog-march him to a drug-store – then, when the blacksmith floored him with a bag of silver dollars, drew his revolver, wounding not only Wiser but two luckless bystanders.

Yet San Francisco's lesson was plain. By the first week in November, only nine days after the ordinance came into effect, the epidemic was already petering out – after a tally of 22,700 cases, 1608 deaths. It was a higher death-rate than Mayor Rolph had forecast in his appeal of 19 October – yet the cases he anticipated had been cut by more than half.

It was the same story in Sydney, New South Wales. Some Australian authorities, like the Chairman of Melbourne's Board of Health, Dr Edward Robertson, approved the mask in principle – 'but any measure to make them compulsory could not be enforced'. But New South Wales' Minister of Health, J. D. Fitzgerald, thought otherwise. At four days notice, Sydney's 700,000 citizens learned that, apart from those surfing on Bondi Beach, any among them who thereafter 'did not wear upon his face a mask or covering of gauze' were offending 'against the peace of our sovereign lord, the King, his crown and dignity'.

And again, the city's example proved an object lesson. Within one week of the edict, maskless Melbourne was recording its 2000th case, of whom 100 had died – while Sydney's total cases did not even equal three-quarters of that death roll.

All over the world, these masks were wondrous to behold. Few carried as grim a warning as those worn in Rockford, Illinois, embroidered with a skull-and-crossbones; most struck an aesthetic note. In San Francisco, fashion-writers noted three predominant styles – the Agincourt, with the snout extending like an old-time French helmet, the Ravioli, a square serviceable slab, popular with policemen, and the Yashmak, in vogue with girl clerks. One Sydney solicitor, not to be outdone, won a magistrate's applause for a mask so large it enveloped his entire face; he explained that in his wife's absence he had ripped out a muslin window-blind and run it up on her sewing-machine.

By common consensus, the prize for originality went to the secretary who sported a mask with horizon-blue georgette wings, plus a pink propeller to ensure that the air kept fresh.

For law-breakers the masks were a heaven-sent opportunity. In Kansas City, one masked stranger, advising grocer J. F. Elsworth that everyone should wear a flu-mask, volunteered the information that a freezing temperature also checked influenza. 'Try the ice-box', he invited Elsworth genially, 'and see if it won't cure your cold.' Prodded with the business end of a revolver, the indignant grocer was forced to comply – later to find twenty-five dollars missing from his cash-register.

To one man, at least, the day he first donned an influenza mask remained the most profoundly embarrassing of his life. Scarcely had he boarded a Newtown tram outside Sydney's Anglican Cathedral, than the Reverend Horace Barder, a young hospital chaplain, became aware that a woman passenger with a fourteen-year-old girl was studying his eyes intently. Suddenly, to his astonishment, she craned closer, matching him against a photograph drawn from her handbag. All at once she explained triumphantly: 'You are my husband. I know you by your brown eyes. You left me ten years ago.'

Then, as the young cleric squirmed uneasily, she hailed the conductor: 'As soon as you see a constable, stop the tram. I want to give this man in charge.'

Near Newtown Bridge, to Barder's relief, two constables did board the tram. At once he protested indignantly: 'I have never seen this woman before.' Nonetheless, the constables decided to make sure. Shortly, the whole masked party –

mother, daughter, policemen, and Barder – stood before the Superintendent in Newtown Police Station.

'He's my husband all right,' the woman never stopped affirming. 'They are my Tom's eyes.'

Now Barder asked her patiently: 'When were we married?'

'Fifteen years ago,' the woman replied.

But, Barder expostulated, at that time he had been a fifteen-year-old schoolboy. Crimson with mortification, the young chaplain stripped off his mask. 'Now,' he demanded, 'am I your husband?'

For some minutes, the woman studied him intently, but finally she conceded: 'You have his eyes and chin, but that isn't Tom's nose.' Suddenly, as the Superintendent made to dismiss the charge, the small girl burst into tears. Between sobs she confided: 'Whenever Mother sees a man with brown eyes, she has him arrested. She always thinks he's Father.'

It was left to the Reverend Barder to sum up the bizarre events of this whole morning with a text handpicked from Genesis: 'The voice is Jacob's voice, but the hands are the hands of Esau.'

For Dr Juan Zamora and countless thousands of his colleagues, the uphill road they trod was made harder still by many unfeeling citizens. These were the men and women who for varying motives impede the rescue work in any great disaster.

As always, there were the militants. At Chekiang, China, high-school students, protesting against the death of one of their number, staged an early version of a 'sit-in' and promptly spread the infection fourfold. On 7 November, Swiss Socialists, proclaiming a General Strike 'to end the rule of the bourgeoisie', affirmed 'Flu Avenges the Workers' – an apt slogan, since 1200 of the security troops called in to maintain order went down within a week.

Worse, by far, were the profiteers; in countless cities, prices soared overnight as the quick-money men moved in to corner vital supplies and medicines. Despite all government efforts to intervene, a householder paid ten shillings and sixpence for a thermometer in New Zealand, and fifteen shillings for a chicken in Rio de Janeiro. All over China, overnight, the price of surgical gauze doubled. Jamaicans were charged a shilling for thirty-six grains of quinine, and camphor had soared to $6.50 a pound in Vancouver, British Columbia. South African oranges fetched two shillings and sixpence apiece, and in Bogotá, Colombia, all fruit was so scarce that one blue-blood offered his genealogical tree in exchange for a lemon.

In Catania, Sicily, housewife Maria Mazzaglia, after buying scarce aspirin powder for her family, was suddenly alerted to the danger and flushed it down the toilet. In the nick of time she had seen the tiny glinting granules of powdered glass with which an infamous druggist had adulterated it.

Those whom one irate Louisiana physician termed 'nostrum nuts' were enjoying their finest hour. Their 'cures' ranged through sacred pebbles from a shrine in Kyoshu, Japan, whose 'divine property' prevented anyone who handled them from contracting influenza, and bottled river water, awash with red mud, in Ipoh, Malaya, to surgical vests which sucked the disease from the body in Nyköping, Sweden. Cranks in North Carolina advocated sulphur sprinkled in the shoes, sliced cucumber bound to the ankles and a potato in each pocket. On a South Chicago sidewalk, two charlatans did a land-office business with a colourless liquor labelled 'Spanish Influenza Remedy', abetted by a turbaned snake-charmer complete with flute and cobra.

Some were more dangerous yet. One gang of unscrupulous girls in Calgary, Alberta, posing as graduate nurses, mulcted their unsuspecting victims of $25 a day. Quacks in Kwangju, Korea, drubbed one patient so mercilessly with clubs to expel the evil spirit that he almost expired under the blows. And in Pokkalik, Chinese Turkestan, Lieutenant-Colonel Percy Etherton, on a British diplomatic mission, was astonished to see a man he knew well treating a long line of sufferers at his market stall, referring gravely to a learned tome.

In truth, the man was a groom whom the Colonel had

discharged for inefficiency, and the tome was a thriller by the Victorian best-seller, Guy Boothby, stolen from his library.

Then there were the few whose flagrant selfishness in the midst of disaster robbed many a doctor of breath. In Christchurch, New Zealand, one woman sent a priority message to Chief Medical Officer Herbert Chesson; would he please send a nurse right away, she wanted her ironing done. One man flagged down a doctor's car for what the medic took to be an emergency call – only to find the man had cadged a free lift to his dentist to have a tooth pulled. Another house sent out a call for a nurse and two oranges, yet to the girl who hurried to the scene the man who received the fruit seemed the very picture of health.

How many, the nurse wanted to know, were ill in the family? 'Oh, there's no one ill *yet*,' the man replied, in the instant before slamming the door.

There was no lack of well-wishers, with advice, either – but to the hard-pressed doctors time was now too precious to waste on amateur theorists. On one single day, more than 300 telegrams reached Major Alfred Friedlander, the bone-tired chief of the medical service at Camp Sherman, Chillicothe, Ohio, specifying sure-fire remedies that would stop the pandemic in its tracks. Most were poultices composed of every known ingredient from asparagus to turpentine – but no less than a hundred of them insisted that the fine steel of shotgun barrels, if placed under the beds of stricken soldiers, would 'draw out' the fever.

The Greek Ministry of the Interior was rash enough to solicit 'useful suggestions' from the public – but in most countries people needed no second bidding. From his town house off London's Park Lane, Lord Dunraven advised British doctors to isolate the lethal miasma arising from the battlefields of Flanders due to French shellfire. Others blamed insects; the British 23rd Division, billeted near the Italian silk town of Arzignano, knew without the shadow of a doubt they had caught the infection from silkworms. Even New York's Dr

Gedide Friedman, who should have known better, solemnly invited his colleagues to consider that the entire pandemic had been started by bed-bugs.

More harboured theories involving diet – everything from poisoned fish to a sugar deficiency. In Washington, the badgered Surgeon-General Rupert Blue, flooded out with reports that the bacteria was being spread by chewing-gum and even aspirin, had to waste precious time calling in samples for his experts to analyse. One offbeat theory was held by a Swedish labourer, convinced the pandemic was due to the pork shortage. Having killed and eaten a thirty-pound sucking pig he called on his doctor to announce himself immune from Spanish flu.

Religious interpretations weren't lacking. For Christian Scientists in New York, there was triumphant proof of mind over matter: if the city's Chinese were barely affected, wasn't it because few of them could read the scary newspaper headlines? To Jehovah's Witnesses, it was the vindication of a prophecy: the 'pestilences and sorrows' of which Jesus had spoken upon the Mount of Olives. From a newly-erected tabernacle in Providence, Rhode Island, evangelist Billy Sunday, onetime White Sox ballplayer, announced his intention of 'praying down' the pandemic in a mammoth month-long prayer session – though victims were being carried head-first from the auditorium as he spoke.

Astrologer Albert F. Porta urged Surgeon-General Blue to consider that the true culprit was the planet Jupiter – its effect on the earth's electro-magnetism had developed a strange and lethal micro-organism. But astrologers in Lagos, West Africa, by contrast, noted that for two years the sign of Leo had been occupied by two 'malefics', Saturn and Neptune, whose vibrations were out of tune. Only the entry of Jupiter into Leo in the latter half of 1919 would rid the earth of the baneful influence.

Nor were the weathermen far behind. In countless households where the inhabitants were still on their feet, a solemn tapping of the barometer heralded each new day – followed by a flood of letters to local health officers from writers signing themselves 'Prophylactic', 'Safety First', or 'Forewarned is Forearmed'. Wiseacres in Quebec blamed the cold rainy summer that had been followed by a warm September; in Europe, they blamed the hot dry summer. Even Britain's fresh air fiend, Dr Leonard Hill, blamed the raw east wind; once it veered to the west, the flu would decrease. This was news to Dr Thomas Finlayson Dewar, Health Officer for Edinburgh; the wind had been in the west in all the weeks that saw the highest recorded death rate in the city's history.

In Frankfurt, Germany, pundits were blaming the unseasonably dry air; their Swiss counterparts put the death rate down to the foggy humid weather. Few could come to terms with the fact that the Spanish Lady was oblivious to climate. In Yozgad, Turkey, British prisoners-of-war, survivors of the siege of Kut, were dying of flu even as the water froze in the lunchtime glasses within minutes of being poured. But in Melbourne they died, too – as the thermometer, on sultry airless days, registered 106°F in the shade.

Yet more dangerous to the doctors than any crackpot theorists were those who failed to grasp that the world was facing but one dire alternative: the choice between life and death. At Camp Sherman, where the laundry was army-owned but civilian-operated, Major Friedlander faced an appalling dilemma one November evening. In all the hospital, not one clean sheet or towel or surgical gown was available – yet in fifteen minutes the laundry was closing for the day, with as little concern as on any weekday in peacetime.

Somehow Friedlander must convince these unthinking men and women that a state of emergency as deadly as any the world had ever known existed right here in Chillicothe, Ohio.

At once, hastening to the laundry, he asked for every worker to be assembled in the dining-hall. Then, tears starting to his eyes, he gave them the brutal facts. So far on this day, forty-five soldiers had died. By midnight, twenty-five more deaths could be expected. Meanwhile, new patients were coming in at the rate of fifty an hour, yet there was not one item of clean linen in the entire hospital.

Pleading with the workers to somehow help right this situation, Friedlander wound up his moving appeal: 'Every man at least has a right to die on a bed with clean sheets.'

It was enough. As the magnitude of the disaster came home to them, the men and women were trooping back to their posts, almost before Friedlander finished speaking. Four hours later, the Army had enough linen to save that day – nor did the laundry fail them again from this time on.

Elsewhere in the camp, Major Carey McCord, the Chief of Laboratory Service, faced a similar stumbling-block in the shape of a by-the-book quartermaster. Almost all the camp's supplies had now been exhausted, yet the Lieutenant, after thumbing laboriously through the Quartermaster's Manual, saw no way he could help. There was nothing in the manual to cover the disaster.

McCord tried one last desperate gambit. 'Lieutenant,' he said, 'the best Army officer is the one who knows when the time has come to disobey orders. Those dead men in the morgue, the sick men in the corridors, are the ones who are issuing orders now.'

After a long moment, 'with an almost symbolic gesture', the Lieutenant shied his manual into a far corner of the room. 'All right, Major,' he said thoughtfully, 'I'll take orders from dead men. What do you want?'

McCord sprang his trap. As of now, he estimated, he needed 5000 sheets, 5000 pillow-cases, 2000 blankets, 500 bedpans, 1000 beds with mattresses and pillows, 500 thermometers, 100,000 aspirin tablets and 2000 hospital gowns. 'What's more,' he added, with what he hoped was nonchalance, 'we need them today.'

Pop-eyed with awe, the quartermaster replied: 'Sir, what you want is an impossibility – so I will do it. But all I can supply now is 100,000 aspirin tablets.'

Conscious that he had just committed the U.S. Army to a million dollars' worth of emergency expenses and supplies, McCord ordered: 'Then comb every city within 200 miles. If it's needed run a special train out here. Sign my name yourself for anything that will be good for those sick soldiers – but get those supplies.'

Across the damp green pastures of Tonder County, Denmark, the wind cut like a scythe from the North Sea. Pedalling mechanically, Nurse Else Dahl stared unseeing at the darkened ribbon of road beyond her cycle's handlebars, a salt rain streaking her face like tears. In half an hour it would be midnight. Then she would reach Ejstrup and home.

Never, she thought, had she sunk so thankfully into a warm bed as she would do tonight. Behind her lay the six most appalling hours she had ever experienced in all her years as a nurse.

From the moment that God had sent her a sign, in the shape of that frantic small-hours rapping at her bedroom window, Else Dahl had not rested. Indeed, when word had spread through Ejstrup district that she had once again donned her white gown, the people had allowed her no respite. Day and night she had toiled unremittingly, pedalling from village to village, from farm to farm, no sooner quitting one case than another supplicant hailed her from the roadside: 'Mrs Dahl! Could you please come and look at our little girl?'

In a way, this non-stop schedule had been a blessing in disguise, for the one thing she had secretly feared – an open rift with Marius – had not come to pass. Never had she crawled into bed earlier than midnight, and often it had been 1 a.m. – just five hours before her alarm clock again clattered out its summons. Working for eighteen hours at a stretch away from home, she had barely exchanged a dozen sentences with Marius since the epidemic began. There had been no time to quarrel.

Nor was there time even to read a newspaper, though she saw at a glance the nature of the challenge she had accepted: the death-roll was mounting daily. There was no longer space for individual obituaries – just a long forbidding list of names.

At first, her life had resolved into a routine that rarely varied. Arriving at a farm-house, she would find all the familiar signs: fever, glazed eyes, hands and faces smeared with blood. At once, brisk and methodical, Else set to work. First, a fire must be lit in the kitchen range and water heated. The next step was to wash and change the patients. Since every home had an overstuffed easy chair, Else would manhandle that into the bedroom, contriving to prop the patient up in it, wrapped in blankets, until she had changed the bed.

Just as she had guessed, not a soul had owned a thermometer, and the first question on every lip was: How much fever do I have? She was grateful now for the practical psychology that years of nursing had taught her. If the fever was slight, then tell the patient the exact temperature – this reassurance alone would help them on the road to recovery. But all too often, the mercury registered 105°F, so Else had learned to smile and say, 'Oh, that's not too bad.'

Almost always, even the hardest-hit patients would relax perceptibly at her words. 'Oh, good,' they would say with a contented sigh, 'then I'll get better,' and Else knew that somehow, despite all the odds, they would.

Everyone, of course, was dosed with her special mixture of boiling milk and soda water, but with luck, before she left, she could coax them to take something more substantial – beef broth, perhaps, or a few mouthfuls of boiled chicken. Already, with solid food in their stomachs, feeling clean and fresh, the temperature subsiding, they had passed the danger point.

Else's last chore was to pile all the dirty clothes to soak in a tub, for while neighbours fought shy of paying calls and endangering their own families they were willing enough to do each other's washing in the outhouse and attend to the livestock. It was all part of a cherished if unspoken rural tradition: as one family fell ill, another was recovering, and they steadfastly took turns to help one another out.

Thus the days had passed, busily and contentedly monotonous, until the nightmare of the attic.

It was the man who collected the milkchurns from the farms who had first alerted her. At Madsen's place, he said, there had been no milk out for two days, and the cows were lowing pitifully in their stalls. It might be that the family were ill, but he dared not enter and nor did the neighbours.

Extracting a solemn promise that the man would find a farm-hand for the milking, Else Dahl pedalled up the miry dirt road to Madsen's farm. Apart from the long drawn out bellowing of the cattle, there was a curious brooding silence. Dismounting, Else entered the kitchen, peeled off her water-proof and donned a medicated mask. It was the sole personal precaution to protect herself against infection she had taken all through the epidemic. Then she climbed the stairs to the bedrooms.

At a casual glance, the case was as routine as ever. Farmer Madsen, his wife, and three children, were all sick in bed, but the fact that they had suffered massive nasal haemorrhages suggested the crisis was past. For more than an hour, Else busied herself with doling out pills, washing, bedmaking, heat-ing chicken broth. From the cowshed came a clatter of buckets and by degrees the lowing of the cattle died down, so the dairy-man had been as good as his word.

She was on the point of leaving, promising to look in again that night – always until her patients were on the mend she had sandwiched in two daily visits – when the farmer's wife opened her eyes wearily. 'Nurse Dahl,' she said, 'I've just remembered. There are eight Swedish workmen in the attic and they haven't been down for two days. Don't you think they must be ill?'

Promising to investigate, Else carefully mounted the steep stairs to the attic. She had no premonition.

Then, as the attic door creaked backwards on its hinges, she felt her spine crawl with a nameless horror. The tiny sloping room had been converted into a primitive billet for workers of the Harte Construction Company, and in each of its four corners planks had been nailed together and packed with straw to form large box-beds. Sprawled out in each bed were two desperately sick men, blond brawny Swedes, their faces matted with the stubble of days, their hands caked with blood and excrement.

The whole expanse of the filthy straw-covered floor was

littered with boots, socks and trousers, piled everywhere in wild confusion, sonorous with flies even in winter, and as Else stared unbelieving at this nightmare tableau the sight and smell of blood and vomit turned her almost dizzy with horror.

Then the long years of training asserted themselves, and she accepted with an unflinching sense of duty that only such skills as she possessed could save these eight men from a death too horrible to contemplate.

Clattering hastily downstairs, she grabbed a straight-backed wooden chair and carried it back to the landing. On to this she piled all the fouled and discarded clothing she could find. Next, hastening to the outside wash-house, she re-filled the copper. Ordinary toilet soap would make no impression on that Augean stable, but in the wash-house too, she found coarse brown household soap, whisking it with water and a brush to a creamy lather. Then, armed with soap and a bucket of hot water, she returned to the attic.

Next, with soap and rags, Else scrubbed each filthy prostrate man from head to foot, carrying fresh straw from the stack in the yard to remake their reeking beds. Now she realised that while they had been issued with blankets and pillows they had no sheets, so once more, promising to return swiftly, she mounted her bicycle. Within the hour, she was back, laden with sheets and pillowcases raided from her own linen cupboard.

Soon each man lay clean and comfortable in cool white sheets, barely capable of speech, yet all of them striving to gasp out some words of gratitude.

Temperatures came next. One of the men was dangerously ill, with a temperature of 106°F, so once more Else descended the stairs in search of a telephone. On the line to Dr Thorup in Kolding, she urged him to send the horse-drawn ambulance as soon as possible.

Though Marius was as yet unaware of it, the man would arrive at the hospital wearing one of her husband's clean white shirts, in order to look as presentable as might be. Reluctantly, Else had abandoned the idea of bringing each of them a shirt, feeling that Marius might baulk at donating eight.

Then, following the ritual milk and soda, she steeled herself to scrub her way across every inch of the sodden planking, returning time and again to the yard with armfuls of filthy straw, ascending again with one more bucket of hot water. Darkness had fallen, and the ambulance had collected the sickest of the men, before she again mounted her bicycle.

Now, pedalling through the freezing darkness, six hours after setting foot inside that stinking attic, Else Dahl wondered. With everything that was in her she had responded to the most fearful challenge that had ever come her way – and though she held out few hopes for the man who had gone to Kolding, the others, she believed would pull through. At dawn, in any case, she would start back all over again to see how they had fared through the night.

Yet still, troubled thoughts kept pace beside her in the darkness. The men had lain for days undiscovered, within yards of the Madsen family, close to death, helpless in a squalor that would have been alien to beasts. Only chance had taken Else to the farmhouse that day – and only by chance had the farmer's wife, so sick herself, recalled their existence.

How many other human beings throughout the world were enduring conditions like this? And how many patients in desperate need of care would remain undiscovered until the end?

CHAPTER NINE

'We're Like Sheepmen Mending Fences'
4 November—11 November 1918

The question that Nurse Else Dahl had asked herself on this
November night was all at once on everyone's lips. Until this
moment, too many nations, whatever powers might rule them,
had stood divided: the haves, tolerably secure in their close-
knit world, the have-nots, whose way of life across the tracks
was a closed book to all.

Now, as health visitors, nurses and volunteers were called
to the sick in houses that had never known a doctor, the full
enormity of the situation came home to them. In almost every
one of the world's capitals, there existed slums that were an
affront to mankind – and if these conditions of life were typical,
hopes of checking the pandemic before it engulfed the world
seemed pitifully small.

Wherever one looked, sanitary ignorance was seen to be
appalling. To an on-the-spot observer, the streets of Kingston,
Jamaica, seemed no more than 'one great urinal'. Inspectors
working under Arizona's State Superintendent of Health, Dr
Orville Harry Brown, uncovered conditions that Brown himself was to term 'a menace to human life' – restaurants with
filthy germ-infested ice-boxes, even a drinking pool for cattle
into which passing trains emptied their cuspidors. Nor did
medical men always set a shining example. In Valencia's
Hospital Provincial, where Dr Juan Zamora had done his mili-

tary training, flies swarmed thickly on the surgeon's arms and neck as he worked in the operating theatre. And in one district of Montreal, health workers consigned all the bed linen of defunct flu victims to be disinfected in a local baker's oven.

Throughout Virginia, unbelieving health officers found that only billboard posters on every city block could drive home to people the need to abandon the use of a common drinking cup – or even to use a handkerchief when coughing or sneezing. For shop assistants everywhere, spitting on a finger to separate wrapping paper – and weighing out food and vegetables with unwashed hands – was the unhygienic norm.

Personal hygiene was a closed book to many. Sanitarians surveying Army camps found that soldiers invariably washed their mess-kits in a communal tub of tepid germ-laden water – using their hands as a mop. At Christchurch Hospital, New Zealand, many patients protested furiously against the rule enforcing clean cotton night-clothes as bed-wear. Many had come attired in a thick woollen shirt worn over two singlets, a chest protector and a cholera binder – and were bitterly reluctant to yield up any garment to authority.

No nation was immune from the shameful revelations. In the same moment that M.P.s in Melbourne, Victoria, learned of 10,000 houses in the city that had no sewage connection, shocked health-workers in Wellington, New Zealand, were finding men and women dying on heaps of sacking in shacks with neither crockery nor furniture – though fur coats and smart dresses hung on nails from the wall. In one Wellington plague-spot, which took two men three days to clear of accumulated filth, they found one bedridden veteran lying helpless with only a whip to keep the scurrying rats at bay. It was small wonder that M.P. Peter Fraser (later New Zealand's Second World War premier) himself down with flu following his tireless work among the poor, raged: 'Half Wellington needs to be rebuilt.'

Volunteers in Cape Town were appalled to find twenty families housed in one stable – or five people crammed into a room no more than six feet high, paying exorbitant rents of thirty shillings a month. But whatever the country, the hotbeds of infection were there. Later Premier David Lloyd George was to admit that if sub-standard housing conditions had not impaired their health, a million more men would have been fit enough to enrol in the British Army.

It was hardly surprising that Indian Army recruiting propaganda stressed that a barracks was a safer place to see out the pandemic than any up-country village – and in one State alone, enlistments soared to 23,000 in the space of a month.

Nation after nation was rocked by the facts now emerging. Swedish social workers told of children who, lacking both clothing and shoes, couldn't even attend the funerals of their parents. One Norwegian nurse, Margit Møller, recalled treating a patient in Naerbø who had lain so long neglected on the only bedding he owned, a pile of newspapers, that flu obituaries for weeks past were imprinted on his buttocks.

'The lesson of the pandemic', claimed the Copenhagen daily *Berlingske Tidende*, 'is to fight poverty,' and it was due to the conditions the pandemic had revealed that this fight could now begin in grim earnest.

One of the strangest life-styles the pandemic revealed was witnessed by Dr Fernando Namora, medical officer for Monsanto, Portugal, high in the Gardunha mountain range flanking the Spanish frontier. From the first, the twenty-four-year-old doctor had known it as a region well below the poverty line – where the peasants staved off griping hunger-pains by imbibing litres of water, with mounds of cooked greenstuff on the side. Only thus, their bellies swollen, had they an illusion of well-being.

Long before the pandemic struck, Namora and his co-workers had become aware of a strange gipsy-looking lad hovering near the clinic – often when the children in the schoolhouse adjoining were being served their midday meal. Once he had smashed a classroom window with a stone, though for the most part he kept a wary distance. But Namora noted that his prime target was the garbage-can –

often scooping scraps into an earthenware dish when he thought no one was watching.

Shocked, Namora had tried for weeks to win the boy's confidence. Once they even persuaded him to accept a meal, but he ate grudgingly, without thanks, maintaining only a tight-lipped silence when questions were put. Who was he? Where were his parents? But the boy, stubbornly, would say nothing. When Namora surveyed him a shade too intently, the boy covered his plate with his arms, as alert to defend his food as a wild animal, the hair tumbling over his freckled face.

In despair, Namora briefed the clinic's laundrywoman, the fount of all mountain gossip, to find out the stranger's identity. But the woman, irked, finally admitted defeat. She could find no trace of the boy, or from whence he came. Meanwhile, the garbage-can was nightly deplenished – even though the clinic's entrance gate was locked after hours.

Then, by chance, Namora uncovered the boy's secret. Returning to his office late one summer evening, he spied smoke filtering through the cracks of a wooden hut not far from the main building. Once it had housed the building materials from which the clinic had arisen, but it had long been abandoned – or so Namora thought. Peering through his curtains, he now saw the boy run from the shelter of a stone wall, seize the tether of a goat which was quietly cropping the herbage, and vanish into the hut.

Still, Namora watched. At last, perhaps feeling the coast was clear, the hut door opened and the boy came out, in company with a stooping gypsy woman, a tall man with a sack slung over his shoulder, and the goat. For the first time, the doctor realised the hut had been sheltering an entire family.

Within days, following careful observation, Namora had unravelled the truth. This was one of the ragged families of itinerant tinkers who roamed these mountains, at intervals invading the towns and villages with their trinkets and tinware. All through the daylight hours, the doctor found, they squatted in the lee of a nearby olive-grove, the father moulding tins with his hammer, the boy watching the right moment to pass him tools and tin-plate.

At intervals, from early evening on, a furtive wisp of smoke from the hut showed they were back in residence – but soon after daybreak they would evacuate it once again, removing even the rags and ashes that might give them away. All through 1918, the nomad life had continued – as if this pathetic parody of a home somehow satisfied their needs.

Then the pandemic struck. For days Namora had no time even to think of the strange visitors, for Monsanto's victims were numbered in hundreds and the clinic's work stopped only at nightfall. But one night, looking up from his desk, he started violently with surprise. A freckled face was pressed silently against his laboratory window. As suddenly, it was gone.

Next day, the boy was awaiting the doctor outside the clinic's gate – sullen, embarrassed, feet planted defiantly apart. Speech-less, he bit his lip, until Namora ruffled his tousled hair and lifted his chin. 'What's the matter?' he coaxed him. 'Don't you feel well?'

'My mother's ill,' the boy muttered, but as the doctor, without waiting, made tracks for the hut, he sprang to block his path. 'She isn't *there*,' he confessed, palpably ashamed that their secret was known.

They found her in the olive grove, propped on a bundle of hay, face burning with fever, her husband kneeling beside her. Even as the doctor approached, she tried to struggle upright and run, but the husband held her firmly in his grasp.

Namora knelt to examine her. One more case of influenza with pneumonia complications, and in her exhausted under-nourished state, there could be only one end. At once, with the boy beside him, he hastened back to the clinic for bearers. 'Your mother's ill,' he told him, more sternly than he intended, but the whole situation distressed him. 'You ought not to have kept her outside in the cold in the state she's in.'

Still the boy's face was hard and tense, until Namora placed a hand upon his shoulder. Then, for the first time, he began to cry. Even in her illness, he said, his mother had struggled to the olive grove each day at dawn. In this way, she hoped, no one would discover their hiding-place and drive them from the only home they had known.

All that night, in the clinic's hospital, the woman raved in delirium. As the dawn broke with a steely pink light over the Gardunha Range, she was sinking fast. Arriving at the clinic, Namora found the boy lying on the steps, where he had bivouacked all night, numb and blue with cold. For the first time he felt hatred come close to driving out compassion. Why hadn't the lad gone away, sparing him this painful encounter?

'Is she dying?' the boy asked. He spoke without hesitation, clinically, cruelly.

'She's very ill,' Namora temporised, conscious of cowardice. 'We'll have to wait and see. But with this illness, you just can't leave a warm shelter and go out into the cold ...'

The morning after the woman's death, Namora found the hut burned out. He stood lost in thought as the mountain wind swirled the embers in grey-red shifting circles, and the smells of charred wood and scorched earth were pungent in his nostrils. Of the boy and his father there was no sign.

Why, the doctor wondered, had the boy started that fire? Was he seeking some kind of revenge for his mother's death? Or was he striving to convey to the comfortable and civilised a message of total rejection: that they, as creatures of the wild, didn't need a house for anything?

The thought was born in Namora with pain: not even to die in.

Five hundred feet below them, the cortège wound like a black cumbrous snake. Faintly, on this Sunday morning, the mountain wind bore the sad sweet words of the *Ave Maria* to their vantage-point below the snow-line. But today, eight-year-old Alfredo Martinelli and his friends were less concerned with the strange antics of the adult world. Today they had a funeral all their own.

For weeks now, the little community of Semogo, high in the

Valtellina range that bordered the Swiss frontier, had mourned its dead like any Italian village. But to the children, who had so swiftly come to accept death as a corollary to life, the daily processions held little meaning. To them, once the schoolhouse was converted overnight into an isolation hospital, 'La Spagnola' meant, above all, precious days of unbridled freedom.

Of course, they had been involved like any villagers, like it or not. When Don Angelin, the sacristan, fell ill, they had all weighed in to help toll the bells – solemn notes for an elderly victim, joyous ones for a young – and the old man had rewarded them with dried chestnuts and candied sugar. They had played doctors, with khaki-coloured gauze masks, and when Alfredo's devout Aunt Emilia, whom the family nicknamed 'the prioress', had talked seriously of Paradise, the children had discussed it, huddled among the larches, and created a Paradise of their own. Above all, it was a kingdom where there were no more winter chilblains, and a rap on the knuckles from the schoolmistress, Signorina Bormetti, was unknown.

But now, for the first time, death had touched them in a painfully personal way. Their pet hare had died mysteriously, and all of them had decided that they, too, must commemorate its passing.

It was only three days since they had found it in a thorn bush newly born and abandoned by its mother, and the determination that it should live had occupied all their thoughts until now. They had fed it on a mush of rye bread and milk, and Alfredo's sister, Ines, had made it a nest of rags, but this morning it had been as still and cold as any 'Spagnola' victim. So now it must be laid to rest, with the same ceremony as the procession winding below.

Alfredo, of course, played the priest, because he could mimic to perfection the way Don Albino walked in his cassock, and Ines and four-year-old Irma played the mourning women. Enrico was Don Angelin, carrying the Cross that they had whittled from brushwood, with the stoup of holy water dangling from his belt. Now, as they kept pace with the adults down the mountainside, their own voices took up the words of *Ave Maria*. Three times, Valentin tolled the little goats' bell that he carried, then the rough plank coffin they had fashioned was lowered into the earth.

Solemnly, Alfredo recited: 'Dormi, dormi, in terra bene-detta. Eccoti l'acquansanta; ti bagnò appena nato, ora bagna la tua cassa.' The dry earth rattled on the wood, and suddenly it was over.

All of them felt sad, but satisfied, too: they knew they would see the hare again. Those whom you loved, Aunt Emilia said, were always awaiting you in Paradise.

To the danger threatening all mankind, the people were reacting each in their own way. Some still stubbornly ignored it, hoping it would go away. Some carried on determinedly. Others reacted with anger or fear – or, with a new conviction of the sanctity of life, became aware, as never before, of the quiet power of compassion.

There were small incidents, trivial in themselves, that were remembered long after bigger events were forgotten. On the Portuguese island of St Vincent, Maria Fernanda Rafael, a soldier's wife, always recalled knocking up a chemist in the small hours of one morning to find the man collapsed upon the floor. Painful as this moment had been, she felt better in the knowledge that as he died in her arms she had been there, to moisten his lips with damp cotton wool until the end.

At Camp Dodge, Iowa, medical corpsman Charles Graham devoted hours to a similar exercise – wetting the lips of a man so sick he was debarred even from fluids with the juice of a freshly-squeezed orange. His true reward came later, when the man recovered enough to thank Graham for 'the best orange I ever tasted'.

This capacity to share another's pain was universal. On a farm near Ermelo, in the Transvaal, landowner William Smuts walked quietly ahead of the waggon drawn by eight oxen, bearing his daughter to her last resting-place, for more than a mile, carefully removing every stone he saw on the way. There was no true logic to the gesture – it was just the one way Smuts could think of to smoothe his beloved daughter's last journey.

Not all derived comfort from humans. Dr Arthur Lee Shreffler never forgot one late night call, at a house in the mill district of Joliet, Illinois: an urgent message had reached him that a small boy was alone there, with both his father and mother delirious in hospital. But on entering the house, Shreffler found no puzzled frightened youngster – only a lad fast asleep beside the stove, his arms tightly encircling a dog which had huddled close to comfort him. 'I always knew a boy should have a dog,' Shreffler commented thoughtfully later, 'but I was never so sure of why as I was then.'

Sometimes, as strangers drew closer together, good was born out of evil. To Ole Nilssen, a young garage mechanic, sick and helpless in a tiny bed-sitter in Trondheim, Norway, it seemed at first that life had never been so bleak; at the first signs of his coming down with it, his room-mate had packed his bag and departed, leaving Nilssen to fend for himself. Then, two days later, a woman living on the second floor, whose name he never knew, knocked shyly at his door and offered her help. Even knowing the nature of his sickness she had no fear of death. 'When we die,' she told Nilssen calmly, 'that is God's decision.'

For the entire month that the youngster remained in bed, the woman was scrupulous to visit him three times a day – washing him, changing his bed, feeding him porridge soup with slices of boiled potato. She brought a doctor to see him, and gradually Nilssen grew stronger, but what touched him profoundly was when the woman, by chance, discovered that his eighteenth birthday was on the way. On the appointed day, the wide-eyed mechanic sat up in bed for a tray dinner to beat the band – rare roast beef with all the trimmings, coffee and cake for dessert, with one lighted red candle flickering in a saucer. Afterwards, alone, thinking back to the birthdays of his child-hood, Ole Nilssen cried.

Some pinned all their faith in their ability to carry on

single-handed – like Jack Alexander, a Goodland, Indiana, farmer, who came down with a mild bout. Ordered by the doctor to go to bed and stay there, the brawny farmer replied, shocked: 'But if I did that, I'd die – so I'll just finish husking my corn.' But most found that in times like these, no man or woman stood alone. Vittore Ferretti, a Milan engineering apprentice, was convinced he would live if only he could keep shaving; even in sickness, there were certain standards a man must observe. On the third day, Ferretti was too weak to make it – but somehow, propped up in bed each day with his landlady's help, he scraped and lathered his way to recovery.

In Cuxhaven, Germany, Marie Benöhr, an officer's wife, had a similar conviction; during a bad bout she had consented to take her meals in bed, but as convalescence approached she told her home-help, Dora: 'This breakfast in bed must stop! From now on I get up.' But despite her determination, she was weaker than she knew, and the food, above all, milk, that would have aided her recovery was hard to come by. It was Frau Nachtigal, the dairyman's wife, who proved her friend in need. 'I dare not give you an extra ration,' she confided in Marie Benöhr, 'but no one can stop you coming to visit me every morning. And in my living-room, you'll always find a big glass of milk.'

Perhaps because of the prevailing fear, there had never been such a time for lovers. Though statisticians in some cities – Auckland, San Francisco – noted that marriage licences were falling off, in other cities they actually increased, as if come what might the young in heart were determined to affirm that life must and should go on.

Nothing, it seemed, could deter them. Pretty Edith McLean always swore that it was a newly-arrived photo of her fiancé, David Bishop, in the uniform of a Gordon Highlander, that pulled her through an attack in Aberdeen – and David attached the same curative powers to the photo of Edith which reached him in a military hospital in Rouen, France. Schoolteacher Ethel Hemus, working as a private volunteer nurse in Okotoks, Alberta, was of necessity confined to her patient's house, but even the rigours of a Canadian winter didn't deter her fiancé, Lewis Rhine, from carrying on the courtship – from the roof of the lean-to that sloped right up to Ethel's bedroom window.

And despite all difficulties, the weddings went ahead. In Budapest, Lance-Corporal Ferenc Sterz did get to marry his Maria – even though the ceremony took place in the Augusta Hospital, with the bridegroom, running a temperature of 105°F, borne into the chapel on a stretcher. But for Ludwig Krutmeijer, in Sweden's Bärlinska Hospital, the union was numbered, tragically, in seconds. Barely had he slipped the ring on Ruth Lundh's finger than Krutmeijer closed his eyes and died.

Few went through a stranger wedding ceremony than Lieutenant Al Haase, of the 77th U.S. Infantry, returning to Chicago to claim his bride, Irene Wehling. No sooner had he arrived at the home of the bride's parents, where the wedding was to take place, than a local ordinance required Haase, Miss Wehling, the Reverend Thomas Dornblaser and the guests to formally don flu masks. 'We have to wear gas masks and many peculiar devices in France,' Haase sighed, 'but civil life seems to be getting just as complex.'

One of the year's most faithful courtships was that of Adolf Ruhrmann, a young fitter in the railways workshops at Siegen, Germany. So proud was he of Anna Reuch, his girl friend, that Adolf bore with fortitude the fact that he almost never saw her. One of the world's first women railway workers, Anna had been appointed *Schaffnerin* (Train Conductor) one year earlier, and often her work took her away from home for twenty hours at a stretch – sometimes on 160-mile round trips to Cologne.

Yet for a glimpse of her, in her smart dark-green uniform, with knee breeches, brass buttons and peaked cap embossed with the German eagle, Adolf would wait patiently for hours on the draughty station platform – solely to accompany her on the five minutes' walk back to her parents' home.

'How can you be so heartless – letting him wait so long in

the cold?' Anna's girl friends chided her, but Anna was un-repentant. She and her father, the postman, were the only breadwinners in a family of eleven, and at nineteen, fiercely independent, Anna was proud of earning even more than her father. She wasn't sure if she could take Adolf seriously. The long hours in the job claimed all her attention – and often, in these days of griping shortage, she went through both day and night shifts with no more sustenance than a salad of cold sliced turnips, dressed with salt and vinegar, and a slice of bread.

One night, coming off shift at 2 a.m., Anna Reuch knew that she, too, was coming down with flu. Her face was burning and she couldn't stop coughing; barely had she reached home than she vomited and collapsed. One of her brothers sent word that she couldn't report for work, and when the stationmaster replied that her pay would be honoured, Anna determined that she must get well as soon as possible. Thus word of her illness reached Adolf.

Two nights later, her sister Martha was returning from work when a ghostly figure loomed from the darkness. It was Adolf. Briefly he pressed a small flat box into her hand. 'Zu Anna, mit Ihren Schmerzen.' 'For Anna, in her affliction,' he said. Then, as silently as he had come, he was gone.

When Anna opened the box, all her doubts were swept away: Adolf, she knew, was the man for her. To ease her 'affliction', the dogged young swain had sought high and low until he had procured her a gift infinitely more precious, in November 1918, than flowers or perfume: a box of throat pastilles.

By Saturday, 9 November, the doctors had to admit it: the pandemic had them baffled. To be sure, many had seen near-moribund patients revive miraculously – but no medical man could with certainty say why. As one disgruntled physician confessed: 'We're like sheepmen mending fences in the hope of keeping wolves away.'

Inexplicably, in some cities, the sickness was petering out as mysteriously as it had struck. In New York, by 4 November, with cases decreasing by 2000 a day, Health Commissioner Copeland had announced all trade and travel restrictions abolished as of now. It was on the wane, too, in Stockholm, Copenhagen and Rome – yet reaching an unprecedented peak in Pittsburgh, Edinburgh, Amsterdam and Rio de Janeiro.

And on 5 November, the Army's Chief of Staff, General Peyton March, cabled the worst news yet to General John Pershing in Chaumont: 'Influenza not only stopped all draft calls in October but practically all training.'

Almost daily, reports of miracle cures and medical breakthroughs flooded in to the hard-pressed flu-fighters. A Salamanca physician claimed to have isolated a virus akin to pneumonic plague. The Evangelismos Hospital, Athens, swore that every case treated with mercury perchloride injections recovered. But with the restricted communications of wartime, such claims were impossible to check. More indicative of the primitive treatment many physicians still favoured was Melbourne Hospital's offer to eager schoolboys: five shillings for every hundred black leeches they could deliver, to bleed the patients back to health.

Since Dr Charles Nicolle and Dr Charles Lebailly had made that historic discovery in the Pasteur Institute, Tunis, bacteriologists everywhere had marked time. At no 2 Stationary Hospital, Abbeville, France, a three-man team – Britain's Major Howard Graeme-Gibson, Canada's Major Frank Bowman and Australia's Dr Ivan Connor – had successfully duplicated the Frenchmen's experiment – but what now? An invisible virus was known to be at work – but with the electronic microscope undeveloped until 1936, no man was any closer to the heart of the mystery.

What puzzled the doctors sorely was the strange immunity that some exhibited. It was logical that those infected in the mild spring-summer wave should go scot-free now, like salamanders purged by fire. But everywhere in the world, it seemed, gas-works employees were invulnerable – as were workers in cordite and poison-gas factories and Cornish tin-miners. British soldiers – though not their German counterparts – stayed clear of it on the Western Front, yet on other fighting fronts were appallingly at risk: almost 10,000 cases in the Italian theatre, more than 2000 in Palestine. No wounded man ever contracted it at Oxford's Southern Base Hospital – and though the staff were dropping as if sandbagged in almost every German sanatorium, consumptive patients were unscathed.

In Florence, Colorado, the immunity of thirteen-year-old Harry Andrews surprised nobody save himself. With school closed down, the lad was earning spending money on the side trapping skunks.

Yet other groups were marked out with the selectivity of a draft board. Parisiennes were harder hit than their menfolk, for the city had three flu hospitals operating for women alone. In Vienna, tram conductors were more at risk than any other occupational category – just like Australian bank clerks. Among twelve million policy-holders with the Metropolitan Life Insurance Company, it was whites, not blacks, the young, not the old, who suffered most.

Nor did money buy an easy way out. One U.S. statistician, Edgar Sydenstricker, did affirm: 'The lower the economic level, the higher is the attack rate' – but in London at least the rich enjoyed no such protection. For the first time in public health records, the death rate was as high in prosperous Chelsea and Westminster as in the slums of Bermondsey and Bethnal Green.

Yet why should the sickness affect so many organs of the body normally untouched? 'No part of the body is exempt,' recorded the appalled Dr Charles Sundell, of Britain's Medical Research Council, for often the disease more closely resembled encephalitis, with the patient lapsing into a coma, for three weeks. *Otitis media*, with the middle ear cavity choked with pus, was another common complication – as was paralysis of the eye-muscle.

From London's Dr Bernard Spilsbury came reports not only of dilatation of the heart but even of fatty degeneration; his colleague, Dr F. Parkes Weber, noted one heart weighing thirteen ounces as against the normal nine. At Aldershot's Connaught Hospital, Major Adolphe Abrahams recorded a cough so intense that it ruptured the muscles of a soldier's rectum. From Delhi to Dundee, retention of urine, due to muscular atony (flaccidity) was commonplace, but more and more were now exhibiting the puffy faces and swollen ankles of acute nephritis – passing only ten ounces of smoky blood-streaked urine a day as against the normal three pints.

Inevitably, the lungs were the organs most vitally affected. Time and again, Major T. R. Little, of the Canadian Army Medical Corps, found patchy areas of consolidation varying in size 'between a chestnut and a hen's egg'; a victim might cough up as much as two pints of yellow-green pus per day. Through his stethoscope, one Welsh country doctor, Dr David Richards, could hear many lungs emit a sound 'like a bank note being crisped in a pocket', and autopsy surgeons were encountering what one doctor termed 'a pathological nightmare'; lungs up to six times their normal weight, looking 'like melted red currant jelly'.

Few faced a spectacle as grim as twenty-year-old Keith Fairley, a final year student overnight appointed Acting Medical Superintendent of a Melbourne emergency hospital: a patient's face so contorted in death that even close friends couldn't recognise him. Only a dentist's positive identification would still their doubts.

Some surgeons, in desperation, now fell back on resection; often pneumonia was degenerating into empyema (pus in the chest cavity around the lungs), and by making a two-inch incision and removing a section of rib, the surgeon could pass in a tube and drain the pus away. For Mathilde Borchert, a twenty-eight-year-old housewife in Göttingen, Germany, it was an operation she would not easily forget. All told, she and three other like cases lay four months in hospital after surgery, at first blowing feebly on children's trumpets to press out the fluid from the pleura – until other patients complained so bitterly of the noise the doctor substituted milk bottles.

Sometimes the patients were wary. Drowsy from sedation,

but still in possession of his faculties, the long-distance swimmer Shier Mendelson spoke up determinedly from the operating table in Toronto's Western Hospital. How long, he asked Dr Abraham Willinsky, was this operation going to take?

Willinsky was reluctant to commit himself. A complicated resection might take an hour and a half: a straightforward one only twenty-five minutes. His expression both pleased and speculative, Mendelson glanced at the wall-clock. 'Would you say,' he bargained, 'that a dollar a minute makes a fair fee?'

A moment, then the surgeon agreed. With all his attention centred on the clock, Mendelson, he sensed, wouldn't even be conscious of discomfort. And soon after, when Mendelson announced triumphantly, 'Fifteen minutes all told!' Willinsky hadn't the heart to go back on the bargain – or to inform his cost-conscious patient that the standard fee for this operation was even then $150.

For one American doctor, there wasn't the remotest sign of a breakthrough. Galling as it was to admit, Dr Joseph Goldberger, of the U.S. Public Health Service, had to confess to nothing less than total failure.

When Surgeon General Blue's emissary had appealed to the prisoners of Deer Island's Naval Prison for volunteers to join the influenza battle-line, he had been truly heartened by that mass-response. Yet as a doctor Goldberger had hoped for something more positive even than a demonstration of spontaneous courage. He wanted results.

Now, in his spartan office on Gallop's Island Quarantine Station, Boston Harbour, Goldberger glanced dejectedly at the reports before him. The 100 volunteers he had selected had first snuffed a pure culture of bacillus into their nostrils – and no one took sick. Next they had been injected with a brew made up of thirteen different strains of the Pfeiffer bacillus. Result: negative.

Their throats had been doctored with the mucous secretions of men already sick – and every man remained defiantly healthy. Seemingly they even thrived on being injected with the blood of ailing men. Finally, in the most deadly experiment of all, they had permitted hospital patients far gone with the sickness to cough in their faces.

For seven days thereafter, Goldberger and his team had watched them closely, but every man, even in the hope of contracting the disease in the service of mankind, remained fit and cheerful.

Were none of them susceptible? Were all of them immune? When the experiments began, Goldberger had at least been sure of how the disease was transmitted from person to person. Now he knew one thing only: he wasn't even sure of that.

Dr Andrew Garvie surveyed the patient in wonder. But there was no doubt about it. This gnarled old soldier, in the Yorkshire milltown of Halifax, was in better shape than the doctor himself – grinning all over his face as he shaved at the kitchen sink, hugely enjoying the doctor's astonishment. Yet three days back Garvie had found him huddled by the fire in the worst physical shape possible, running a temperature of 103°F. But when the doctor prescribed bed, the man shook his head. 'Aw mak nowt o' bed,' he replied stubbornly, 'Aw'll cure mesen.'

Now, for the record, the old man let Garvie in on the secret of his inexplicable recovery. Far from going to bed, he had gone, instead, for a five-mile walk – but next day, though feeling 'stiffish', he was no better. Plainly, drastic remedies were called for, so this time, after trudging for eight miles, he had wound up in a pub and downed fourteen gins in a row.

'Aw kept a' callin',' he summed it up, 'and they kept a' bringin'.'

As Dr Garvie had to confess, it was no lone example. All over the world, some few favoured by fortune were defying not only all medical prognoses but the worst the pandemic could do – and, against all the odds, surviving.

Sometimes sheer excitement seems to have turned the scales. In her parents' Milan apartment, typist Maria Wittgens had lost all heart for life, when suddenly her brothers burst into her sick-room: the Austrian-held cities of Trento and Trieste had fallen to the Italians. At once, before her mother realised what she was doing, Maria, a fanatic nationalist, had slipped from bed, dressed, and was running joyously through drenching rain across the city, shouting, 'We have taken Trento and Trieste,' to every passer-by she saw. Next morning, fever abated, cough gone, she returned to the office.

Anger, too, was a potent cathartic. Hans Valdemar Thousing, an egocentric pharmacist, took to his bed in Maribo, Denmark, and summoned the doctor, but after twenty-four hours the man arrived to find Thousing better. All night he had so sweated with rage at this lack of prompt attention that the fever had quite dispersed. And in the Yugoslav village of Sadici, headman Emin Sadimly was so incensed when thirteen invalids in his care refused to eat the food he had prepared for them – a spicy ragout of smoked sausage, sauerkraut and red peppers – that his ire proved unwittingly therapeutic. As he laid about him with a bamboo rod all of them fell to eating as if their lives depended on it – and next morning, to their undying astonishment, found they had turned the corner.

Some were luckier than they knew. When Louis Bouvier, an eighteen-year-old novice, hastened home from the seminary at Rennes to care for his mother, his brother and his father, the cobbler, he found things in the Breton village of Marcillé worse than he had thought possible. At once plump little Dr Raskol had broken it to him: his father could not last the night. 'Even so,' he added, 'go to the chemist and get this prescription made up.'

What alarmed Bouvier was that no sooner had his father taken his first doses of the medicine than raging delirium set in – 'a veritable witch's sabbath'. Rampaging through the house like a sailor on the town, the cobbler stripped away all his bedding, invaded his distraught son's room and took over the lad's bed instead. In the morning, Dr Raskol arrived to find Louis dozing uneasily by the fire. 'Is he dead?' the doctor asked. 'No,' said Louis, mystified. 'He's sleeping.'

And the cobbler slept all that day – waking only on occasion to forcibly demand more medicine; so much did he relish it that when Louis' grandmother brought him instead a cup of the milk that was his staple drink he struck it indignantly from her hand. Thus, for ten days, the uneasy farce continued.

Only then, with his father on the road to recovery, did Louis and Dr Raskol, putting their heads together, unravel the simple secret of the cobbler's cure. The medicine, Raskol confessed, did have a calvados (applejack) base – but this in itself could hardly have produced such results. It was the hard-pressed pharmacist who had brought this about; misreading the doctor's prescription he had labelled the bottle not 'One spoonful every three hours', but 'Three spoonfuls every hour'. For ten days, Bouvier senior, virtually a teetotaller, had, with his son's involuntary aid, been on a jag that would have done credit to a Viking.

At Hampstead Hospital, North London, one dog-tired nurse as innocently wrought a miracle as great. So moribund was her patient that the man had turned a livid shade of purple, unable to swallow or even breathe properly; to supply him with essential oxygen, Major William Byam, who headed the unit, had inserted two huge hollow needles in his chest, into the loose tissue lying between the skin and the muscles of the chest wall. To these were attached long rubber tubes leading to an oxygen cylinder.

Unknown to Byam, the night nurse spent the afternoon having a tooth pulled. Arriving on duty, still tired and drowsy with the dentist's gas, she checked the cylinder was full, sat down beside the bed – and fell asleep.

Hours later, she awoke in horror to find her patient unrecognisable. Now the man seemed like nothing so much as a fully-inflated balloon – his whole body so tight with oxygen that even the pressure of a finger could not prise open the swollen eyelids. All unknowing, the nurse had slumped forward on to the valve controlling the oxygen flow, turning it to full.

To Byam, arriving hastily on the scene, the man's whole skin crackled beneath his hands 'like pressing on a lemon sponge pudding'. By now, the vast cylinder was quite empty of gas, all of which had been forced under the skin at pressure, much of it into the bloodstream. Yet from this moment the man began to turn the corner; he left the hospital fully recovered.

For Professor J. B. Haldane, the famous physiologist, this was additional proof of a theory he had long nourished : almost every case of Spanish influenza could have been saved if enough oxygen had been forced into the circulation. But thus far, Haldane confessed to Byam, he had found no one, either doctor or patient, bold enough to put this theory to the test.

Given a malady so lethal, did the mind truly possess sufficient power to heal the human body? At least one doctor, Captain Philip Gosse, of the Royal Army Medical Corps, thought it might. At King George's Military Hospital, Poona, India, Gosse had one morning stopped by the bedside of a mortally sick soldier. From the case-sheet, he saw that this was a private in a Somersetshire Territorial Regiment, in civil life a porter on the Great Western Railway. Now, stricken with double pneumonia, his life was numbered in hours.

Bending close, Gosse asked the man where he lived. In Stogumber, the man whispered back, with his mother. For Gosse, all at once, the years fell away, and he recalled how, as a boy, on summer holidays, travelling between Taunton and Dunster, he had marvelled at the broad Somerset accent of a porter who used to call out the list of stations on this very line.

In the faintest of hopes that it might revive the dying man, Gosse, assuming as authentic a Somerset accent as he could, recited that litany now : 'Norton Fitzwarren, Bishops Lydeard, Crowcombe, Stogumber, Stogursey, Williton, Watchet, Washford, Blue Anchor, Dunster, Minehead.'

Now an astonishing thing happened. At the name 'Stogursey', the dying man, with a supreme effort, contrived to raise his head from his pillow. His whisper was quite distinct and contemptuous : 'Stogursey b'aint got no station.' Then he fell back exhausted – but already, Gosse fancied, some of the dull leaden pallor had left his face.

A few hours later, the ward sister hurried up to Gosse. Would he mind calling over those stations again? It seemed to have done the patient good. Nothing loth, Gosse once more intoned that list of names – careful this time to omit Stogursey, too negligible to rate a railway station. Now the soldier smiled.

For several days yet, the man's fate hung in the balance, but each day, by degrees, his hold on life grew stronger. Not, Gosse thought, due to any medical skill of his, or drugs, or even nursing, but because of those familiar names from a lifetime ago which the Captain, night and morning now, was solemnly reciting beside his bed: 'Norton Fitzwarren, Bishops Lydeard, Crowcombe, Stogumber, Williton ...'

Outside Company K's Orderly Room, in the French village of Culey, Private John Lewis Barkley grappled with the problem. Pacing the glistening cobblestones of the street, his friend 'Jesse' James beside him, he couldn't seem to take it in. For both men, if they felt so inclined, their fighting war was over.

Within hours of reporting back to his outfit after the worst bout of sickness he had ever known, Barkley had been sent for by the company commander. There, in the Captain's ante-room, he had been re-united with Jesse, who had received an identical summons. Astonished, they heard the Captain announce that both of them, for their dash and initiative during the drive on Cunel, had been selected for officers' training school. Their decision must be reached that day.

To Barkley, now, the proposal seemed strangely remote from reality. From the moment he had fallen sick in the farmer's barn nearby, he had lived as strange a chapter of events as any that had befallen him – one that had brought the lone Missourian a stage further towards his fellow-men.

Days back, it was the taste of rum on his palate, warm, oily and somehow comforting, that had once again brought him fully awake. Blinking, he strove to orient to his surroundings: a low-ceilinged room in what seemed to be a farmhouse, flooded with wan November sunlight. Beside the vast feather-bed in which he lay, a sturdy good-looking peasant girl, holding a steaming jug of hot toddy, was smiling down at him. All at once, Barkley remembered. It was this girl, aided by one of his buddies, who had carried him from the barn.

Then, seeing recognition dawn in his eyes, the girl had called to someone out of sight. By degrees, as timidly as if it was a stranger's house they were entering, the whole family tiptoed in to view this emaciated young American who had so abruptly entered their lives: the mother, in a widow's rusty black, a feeble old man, her brother, and the girl's two small children.

Weak as he was, Barkley was concerned. Unless someone had thought to report his collapse, the company might have posted him AWOL. How long, he asked anxiously, had he been here? Smiling uncertainly, the family exchanged baffled glances. Now he realised their English was as non-existent as his French, but all at once the old man had a brainwave. Hastening from the room, he returned with a French–English dictionary. Though it wasn't easy, Barkley worked it out finally. He had been here, unconscious and in delirium, for two whole days.

Now memories of that sacred pact returned to him. 'Nigger' Floyd had gone down the line, but there was still Jesse to rely on him. For the first time he realised he was enveloped in a cotton nightshirt six sizes too large for him. 'Where are my clothes?' he asked – then, seeing the puzzled stares, he hauled himself upright in bed, pantomiming the action of putting on a coat and buttoning it. 'Clothes,' he kept repeating urgently.

'Ah, clothes!' Madame replied, delighted to have broken through the language barrier. *'Non, non!'* The last thing Barkley recalled was her pushing his head firmly on to the pillow. Within seconds he was asleep again.

It was night when he woke once more. But now, to his acute embarrassment, he found the women had pulled aside sheet and blankets, stripped off his nightshirt, and were bathing him as lovingly as if he was a baby. Scarlet with shame, Barkley seized a sheet, striving to cover his nakedness. As calmly as if he was a troublesome infant, the women tossed it aside, continuing to sponge and soap him. Again he grabbed the sheet – and again they defeated him. Finally, he gave up. In any case, he realised, he was so weak the girl alone could have handled him with ease.

Then, too, despite his previous determination to stick out the fighting with his buddies and spurn all medical attention, he had to acknowledge that this aspect of war was pleasant indeed.

Ever since arriving in France, Barkley had grown to like the French more and more; there had been Jeanne, the little peasant girl at Bricon, who had taken him home to meet her parents and made him superb salads and omelettes. To the doughboy it seemed wonderful that she never once found his stuttering funny; only later did he realise she thought it was all part of the strange language known as English.

Now, as these kindly Samaritans cared for him as one of their own, he warmed to them even more. The bath over, they gave him an alcohol rub. They washed his head, anointing it with some kind of ointment, then sprinkled it with white powder. Then they changed his nightshirt for a suit of pyjamas.

It took much thumbing through the pocket dictionary, but Madame finally managed to explain that the pyjamas belonged to one of her sons, who had been killed during the war, but now Fate had sent her another son instead. Barkley was too moved then to find words to thank her.

Then, wrapping him in a blanket, they had lifted him as easily as if he was their child, carrying him to a big armchair by the fire. They placed his feet in a crock of hot water, and something else that smelled like whisky. Finally, piece by piece, they fed him the breast meat of a chicken.

'Capon!' the widow said, and when Barkley looked askance, the woman made the motion of lifting something very heavy, then blew out her chest and thumped it. Everyone laughed, and Barkley, though he only half-understood the joke, was so happy that he laughed too.

Supper over, Sergeant Mike De Angelo, of Barkley's unit,

who knew a little French, joined them, and with the aid of the old man's dictionary they managed somehow to sustain a conversation. All the time the women were adding more hot water to the earthenware crock, and every so often they fed him another hot toddy. At nine o'clock, when they put him to bed, Barkley not only felt that he owned the world but something more important by far. He loved it, too.

After this, the days had passed as in a dream. For the first time in years, Barkley felt part of a family, at one with mankind. The women fed him on omelettes and broths and salads, and doctored his head and feet. And when, finally, he insisted on getting up and dressing, he didn't even recognise the clothes they brought him. His uniform had been so carefully washed and darned and patched and pressed that General Pershing's batman couldn't have done better. His shoes had quite fallen apart, so the old man pressed on him a pair of slippers.

It had been hard to explain that duty called him to the front, so Barkley at first mimicked an infantryman slow-marching, and then blew *tat-tat-tat-tat*, as if he had a bugle. '*Oui,*' they said then, '*oui, oui*' and all three had hugged him as if he was their beloved son and the children had cried.

Now, for both him and Jesse, had come this sudden bombshell of the officers' training school and it called for a swift decision. A unanimous decision, too, because whatever happened they were going to stick together.

But somehow, try as he might, Barkley couldn't reconcile himself to the idea. A man who had single-handed stalled a German advance, survived the embrace of the Spanish Lady, and known the selfless love of an anonymous French family would somehow at such a time seem out of place behind the lines.

Abruptly, he summed up what both of them felt: 'Hell, let's pass it up. One more good fight is all we're likely to see before the war is over.'

Faster and faster, the white horse covered the ground, streaking like a thoroughbred through the cork woods. Fleetingly,

Dr Juan Zamora knew fear; so headlong was their pace that any one of the overhanging branches now swooping close seemed likely to dislodge him. Beside him, his new found friend, Captain Pascual Cervera, shot him a troubled glance. With every yard of their breakneck ride, the roar of the cannon came nearer.

Days earlier, arriving in the city of Algeciras following his decision at the Ministry of the Interior, Zamora had reported officially to General Villalba, Military Governor of the Gibraltar region, and Dr Blanco, the Chief Medical Officer. Both men, after welcoming him warmly and fixing him quarters at the Hotel Sanchez, had seconded to him Captain Cervera, a young naval officer, to act as guide and escort through the unfamiliar terrain.

Then, towards 11 a.m., on this sunlit November morning, as the two were attending a health conference at a rural town hall, the sound of cannon fire had rumbled like a summer storm. At once, Cervera had started to his feet. Only recently, the batteries of Gibraltar had fired upon a German submarine in the Bay of Algeciras, and some shells, falling short, had landed in the city, close to where Cervera's wife and children were living. Now the Captain begged to be excused – and Zamora had decided to join him.

Mounting their horses, the two men had begun this frantic race to the nearest half-way house where they could obtain up-to-date information: the hunting lodge of Cervera's friend, the Duke of Medina Celi. In what seemed like minutes, they were clear of the woods and clattering across the cobbled courtyard. Hastening through the main door, Cervera begged leave to use the telephone, then gave an Algeciras number.

At once, hearing his wife's voice up the line, he enquired anxiously after her safety. Satisfied, he nodded – then Zamora, watching, saw his jaw drop incredulously. He swung round to the doctor. Tears in his eyes, he stammered out: 'Those were victory guns we heard. They have signed the Armistice!'

CHAPTER TEN

'Nothing but Kisses since Breakfast'
11 November—30 November 1918

The world had waited for this moment. For four years, three months and five days, it had been the greatest of all imponderables: an unknown date to be circled in red on a calendar as yet unprinted. Now, on this drizzling November Monday – at the eleventh hour on the eleventh day of the eleventh month – it came. For one brief but foreseeably fatal moment, the people relaxed their vigilance: caveats, all prohibitions concerning public gatherings, the do's and don'ts of hygiene, were cast aside. In one wonderful and joyous explosion of emotion the world went mad.

For three days, at topmost level, it had been a foregone conclusion. At 9 a.m. on Friday, 8 November, five emissaries of the German Armistice Commission had trudged disconsolately in their rusty black suits up the tracks of a railway siding near Rethondes, deep in the rain-lashed Forest of Compiègne. Around a long bare saloon table, in a train drawn up alongside their own, the Allied delegation awaited them. Thin and stern in horizon-blue, Maréchal Ferdinand Foch, Commander-in-Chief of the Allied Armies in France, rapped out to the interpreter beside him: 'What has brought these gentlemen here?'

It was a rhetorical question. All over Germany, the words of Woodrow Wilson had sown revolution like dragon seed. In the great naval base at Kiel, the sailors had mutinied and taken the city, marching under red flags. There were red flags, too, sprouting like minefields, in Hamburg and Bremen, Stuttgart, Cologne and Munich, as regiment after regiment mutinied and workers and soldier councils took over. On 8 November, still shakily convalescent from flu and despairing of ever inducing Kaiser Wilhelm to abdicate, Prince Max of Baden had brought the war to an end by prematurely announcing that abdication from the balcony of Berlin's Chancellery.

Two days later, when the Kaiser had fled across the Dutch frontier to seek sanctuary in Holland, the new German Chancellor, Social Democrat Friedrich Ebert, cabled the anxious emissaries at Rethondes: 'You are authorised to sign the Armistice ...'

But in the wild delirium that seized the world, such high-level consultations were ignored. Laughing, weeping, dishevelled, often tumbling straight from a sick bed, the people spilled into the streets, incoherent with emotion. On Paris's Rue Royale, an overwhelmed doughboy, beset by a throng of laughing *midinettes*, urgently begged off: 'What I want is food! I've had nothing but kisses since breakfast.'

In many cities there was initial disbelief. In London, the people were alarmed: for the first time in six months, the maroons that betokened an air-raid warning boomed up from police and fire-brigade stations all over the city. Then, as the first newspaper contents bill seen in years loomed outside Westminster Bridge Underground Station – 'FIGHTING HAS CEASED ON ALL FRONTS' – and Big Ben, after four years of silence, told noon, London, too, went wild.

At first it seemed that many had become armoured in endurance; almost with obstinacy the people resisted the invitation to rejoice. At Rossall School, near Fleetwood, on England's north-west coast, a sick-bay of flu-stricken boys received in glum silence the matron's news that the war was over. But later that day, when she returned to announce, 'Boys, I regret to tell you your headmaster has been stricken by the prevailing epidemic,' they cheered until the rafters rang.

It was no morning for late sleepers. The iron music of the

nineteen-ton *La Savoyarde,* largest of all the bells of Sacré-Coeur, early brought Parisians scrambling from their beds. On Toronto's Yonge Street, sirens brayed for twenty-four hours non-stop, and normally sedate adults beat frantically against iron telegraph poles with crowbars. In New Orleans, every vessel in port responded to the injunction of Dock Board Superintendent Hayden Wren, 'Blow whistles – peace is declared,' and at this same moment the locomotives in the freight yards cut loose with their whistles, too. On Canal Street, motorists, not to be outdone, jammed down their gong-buttons; soon the lilt of calliopes and 'rebel yells' were adding to the indescribable tumult. On a Victory Parade float, one slogan took thought of an old familiar: 'Spanish Flu – Germans Flying.'

At Red Cross Evacuation Hospital no. 8, near Verdun, France, one American Army nurse, awakened by the most tremendous barrage she had ever heard, remarked wryly: 'That sounds like peace.'

Some gave thanks more soberly. Outside London's Mansion House, a vast crowd, as if impelled by an unseen force, broke spontaneously into the *Doxology,* accompanied by a Salvation Army band, and everywhere people wept unashamedly. On the hospital ship *Aeolus,* two days out from St Nazaire, a thousand men and women – coal-grimed stokers, white-clad Red Cross workers, hobbling men with wound chevrons on their sleeves – raised their voices as one in 'Praise God from Whom all Blessings Flow'.

Everywhere there was wild ebullience; as millions saw the dawn of a new age, customs and conventions melted away. In London's Chancery Lane, a portly bobby on point-duty partnered one cheering typist after another in a whirlwind polka – poker-faced from first to last. From the wings of the Folies Bergère, to the pounding applause of the crowd, came a pirouetting line of chorines, unfurling first the Tricolour, then the Stars and Stripes and the Union Jack. It was no day to stand on ceremony. In the faded ornate lobby of Shepherd's Hotel, Cairo, a remonstrating manager was bundled up in a carpet and parked in a quiet corner, prior to a pitched battle with pillows and pot plants between Britons and Australians.

Only the sight of a lone doctor, bag in hand, shouldering through the press, reminded people in a score of cities that not all could relax their vigilance.

Hourly, the frenzy redoubled. Outside Buckingham Palace, an uproarious mob of Canadians milled among the potatoes replacing the geraniums of peacetime at the foot of the Victoria Memorial, saluting the beaming King George V with a song that hymned the Kaiser's downfall:

> Rah-rah-rah!
> Rah-rah-rah!
> This-is-the-end-of-Bill-Kaisah!

Even those with least to rejoice were still rejoicing. No man who witnessed it ever forgot the spectacle of a red London omnibus threading its way down Regent Street in pelting rain, its top packed with wounded soldiers in hospital blue, chorusing 'Tipperary', beating time on the sides of the bus with the artificial legs they had detached.

Some were in defiant mood. Outside the Brasserie de la Haute Marne, near General Pershing's Chaumont headquarters, most gave a discreetly wide berth to the stocky little American corporal alternatively brandishing a bottle of brandy and a fist at every officer he saw.

For others, the Kaiser was the scapegoat. At Tientsin, China, his metal statue, known to all as 'Tin Willy', was dragged from the former German Concession and hauled in triumph through the streets. On the Kennebec River at Gardiner, Maine, his life-size effigy was thrust atop a monster bonfire by one too-eager citizen who was dragged clear of the blaze by his coat-tails.

There was disillusion, too. For most Russians, the Armistice was only a name for what had happened in the west; there was hunger and terror and the Spanish Lady in Moscow, the White Army of Denikin in the South, the White Army of

Kolchak and Japanese and American troops in Siberia. In Berlin, it was the Red Flag that flew free above the Kaiser's former palace, and the Iron Crosses of embittered officers littered the streets like horseshoes.

A few had very private emotions. In Hesdin, France, Major-General Sir Wilmot Herringham, Consulting Physician to the British Forces Overseas, thanked God simply: 'I shall never see a wounded man again.' For Private Alan Tucker, of Britain's Army Service Corps, it was a moment too complex for words. Following the funeral cortège of a favourite girl cousin whom the flu had claimed through the streets of Bristol he felt only grief. But all at once Tucker knew a guilty lightness of heart, for Union Jacks were fluttering from every bedroom window, and people were dancing in the side-streets.

The news came late to some. It was 9 p.m. in Culey, France, when the village suddenly erupted into wild commotion. As if possessed, old men and women were running from their houses, shouting, '*Vive la France! Vive l'Amérique!*' 'Seems like everyone in town has gone nuts,' John Lewis Barkley told 'Jesse' James.

It didn't even convey anything when a running doughboy yelled out that the Armistice was signed. Not for the first time, Barkley was conscious that he'd spent more hours up Scalybark Creek than ever he had in school. 'What's an Armistice?' asked the boy from Holden, Missouri.

At Carlstrom Field, Arcadia, Florida, his last port of call before demobilisation, Lieutenant Charles Clapp couldn't determine whether he was suffering yet another bout of flu or a Grade A Armistice hangover. But at least, following a barrage of letters, cables and roses, Margaret had agreed to marry him, the present peak of his ambition. Between drinks, Clapp even felt a certain sense of letdown. He was nineteen years old, engaged to a girl he hardly knew, and fully trained as a pursuit pilot. But now there was no longer an enemy to pursue.

In the camp hospital at Bramshott, England, Lieutenant Arthur Lapointe had mixed feelings. In some ways, he felt cheated; he was now too ill with rheumatism to thrill to the blare of bands, the throb of drums, to join in the triumph he felt was his to share. At least, he thought bleakly, it means an end to the butchery – and above all, a speedy return to St Léandre for the family still hadn't written.

For Tersilla Vicenzotto, rattling slowly south-west from Padua on yet another jampacked troop train, there was no sense of rejoicing – only an ineradicable bitterness that San Antonio had rejected her appeal and brought a precious chapter of her life to a close. For insane minutes, she had even felt an impulse to leap from the high bridge spanning the River Po as the train moved south from Bologna. Then she stifled it: from now on, her life lay in Pisa, where Antonietta, four, Angelica, two, and Dora, one, awaited her.

These were exceptions. For millions throughout the free world, the happy screams of the crowds went on all through that day and far into the night – as Eugenie Leonard recalled it in Denver, Colorado, 'with masks and discretion thrown to the wind'. On countless thousand streets, the Spanish Lady moved unseen among throngs such as telephonist Ida Reilly saw on Auckland's Queen Street: 'one mass of laughing, crying, coughing, spluttering, so desperately-ill people'.

At a cost of ten million dead, the war was over, but for doctors, nurses and volunteers everywhere, another greater battle was now beginning.

In the panelled committee room of the Royal Society of Medicine, at 1 Wimpole Street, London, Sir Arthur Newsholme had done what many a top official uncertain of his ground had done before him. He had called a conference to justify his inaction.

On Thursday, 14 November, for the second night in succession, seventeen prominent medical men had told of their varied experiences in combating the pandemic to date. General William Thayer, of the U.S. Army Medical Corps, marvelled all over again at the suddenness of the onset. Sir Bertrand (later Lord) Dawson had yielded the floor to Dr Bernard Spilsbury,

Britain's foremost pathologist. Dr Leonard Hill had stressed the virtues of fresh air – as forcefully as Dr Edward Turner had stressed those of aspirin.

But all these views were secondary to the tenor of Newsholme's prolonged apologia to his peers: there was nothing useful to be done, and thus he had done nothing.

For the first time he confessed his crucial decision, taken as far back as July, that the Local Government Board would issue no warning either to local authorities or war-plants. No one, he maintained, could have predicted an autumn outbreak with certainty – and even had it been possible, the war effort took priority.

'Some lives might have been saved,' he conceded, 'spread of infection diminished, and suffering avoided if the known sick could have been isolated from the healthy. But it was necessary to carry on.'

From down the conference table, epidemiologist Maurice Greenwood put in the first disclaimer. Such an outbreak, he said, should have been regarded as likely to recur – and as medical adviser to the Ministry of Munitions he had long expected it. The managers of the Ministry's hostels for munitions workers had early been alerted to remove all suspect cases to hospital without delay.

Sir Arthur was unconvinced. 'I know of no public health measures,' he affirmed, 'which can resist the progress of pandemic influenza.'

Some murmured their dissent. Only that week the powerful *British Medical Journal* had taken Sir Arthur roundly to task for his long-standing inertia. 'To instruct local authorities at this late date to take precautions,' scoffed their editorial, 'is putting the cart before the horse.' But Sir Arthur was unrepentant. Further than this vague and unspecific counsel, even though peace had been declared, he would not go. Ignoring the energetic measures of Dr Woods Hutchinson in San Francisco, Minister of Health J. D. Fitzgerald in Sydney, and Commissioner Copeland in New York, he asked the committee: 'Are we prepared to pay the heavy price in personal restrictions which prevention will necessarily imply?'

Now another point arose. Large quantities of mixed vaccine, the *Journal* stated, were being prepared for the Army and the Navy – 'but we have yet to learn that the Local Government Board is taking the same course'. Perhaps Sir Arthur could enlighten those present? Newsholme could. 'The utility of prophlylactic vaccine,' he said blandly, 'remains to be demonstrated.'

At once, delegate after delegate gave him the lie. Vaccine treatment, claimed Dr Harold Whittingham, of the Royal Air Force Central Hospital, had already banished the symptoms from 150 cadets whom he had treated. At Fulham Military Hospital, chimed in Dr William Carnegie Dickson, 500 cases had been inoculated and only two had even felt unwell. And at Greenwich Royal Hospital School, as Surgeon-Captain Percy Bassett-Smith, R.N., pointed out, 1000 boys inoculated had remained immune – though the riverside suburb was a hotbed of flu.

A pause, then the Royal Society's President, Sir Humphrey Rolleston, later Physician-in-Ordinary to King George V, summed up what all of them felt. 'My own feeling,' said the mild-mannered Sir Humphrey, 'is that the protective inoculation may be of use, particularly in young people, in preventing the severe complications to which the mortality is due.'

For Sir Arthur Newsholme, this courteous yet damning statement was the final indictment of four months total dereliction of duty. For 228,000 Britons, it was now only an academic medical foot-note, a bitter and belated epitaph for the many who need never have died.

Her eyes blinded by tears of joy that coursed slowly down her cheeks, Mrs Josephine Pritchard celebrated Armistice Day, 1918, in as restricted a fashion as any woman alive. Prostrate with flu in the bedroom of her parents' house in Bloemfontein, South Africa, the victory music she heard was the voice of her husband, Reginald, with their two children, Tony and Betty, raised in a joyous chorus of 'God Save the King' from the

garden outside. To thank them for that concert, she adopted
the means that the Pritchards, with four of their number down,
often used nowadays – tucked a message in the collar of Sixpence, the family's curly black mongrel, who trotted from
sick bed to sick bed.

As 11 November drew to a close, millions of families were
in this same plight – and more were destined to be. For doctors
everywhere, this was the bitterest irony: the climax of the war
to end all wars, in bringing the people closer together, had
ushered in the greatest medical holocaust in history.

Wherever the rejoicing had been greatest, the mortality
graphs were now like skyscrapers, towering above all else.
Within nine days, Hamilton, Ontario, had reported 350 new
cases. In flu-free Cockermouth, Cumberland, in England's
north-west, one crowded church service of thanksgiving was
enough to infect almost every household in town – and this
week, too, saw Britain's deaths soar to more than 19,000. Over
17,000 doughboys died in France – and one American state
alone, Louisiana, reported 350,000 cases.

Now, as never before, entire households were stricken. All
nineteen members of one family came down in Budapest. Engineer Henrique Pieper and his five-strong brood, helpless in
their Rio de Janeiro apartment, communicated like prisoners
on Death Row on the night before an execution – rapping on
the adjoining walls to check each other's wellbeing. And Dr
William Peters, Health Officer for Cincinnati, Ohio, recalled
that the General Hospital alone cared for 151 families – of
which every member had been sick.

In fact, they were lucky. Few, by mid-November, could
expect such specialist care; daily, doctors and health workers
saw the measure of the crisis. Trudging the fog-shrouded streets
of Stepney, East London, Dr Harry Roberts jingled like a lock-
smith; always his pockets were stuffed with the latch-keys of
houses where everyone was laid up. Typical was the sign on a
door in Hailsham, Sussex, England: 'Walk In – Don't Knock
– All In Bed.' Volunteer Elsie Cleland, checking houses in
Hopewell, Virginia, obediently answered one shrill-voiced

summons to come in – then realised with horror that the family parrot was the only living thing left in the house.

In Washington, D.C., Health Commissioner Louis Brownlow had a call from a distraught woman explaining that she shared a room with three other girls. Two were dead, one was dying, she alone was well. Alone and nursing his sick wife, Brownlow called the police. Within a few hours, a laconic Sergeant phoned back his report: 'Four girls dead.'

All over, the cries for help took on unique forms. Victims as far apart as Sydney and Brisbane used reversible fourteen-inch square cards: one side signalling 'S.O.S.', the other, 'FOOD'. In Asunción, Paraguay, it was a white flag fluttering from a window; a red flag in Kimberley, on the Rand, and makeshift flags included neck-ties, hot-water bottle covers, even a pair of red bathing-drawers. But often involuntary distress signals were as effective. In Bethlehem, Pennsylvania, milkmen finding yesterday's delivery still on the doorstep had orders to break down the door.

For country dwellers, it was a nightmare problem. South of the Crocodile River, the Bushveld was as still as a petrified forest; only the once-daily cry of 'Are you still alive?' echoing weakly from farm to farm, broke the absolute silence. Those who lived beyond hailing distance found only drastic measures saved them. In New Zealand's Taranaki dairy country, one bachelor farmer drew attention to his plight by driving off his entire herd of cattle; neighbours interpreted the message and he recovered. At Getan, deep in the forests of Sweden, another farmer conceived the idea of a distress beacon, setting fire to his piled winter kindling. Help arrived just in time to stop him being cremated alive.

Cut off in their isolated worlds, each family did its desperate best. Almost everywhere, it was the mothers who bore the brunt. A few, like Effie Burton of Taranaki, New Zealand, fell back on practical training; a one-time nurse at Guy's Hospital, London, she drew up a hand-written health programme which embraced twice-daily gargling with Condy's Fluid, screened verandahs to serve as isolation wards for her sick, and the spraying of all drains with kerosene. But more, like Mary Downman, in Comet, Queensland, had only maternal instinct to guide them. When a doctor warned it would be fatal for little Esther to kick aside the bed-clothes until her temperature dropped, Mrs Downman lay along-side the child for two days and nights to keep them firmly secured.

Some, aware that isolation spelt only death, embarked on a heroine's journey. To reach the hospital at Chapleau, Ontario, one Indian squaw, whose brave had died, paddled her canoe with her two surviving papooses, thirty-three miles down the Kapuskasing River. Although sick herself, she told Hospital Superintendent Dr J. J. Sheahan, she had portaged the canoe over six miles of rugged terrain, so intent was she on seeking the white man's medicine.

Sick or no, they were determined to keep going. In Durban, South Africa, Johanna Nienaber, though desperately ill, crawled to the kitchen on her hands and knees to brew soup for her stricken family – then crawled painfully from bed to bed to feed it to them by the spoonful. Always it was the family who came first. When the local midwife for Springfield, Colorado, Ma Perkins came down with it, she carried bedding, food and water to the storm cellar and isolated herself like a pariah – refusing to allow her children near until she was out of danger.

Without benefit of doctors or medicaments, most fell back on home remedies – recipes prized as infallible standbys, handed down from generation to generation. Few survivors but cannot recall their mother's insistence on salt water snuffed up the nose, the teas concocted of violet leaves, elder blossom or peppermint – or their abiding faith in goose grease poultices or a bag of asafoetida, a resinous, garlic-scented gum, hung round the neck. Hundreds like Margaret Cragg, of Gerald, Saskatchewan, swore by a shovelful of hot coals sprinkled with sulphur or brown sugar, which enveloped every room in a noxious blue-green smoke. When George, her husband, asked if it could possibly help, Mrs Cragg, with the air of a woman pressed beyond all endurance, replied: 'I don't know – but you've got to do *something*!'

Not many favoured an inhalant so toxic as the preferred nostrum of housewives in Kampala, Uganda: a steaming bowl of eucalyptus and whale-oil.

Many, with more logic, pinned their faith in onions and garlic, since esteemed by many doctors as a powerful antibiotic. In Charleroi, Pennsylvania, Rose Pardiny, a grocer's wife, served up onion omelettes, onion salads and onion soup with every meal, and not one of her eight-strong family came down. At the Chambers' family farm in East London, Cape Province, even the three terriers, Jacob, Midge and Jetty, solemnly lined up for their daily tablespoon of garlic tea. Few settings were a likelier flu-trap than Signora Maria Casa Nova's boarding-house for miners in Diamondville, Wyoming, yet every boarder escaped scot-free. When puzzled health authorities called to enquire her secret, the beaming landlady led them to her store-room piled with 100-lb. sacks of the garlic she had fed her guests three times a day.

The same specific saved the life of four-year-old Ruby Driscoll in Portland, Oregon. Though the child was unlikely to survive the night, Minnie, her mother, not only dosed her with onion syrup but buried her from head to foot for three days in a glistening bed of raw sliced onions. The doctors had despaired of her life, but Ruby recovered.

Try as they might, the strain, for many mothers, proved too great. Almost without warning, the father faced a crisis: his household was a fortress he alone must defend. Some showed more rough-and-ready zest than expertise. To the horror of his family in Edenton, North Carolina, farmer Jack Jordan had only one yard-stick to test the temperature of soup: dipping his elbow in the cauldron, even when fresh from his morning chore of tending the chickens and hogs. Coppersmith Henry Loida, in Fornfelt, Missouri, ran the whole gamut of domestic misfortune – from seasoning the chicken broth with ginger instead of pepper to bleaching his wife's favourite checkered dress a sickly shade of oatmeal. Shipyard worker Alexander

Riddle, in Sunderland, on the Wear, elected to give his invalids a treat of home-made bread, then, incorporating a whole pound of yeast to a stone of flour, blew the oven-door off its hinges.

Few started so low down the ladder of knowledge as Cape Town's Ernest Wassung, who tiptoed to his wife's sick bed to solve a major domestic mystery: 'How do you make a pot of tea?'

More learned the hard way – every skill from infant care to plain home-cooking. Even doctors learned facts never taught in medical school. In famine-ridden Kiev, where 700,000 were down with flu, Dr Herbert Swann, a twenty-four-year-old Englishman attached to the Red Cross Hospital, had all the medical knowledge necessary to treat his Russian wife, Naguimé – but to act as her night nurse through staff shortage was something outside his experience. Nor had the curriculum at St Mary's Hospital, London, taught him to barter his under-pants in return for scarce milk.

At Cavaillon, France, Railwayman Régis Chareyre's care for his nineteen-year-old daughter, Marie, cost his own life. Daily, pallid with fatigue, he made the incisions and applied the suction-cups, and these, with the nasal haemorrhages she suf-fered, pulled her through. But when Chareyre in turn fell ill, the stationmaster, his staff depleted, sternly refused him sick-leave. His last words to Marie were: 'If only I could have bled like you.'

And other fathers, despite inexperience, achieved therapeutic miracles. One Wisconsin stonemason, Charles Heiser, not only nursed his wife, Serena, and three children but single-handed weaned their six-week-old baby, Elsie. Banker John Clark Naylor, in Clifton Hill, Missouri, converted both living-room and dining-room into 'wards' for his invalids, time schedules and packages of medicine pinned as precisely as a monthly statement to window drapes nearest the beds. Schoolteacher Edwin Whitcher made it all seem a game for his three children near Knysna, Cape Province; each evening, enjoying a glorious romp under a living-room tent mocked-up from blankets, they were barely conscious of inhaling steam from a bowl of menthol solution. Antique dealer Frederick Seacombe, in Deptford, South London, unable to lay hands on one hot-water bottle, literally baked the flu from his wife and daughters by clapping hot enamel dinner plates to their chests and backs.

'We've come through the Zeppelin raids,' Seacombe announced indignantly, 'I'm not going to lose my family now.'

Retail grocer Philip Ruehl, in Milwaukee, Wisconsin, felt the same determination – though the shock-therapy he gave his eighteen-year-old son, Ray, was drastic indeed. When the lad became so weak he could stomach no food for two weeks, Ruehl senior propped him up in bed and sent a man-sized slug of whisky jolting down his throat – inducing a convulsion so violent Ray spun from the bed, hurtled across the room and hit the wall unconscious. Yet within minutes, he was drenched in icy sweat, his fever miraculously broken.

It was hard for the children, too. Some were too small even to comprehend the disaster; they cried for the world they had known. In Newmarket, England, four-year-old Pat Russell wept uncontrollably; the sight of her mother's crisp white blouses dyed a funeral black seemed sadder than the loss of an uncle she had barely known. It was the same for five-year-old Veronica Schroeder in North St Louis, Missouri. Every other day, the little old ladies living next door had given her five cents to fetch a loaf of Bond Bread; now the grey crepe bow above their door knocker told her the worst. Something of her youth had gone for ever.

At times they felt bitter resentment. In Kiev, Nelly Ptaschkina, a fourteen-year-old schoolgirl, appalled by the mounting death rate among her friends, confided in her diary: 'It is particularly sad when it is the young who die. The old people have had their time; but these are only on the threshold of life.'

Yet many, of necessity, came of age overnight. One ten-year-old Texan girl cared for her mother, father and four brothers and sisters – though she needed the help of an orange crate to reach the sink when she did the dishes. In Morgantown, West Virginia, Josephine Ferrara speaks for a whole generation for whom the pandemic was a forcing house: 'We were never children but adults.'

Hundreds were the sole mainstay of their families. Nine-year-old Betty Alexander and her brother Alec, aged ten, took over and ran the family farm on Bruny Island, Tasmania. In Coutts, Alberta, Emma Theodorovich, eleven, cared for a family of six, secretly relieved that one pot of chicken soup lasted them two days. 'As weak as a rat', his bowels constantly failing him, eight-year-old Larimore Cooper still learned to poach eggs, make toast, wash dishes and scour chamber-pots when his parents fell sick in Sparta, Tennessee.

When his newsagent father died in Pentonville, North London, ten-year-old Bertram Copping was all of a sudden the man of the house – arranging every detail of the funeral, joining every food queue he saw, fiercely proud to get potatoes at a bargain price, totting up each day's takings for his mother and filling in order forms after a long day at the local grammar school.

Some laboured as hard for others. For more than two weeks, eleven-year-old Pieter Retief daily walked a mile and a half to the hospital in Lichtenburg, Transvaal, balancing on his head an earthenware crock of home-made bread his mother had baked for the patients. To set it down and pause for a rest would have been fatal; the crock was so heavy he couldn't lift it. And at one Mowbray, Cape Town, soup kitchen, Supervisor Winifred Currey, challenging a latter-day Oliver Twist, who had queued for soup too often, uncovered the sober truth. For nine stricken people in two households, this hard-pressed ten-year-old represented their only hold on life.

Yet for every family sustained by one valiant member, ten went unaided until too late, as statistics now made plain. By Sunday, 17 November, appalled health authorities for the first time, totted up the pandemic's colossal cost to date. Within twelve weeks, six million had died.

Soon there would be no way to bury the dead.

All that night, to the east of Paris, the hearses rumbled by on the Avenue Jean Jaurès, their heavy iron wheels shaking the bridge that led to the Pantin Cemetery. From his vantage point on the embankment, railway worker Pierre Fournier watched the endless defile, the horses silhouetted like black centaurs against the sky, and held his breath. It was, he thought, like that other age of mortality Paris had known, when the day-long rattle of the tumbrils symbolised the rule of Madame Guillotine.

Now the contrast was in the secrecy. No longer were the dead paraded in broad daylight to make a Parisian holiday. To avoid alarm and despair among the population, they were buried by night.

Though Fournier could not know it, these anonymous Parisians at least had the privilege of burial with due ceremony. Day by day, throughout the world, the orderly process of death and interment was breaking down. The death rate was sur-passing any country's capacity to keep pace.

In some cities, like Montreal, the Army, to the end, staged ceremonial funerals, with full military panoply : gun carriages, drums bound in black cotton, a guard of honour with fourteen men. But most victims made their last journey more humbly – on bread-carts, wheelbarrows, bullock carts, even garbage-trucks. Not every cortège reached the graveside without in-cident. On one Barcelona street, the driver, smitten with Spanish flu, toppled from the hearse as if struck by lightning, dead before he even touched the ground – and in the ensuing panic others, too, fell dead. It was a lone policeman tethering a rope to the horse's neck, who led the hearse to the cemetery.

Everywhere, try as they might, the men in charge found the organisation breaking down. In Philadelphia, after 528 had died in one day, the Reverend Dr Joseph Corrigan, director of Catholic charities, took a convoy of six horse-drawn waggons and one truck on a twenty-four-hour search of the abandoned dead, combing back streets and alleys, forcing door after door. Yet the net result was 200 bodies piled in a morgue built for thirty-six – in conditions so primeval even veteran embalmers refused to work there.

Many lay unburied for five days on end in the country villages outside Athens; even in Pittsburgh coffins were stacked, a week at a time, for more than a city block. Farmers in Norway's far north, where the earth froze as hard as a barn door, resorted as always to a macabre stratagem: their dead were strung in the trees like scarecrows until the spring thaw. And in Rio de Janeiro, one householder, pleading with the fire brigade men to remove his dead brother, found them adamant – there was no room on the death-cart.

When the man pleaded the corpse was five days old, the fireman offered only one solution. They would take his brother – and leave a stranger who had died more recently.

On every hand, the shortages were pitiful – of wood, above all. Those who were fortunate buried their dead in plain unvarnished boxes – often fashioned from doors, floorboards, and in Japan, from old saké barrels. Even in timber-rich Sweden, a dearth of nails decreed many went without coffins; in scores of countries the dead were interred in cardboard boxes, sheets, blankets, or paper shrouds, piled in mass graves. Nothing spotlit the grim economics of death more clearly than the appeal of Montreal's Ormiston Roy, Director of Port Royal Cemetery: would relatives in this time of crisis please refrain from using outside casings? The reason was simple: an outside shell meant an extra three tons of earth, and five men to lower the coffin instead of two.

It was the same all over the world. On the tiny island of Mauritius, in the Indian Ocean, one coffin changed hands on the black market three times before even finding an occupant. Undertakers in Cuxhaven, Germany, would loan coffins, but not sell them; following its journey to the churchyard, for appearance's sake, the coffin was returned, to be used again. One man, scouring Bogotá, Colombia, for a casket, finally ran one to earth in a funeral parlour – but the assistant, regretfully, shook his head. It was reserved for the undertaker, who had died that morning.

As scarce as wood was manpower itself – the men to dig the graves, the clergy to conduct the funerals. One Warwickshire village carpenter not only made forty coffins but conducted every service himself. To dig a grave might take eight hours, and ten-year-old Lenorah Ashley, in Huddersfield, Yorkshire, always held fast to one memory: taking the nightly dinner-pail to her policeman father who helped out in village church-yards for miles around. At Maitland Cemetery, six miles out of Cape Town, it was the mourning relatives who dug the graves; often others sought to take over their plots by force, and there were savage battles with spades and mattocks across the piled earth.

American soldiers, British Tommies and park-keepers, Austrian prisoners-of-war, all were called in to help, and even Brazilian convicts – who, despite working at night under powerful arc lights, didn't scruple to first prise loose a victim's gold teeth.

Even burial space was at a premium, as property-owner Charles Swancott, in Sydney, New South Wales, discovered to his chagrin. At the height of the pandemic, the public-spirited Swancott recalled that years earlier an uncle had purchased some plots in Rookwood Cemetery, none of which had ever been used. Promptly, seeking out a local undertaker, he offered every plot free of charge to help lighten his burden.

Forty-eight hours later, the disgruntled undertaker reported back: the plots were no longer Swancott's to offer. Rival under-takers had, without scruple, annexed them weeks ago for clients of their own.

Outside the house, Dr Juan Zamora paused. The November night was sharp, yet he was sweating. In truth, he thought, this diabolical sickness had a chameleon quality, able to assume any one of a dozen different guises. In the most hair's-breadth case he had yet attended, he had barely managed to save the patient from a death too fearful to contemplate.

Within days of his arrival at Algeciras, Dr Blanco had despatched Zamora to take sole charge in Facinas, a small vil-lage close to Europe's most southerly town, the tuna-fishing port of Tarifa. With a mounted escort of border police, who guided him from house to house, Zamora set to work.

At the outset, he had been troubled in divergent ways by two of the first cases he had attended. One was the wife of the village medico, Dr Poyato, who was himself laid up. But Señora Poyato had been far more gravely ill, and she had known it. 'Please, Doctor,' she begged, as Zamora made ready his hypodermic, 'don't give me an injection. It's useless. Don't you see the Holy Virgin is coming for me?'

She had been pointing at the bedroom ceiling, in the absolute certainty of her vision, as Zamora slid the needle into her arm. Deeply disturbed, he had felt that her apparition possessed more power than any medical skill of his, for she was dead within hours.

Days later, he had been called to a thin nervous well-to-do woman who insisted she was dying. At first glance, her extreme cold, the chattering teeth spelt nothing but the flu that had stricken her family, but Zamora's thermometer told another story. Her temperature was normal. Sheer terror had brought about a panic state in which her body could simulate every symptom but the one that counted.

Always inimical to hypochondriacs, the practical strong-willed Zamora had but two prescriptions: a bromide syrup to calm her nerves, a forthright injunction to get on her feet and nurse those who needed her help.

Over late dinner at a nearby *posada*, Zamora was mulling over these widely-differing cases when a messenger arrived. A young man he had attended that morning for pneumonia had died. Would he please issue a death certificate at once?

Automatically, Zamora fumbled for his pen – then something stopped him short. It was the sixth day of the patient's illness – and somehow he had not expected the crisis until the following day. In these chaotic weeks, the young Spaniard knew, many exhausted doctors were signing death certificates as readily as prescriptions – often to lessen the family's grief by enabling the body to be removed at once. Now a strange intuition warned him: see the patient first.

Minutes later, he reached the house. It was small wonder the family suspected the worst: the man had reached the stage which doctors call 'apparent death'. He was as cold as a stone. There was no pulse, no respiration. Yet to Zamora the sodden nightshirt was evidence that not long ago he had been sweating freely in the throes of a 103°F fever. What the doctor now suspected was that hypothermia – a rapid lowering of the body temperature – had brought about a cardiac stoppage.

Calmly and surely, Zamora went to work. First a brisk friction massage, concentrating on the region of the breast-bone. Then injections of caffeine and adrenalin – both intravenous and intramuscular. Calling for mustard poultices, hot coffee and cognac, he next applied artificial respiration, using the Schafer method – kneeling astride the patient and compressing the lower chest rhythmically fifteen times a minute. Now, as a servant arrived with the stimulants, Zamora applied poultices, piled the man with blankets, then dribbled alternate doses of scalding coffee and fiery spirit between the livid lips. A shot of glucose serum followed.

Within ten minutes of this high-pressure treatment, Zamora noted the first faint, almost imperceptible flutter of the eyelids. Expert fingers detected the uncertain rhythm of a pulse returning to life.

Now, on the front doorstep of the house, Zamora had halted. Inhaling the salt air wafted on the night from Tarifa, he gave silent thanks to God. No doubting now that the man would recover. But only Zamora's faint and niggling uncertainty, in the moment of reaching for his pen, had saved him from burial alive.

Almost everyone had heard the stories. Some dismissed them as pure fiction. Others gave credence to the rumours that 'hundreds' were buried alive each week, which was certainly an exaggeration. Yet most doctors recognised that this state of 'apparent death' was a disconcertingly common feature of the sickness. Nor could it be denied that hundreds were buried weekly, if not alive then at least without any death certificate. In this fantastic mass-production of burial, there were just too few doctors to attest the deaths.

There were many narrow escapes. Neapolitan Giovanni Campanella awoke with the feeling that the world was closing in on him, as indeed it was; as he came upright to thrust aside the lid of his partially-screwed-down coffin in the local Campo Santo, the mourners took to their heels. One sick native chief in an African kraal even closed his eyes and feigned death – anxious to see how grievously his wives would lament their dear departed. Before he realised it, he had dozed off – waking to fight his indignant way from the crudely-carpentered box.

Never had vigilance been so necessary. It was a watchful undertaker, carrying three-year-old Robert Coulter to a waiting hearse in Wellington, New Zealand, who saved the boy's life. Robert's certificate of death was already secured in his pocket – yet as he glanced compassionately down at the mite's discoloured face, the undertaker, in the nick of time, heard the faintest of sighs.

On Milner Road, Woodstock, a suburb of Cape Town, office worker Kate Le Roux saw a sight she was never to forget: from a double-storeyed apartment house owned by her friends, the Jones family, a waggon loaded with coffins had just pulled away. As she watched, the truck jolted over a pot-hole and with the sudden impact the topmost coffin tilted drunkenly to the left. Next instant it toppled and fell, smashing to matchwood on the pavement below.

To Kate's horror, the corpse cried out like a man awaking from a nightmare, then scrambled shakily to his hands and knees. Hastening forward, Kate and some bystanders helped him to his feet. It was one of the Jones's lodgers, Mr Irving, who lived on to tell of his nightmare escape for another fifty years.

There were other, grimmer endings. When a doctor pronounced Clara Garduno dead in Las Vegas, New Mexico, the Health Department insisted she must be buried as soon as possible. Despite high fever, Frank, her husband, staggered from bed to help – and to beg a favour of the undertaker. Two of their three children were so sick they would die before the day was out. If the grave was left uncovered, their coffins could be placed with their mother's.

It was Helen, the baby, who died first, and once again Frank Garduno made an unsteady pilgrimage to the cemetery. On impulse, he asked for his wife's coffin to be opened to take one last look. Nor could he ever blot out the sight that met his eyes: Clara now lying face downwards, her long dark braids twisted between her fingers, in silent testimony of the agony she had undergone.

It wasn't always accidental. On a Kenilworth, Cape Town, side street, Driver Richard Brown, at the wheel of a Council death cart, heard a sudden frantic drumming above the engine roar. For a moment, he and his mate looked at one another bemused. Both men, though far from incapable, were moderately drunk. To keep them from quitting, the Council allowed as much free brandy as they could drink a day.

Now, stalling the truck, Brown and his mate walked thoughtfully round to the rear. There were many crude black-painted boxes stacked one on top of the other. The shouting, they could tell, was coming from a box halfway down the pile: a man they had crated themselves. He had seemed very dead when they found him in the tenement, twenty minutes back, but of course there had been no doctor to consult with.

The two men looked at one another. He was the worst man in all that neighbourhood – a loafer, a drunkard, a wife-beater, a man for whom no one in their coloured community had anything but deep contempt. 'I reckon,' said Brown slowly, 'ain't no one going to miss him.'

His mate nodded solemn agreement. They climbed back into the truck. It ground away down McKinley Road, the long trailing cries fading into silence as it went.

At 4.40 p.m., Dr Nathaniel M'Connell was almost certain of success. It had been the longest tensest week he had ever lived through, but it was almost over. Soon, with the Reverend John Gailey at the graveside, Mary Jane Reid would be buried in the churchyard of the little Presbyterian Church at Ballysillan. With her would die the secret M'Connell had striven so tenaciously to preserve.

True, the last thing M'Connell had anticipated was a post-mortem and an inquest. The girl's mother must have confided her suspicions to others. But again M'Connell had been one move ahead, though the question of ethics might cause some raised eyebrows at a Medical Council. Indeed Professor William St Clair Symmers, of Queen's University, had seemed taken aback, arriving at Belfast's City Morgue to conduct the post-mortem, to find M'Connell already there.

It was more usual, he told M'Connell curtly, for a doctor in his position to have two medical representatives present. They could make observations, but not, of course, touch the body. For the doctor concerned to attend the post-mortem was un-orthodox. M'Connell was disarming: in such a time of stress he hadn't found any practitioners who could spare the time.

'On the Sunday morning,' he volunteered, 'the girl was, in my opinion, dying from influenza and acute gastritis. I had curetted her for a haemorrhage the previous Friday.'

Professor Symmers had kept silent. There was no indication as he later told the Coroner, that the girl had ever had in-fluenza. He found no trace of cyanosis or lung complications of any kind. Gastritis, too, seemed out of the question. Death, as he saw it, was due to peritonitis, caused by a recent perfora-tion with a blunt instrument – certainly not more than two days before death. But to M'Connell he said nothing of this.

Now Dr M'Connell was anxiously awaiting the results of the inquest. It was to begin at 4 p.m. this very day. Almost certainly, he thought, the Coroner would support the con-clusions of a medical man with twenty years' practice in Belfast.

A knock at the surgery door interrupted his train of thought. It was dispenser David Thompson, announcing District-Inspector Ross. The Inspector came directly to the point: 'Nathaniel Osborne M'Connell, I arrest you for the wilful murder of Mary Jane Reid....'

At 4.50 p.m., Dr M'Connell knew he had lost.

In vain, Lieutenant Hector MacQuarrie strove to ignore the

shouting. It jarred against his ears, on this overcast morning of Wednesday, 27 November, at the onset of Tahiti's rainy season, as painfully as a fist against a cheekbone. But it was fruitless. 'She's as heavy as lead, Mac,' the voice came gratingly. 'A good woman, but my God, she's heavy!'

They stood grouped in a circle on the little square outside the French Protestant Church. Already, the clergyman had read the service, and slowly, with immense effort, the coffin was being carried to the hearse. Glancing upwards, Mac-Quarrie, for the first time, took in the driver's identity. It was Vava, the deaf and dumb servant from the Hotel Tiare, who, in the words of one Tahitian, had worshipped 'Lovaina' Chapman 'as mother and God'. This morning his broad sullen face was crumpled with grief. Lovaina was dead – first victim of the sickness that the jungle telegraph, the 'coconut radio', called the *hotahota*.

Even now, MacQuarrie could not comprehend it. To him, as to many others, Lovaina had been the soul of Tahiti: friend alike to princes and poets, pearling skippers and beachcombers. The day she died, it was as if a cloud had passed across the sunlit reef.

'D'you hear, Mac?' the voice was once more assailing his ears. 'She's as heavy as lead.'

It was Henry, Lovaina's nephew, one of the four pall-bearers who was hailing him so persistently. He had, MacQuarrie saw, tried to stifle his grief with sugar-cane rum, and it was easy to forgive him. This morning, the small group of men and women who had gathered to say goodbye to Lovaina were weeping openly. All Papeete would have attended this service, had not half the town been down with sickness.

Now, slowly, the procession wound up the steep hill towards the cemetery – silent save for Henry's persistent shouts of 'My God, she was heavy.' At one moment, as if to bear him witness, a trace in the harness snapped and the hearse teetered perilously, but MacQuarrie and the others lent the support of their shoulders and by degrees, as Vava mastered the plunging horses, they reached the graveside.

Already, resolutely ignoring the nephew's drunken im-
portunities, MacQuarrie was thinking ahead. At last, it seemed,
his chance had come to repay the Tahitians for the life they
had restored to him. Automatically his hand reached out to
drop a last token of his regard, a single red rose, on Lovaina's
coffin.

In this moment, his mind had recalled a proverb as old as
Tahiti itself: 'The palm grows, the coral spreads, but man
departs.'

'We *must* do something!' Above the steady whirring of the
electric fan, the voice of Thomas Layton, United States Consul-
General in Tahiti, angrily broke the silence. From the nine
men gathered later that day in the office of the Director of
Public Health, Dr Allard, came a low murmur of assent.

It was a breathless afternoon. The hot sweet smells of copra
and tiare blossom vied for mastery on the warm lifeless air.
Yet the situation in Papeete was now so desperate as to preclude
all thoughts of a siesta – rendered the more so by the near-
paranoid behaviour of the Governor, Gustave-Henri-Jacques
Julien.

Ranged round the colonial doctor's desk were the few men
remaining in the town who stood, whatever their creed or
calling, for a policy of concerted action: Monsignor Hermel,
the Roman Catholic Bishop, the Mayor, Lucien Sigogne, the
Reverend Ernest Rossiter, of the Mormons' Tahitian Mission,
Alfred Rowland, Associated Press correspondent and U.S.
Vice-Consul and a handful of other officials. Only MacQuarrie,
withdrawn and apart, seemed a delegate without portfolio.

Rankling in every man's mind was the bitter knowledge that
only Governor Julien's overweening vanity had unleashed the
pandemic on Tahiti. When eleven days back, on 16 November,
the s.s. *Navua*, 2930 tons, had arrived from San Francisco with
supplies, her Master, Captain John Doorly, had reported
'several acute cases' of Spanish flu aboard. Yet Julien had
granted the ship free pratique – placing no restraint on communication with the shore.

Two days later, seventeen members of her crew were down. Still, incredibly, the Governor gave no order.

A courtly ineffectual peacock of forty-eight, Julien had been four years Governor of Tahiti. Although the red ribbon of the Legion of Honour adorned his immaculate white uniform, his main distinction was as a linguist: no man was more versed in the language and customs of Madagascar, on which he had written the standard work. Yet to date Tahiti had given him scant chance to do more than issue placid daily bromides on the course of the war. Now he saw his chance.

Paramount in his mind was a determination that Tahiti's victory celebrations should eclipse anything staged by a French colony anywhere in the world. Like a new-rich host intent on showing off his treasures, he ordered victory services to be held in Papeete's three churches – and, as fitting climax, on 23 November, a monster banquet, in the old barracks on the coast road, to celebrate the Allied triumph.

To that banquet the gregarious warm-hearted Tahitians had flocked, by gig, on horseback, or on foot, from islands far and near. Island tradition knew no such word as gate-crasher; all were welcome if a party was afoot, and the guests were numbered in hundreds, to enjoy the choicest Tahitian delicacies culinary skill could devise. Raw fish marinaded in lime-juice gave place to curried freshwater shrimps, to sucking-pigs barbecued whole over hot embers. Toasts were drunk both in gallons of beer and in the rarest wines of France that the Governor had reserved for the occasion. As guests of honour, the officers and men of the *Navua* mingled freely with the islanders, and as feasting gave place to dancing the sound of guitar and accordion music was plangent on the soft blue night.

For Hector MacQuarrie, only one factor had marred the evening's pleasure: Lovaina, troubled with a bad cough, had thought it imprudent to risk the night air. The young New Zealander had missed her unrestrained mirth, the sparkle of her warm brown eyes, but he felt no premonition. Only later did he learn that Lovaina's last visitor before falling sick was

the Chief Engineer of the *Navua*. As always, before taking his
seat on the camphor-wood chest, he had kissed her on the
cheek.

Within days, as the villagers departed to their homes, the
disease was sweeping the Society Islands like a typhoon. Mac-
Quarrie's first intimation had been an occasion as mundane as
the non-appearance of his laundry: together with Wong, his
Chinese servant, he had cycled into Papeete to find the laun-
dress and all her family sick. Next day, Wong, too, was
missing. Again MacQuarrie had cycled to market, but few
Chinese were there. Apart from potatoes and a few eggs, there
was nothing to be bought. The butcher was ill; there were no
policemen. Then Lovaina had died.

Even now, the Governor made no move. It was Captain
Doorly, himself falling sick, who had made his own decision
to move the *Navua* to mid-harbour and anchor there, but it
was now too late to save Tahiti.

This morning, 27 November, Consul Layton himself had
paid a call on the Governor. He begged Julien to let him appeal
to the State Department for whatever help the United States
could afford. But to his consternation, the Governor refused
to acknowledge that any epidemic existed. The disease, he insisted, was 'of a benign form', and only the old were dying.
For a French representative to appeal, even indirectly, to the
United States would be to forfeit all self-respect.

Layton had driven home his point. Even Dr Allard, who at
first had played along with the Governor in minimising the
gravity, admitted that medicines were pitifully scarce. If not
the United States, then why not New Zealand? Grudgingly,
the Governor had given his assent.

Now Layton was reporting to the men assembled in Dr
Allard's office the almost total failure of his mission. Only one
thing, he affirmed, now remained to be done: they must,
within bounds, take the law into their own hands, organise the
town into districts, and somehow keep the situation under
control until New Zealand sent help.

*   *   *

More than 2000 miles away, in Suva, the capital of Fiji, the Superintendent of the Pacific Cable Board was just then scanning a bleak and final message from the Secretary of Telegraphs, Wellington, New Zealand: OWING TO INFLUENZA EPIDEMIC PAPEETE UNABLE WORK WIRELESS STATION. MESSAGES FROM PAPEETE MUST NOT BE ACCEPTED UNTIL FURTHER NOTICE.

Back in Papeete, Governor Julien was as yet unaware that both radio operators maintaining the island's frail link with other communities had fallen sick. Consul Layton's message had never even been transmitted.

Tahiti was cut off from the outside world.

At sunset the wavelets lapping the shore abutting the Hotel Tiare's annexe were maroon-coloured. In this moment, the lagoon itself was dark. Slowly, minute by minute, maroon faded to pink; further out still, the sea became golden, streaked with rose-pink bars. Ten miles distant, the peaks of Moorea were tipped with gold.

The man lying at the edge of the lagoon was burning with fever, but mercifully he felt the salt water cool his whole body. To his ears, as he reclined, there came the plodding echo of a horse's hooves. Then he remembered. Always at this hour, Vava, 'the Dummy', brought the old horse that drew Lovaina's chaise to swim in the lagoon.

Abruptly, the golden light left the water's surface; once again it was burnished blood red. Idly, the sick man watched Vava go. Tonight he saw, the Dummy was bound further afield. He had ridden the horse straight out into a sea of bronze, and kept on riding, towards the reef. Soon only the horse's neck and mane were visible above the waves.

Still the man watched, but now the sun was below Moorea. It was night. He could not see Vava at all.

The mission bell was tolling. In the icy Labrador night, the notes carried a long way over the still water. Light streaming from the church porch laid a ladder of gold across the harbour, to where the mission barque *Harmony* lay at anchor. Lanterns cast flickering pools of light on the frozen pathways, and there was the shuffling sound of many feet. As always, when the *Harmony* made ready to depart, the Eskimos of Hopedale were flocking to church for a service of thanksgiving.

In a moment, the porch door was closed. A neatly clad Eskimo woman walked gravely to open the preacher's door. Once again, the Reverend Walter Perrett faced his congregation ranged on the benches before him, in their white calico smocks and seal-skin kneeboots. At the harmonium, the organist's hands strayed softly over the keys. Then the magnificent thunder of a chorale flooded the little pitch-pine room.

Never had Perrett offered a prayer of thanks to God as fervently as he did tonight. After weeks of suspense and anxiety, his fears concerning the *Harmony*'s fate had been proven groundless. More and more, as the days passed, Perrett had been tormented by the thought that the barque's crew had come down with Spanish influenza – or that some settlement along the way had been fatally stricken. Now, at long last, with the *Harmony* in port, Captain Jackson had set his mind at rest.

Owing to bad weather, the *Harmony* had left St John's later than anticipated, and at Nain, which lay ninety miles from Hopedale, an outbreak of measles had meant a scarcity of menfolk to unload the cargo. But of Spanish flu, apart from one suspect case aboard *Harmony*, there had been no sign. Hebron and Okak were still unaccounted for, but Perrett was less troubled now.

All had been well at Okak, as October dawned, for the entire week the *Harmony* had been in port, so Perrett reasoned, all must still be well. Once she departed, Okak could have had no contact with the outside world at all.

Almost 200 miles north-west of Hopedale, the village of Okak was silent. Among the frost-scoured acres of the settlement, ridged and hummocked like a lunar landscape, nothing stirred. Only the dogs were alert and listening.

There were many dogs and all of them were puzzled. The village's population numbered eighty men and it was only a poor man who kept a minimum of three dogs; most had a team of at least a dozen. Now, in the lees of scores of wooden huts, they huddled waiting: a killer pack, almost 500 strong.

By instinct, the dogs knew that only in summer did they forage for themselves. Then, in the shallow waters of the bay, they used paws and teeth to catch and devour the slow sculpins or frog-fish. But now it was winter; the bay was frozen over. By custom, it was the men who fed them then, four times a week in all.

It was a task even veteran hunters like Little John or Big Josef approached with caution. Any man moving imprudently among them without a whip in his hand was engulfed within seconds in a snarling fighting mass. Always ravenous, the dogs would eat gloves, fur hats, even Sunday boots. A wise man stood well clear when he threw their meat on the snow. At first there was a cautious pricking of ears, a lolling of tongues, then, with one mighty bound, the dogs were on to the food, yelping, snapping, snarling, guzzling, bolting the frozen meat, bones and all. The only way to get enough, ever, was to be faster and meaner than the next dog.

Now the dogs were crazy with hunger. It was many days, not long after the *Harmony*'s departure, since Big Josef or any of the men had appeared to feed them all. At the same time the age-old paleolithic instinct of the wolf told them they were in the presence of death. All round them, close at hand beyond the flimsy windows, lay human carrion.

All at once, they began a strange ritual. At first they whined softly, padding in small circles, each dog a separate entity, goaded by its own hunger pangs. Little by little, they gathered outside each hut, a tight compact group, each dog weighing upwards of sixty-five pounds. Now they squatted on their haunches. Dog after dog was breathing strangely, a queer unearthly whistling sound.

It was a sound the Reverend Walter Perrett would have recognised instantly. Time and again he had heard it during his years of exile: the noise the dogs never failed to make when feeding-time was near.

Lieutenant Arthur Lapointe awoke trembling. Fearfully, bathed in icy perspiration, he struck a match, groping for his wrist-watch. It was 3 a.m. on Saturday, 30 November. Dimly, the wavering light picked out the shapes of other truckle beds, which in its way was reassuring. He was still here, in the Officers' Ward of Bramshott Camp Hospital. It had been only a dream after all.

Yet a dream so vivid that even now, petrified in the darkness, Lapointe lived a waking nightmare. Five days earlier, he had at long last received a letter from home – one which had plunged him into black despair. One of his elder brothers, Guillaume, was dangerously ill. 'When you get this,' his mother had written, 'he will probably have passed away.'

For five days, a terrible sense of impotence had tormented Lapointe, both sleeping and waking. Four thousand miles from St Léandre he could do nothing but wait helplessly, unable to fly to them as he so much yearned to do. Now, in the small hours of this night, he had been wholly convinced that his youngest sister, Martine, stood before him, dressed in deepest mourning. Silently, taking him by the hand, she had led him to a row of graves, and one after another named his brothers and sisters as the occupants: Alphonse, Delphine, Guillaume.

In the dream, Lapointe recalled now, he had been pitifully grateful that at least Martine, his favourite sister, had been spared. 'No, Arthur,' she told him gently, 'I, too, am dead. God in His Mercy has allowed me to spend this day with you.' Then, like a wraith, she had faded from sight.

Now, five hours before dawn, Lapointe knew that sleep would not come again. Alone and awake in the darkness, he fought a personal war more painful than Ypres or Petit Vimy, more bitter by far than Lens or Neuville Vitasse.

CHAPTER ELEVEN

'There are Only Men who Suffer'

1 December—9 December 1918

By Sunday, 1 December, a month before the troubled New Year of 1919, one group among the world's population stood in greater peril than any other. All of them had one physical condition in common, and neither race nor creed nor colour nor wealth could guarantee them immunity. They were pregnant mothers.

Everywhere doctors recognised these women, at any age from puberty to the menopause, to be more at risk than any other group. Since the menstrual cycle was interrupted, none of them could hope for the merciful haemorrhage which might have eliminated toxins from the system. For such women, stricken by flu, abortions, miscarriages, and premature labour were commonplace – often, noted Dr George Kosmak, a New York obstetrician, with a devastating mortality rate of seventy per cent.

They faced many agonising decisions. In Milan, Michigan, Elsie Lee, a twenty-three-year-old farmer's wife, was too weak to share in the consultation that took place one overcast morning in the corridor outside her sickroom. Almost nine months pregnant, she was sinking fast, and it was Philip, her husband, and her father, Sam Ash, who now conferred gravely with the family physician, Dr Kenneth Noble.

'It's Elsie's life or the child's,' Dr Noble told them. 'I know it's a hard decision, Phil, but it's up to you.'

Why us? Philip Lee wanted to cry out. Was taking an unborn child's life something he had any right to decide? It
would never know, of course, that the doctor would terminate
its life with an injection of pituitrin, yet even so ... Already
the Lees had Kenneth, aged two, but like many fathers, Philip
had set his heart on a daughter. They were almost certain that
this time it would be a girl, and they had the name already
chosen: Thelma. For long minutes, Philip Lee bowed his head
in silent struggle. 'Save Elsie, Doc,' he said finally.

Thelma Lee was stillborn three days later to a mother who
was by then 'too weak even to tear an envelope open'. But Elsie
Lee lived on to bear five more healthy normal and responsive
children, to atone for the child the pandemic had claimed, and
never, in their conscious minds, did they question the logic of
Philip's decision. Only sometimes, in the silence of the night,
they would wonder.

On another farm, in Kirklin, Indiana, twenty-four-year-old
Sibyl Clark was battling for her child's life. The flu had struck
her down a week earlier, but she knew one thing: as of now,
the child was alive. She had felt it kick inside her, an independent being asserting its lusty right to existence.

Convinced she must somehow keep moving, Sibyl Clark
struggled doggedly from her sick-bed. Clinging for support to
the dining-room table, she walked in slow relentless circles,
staggering, resting, walking again. Abruptly, at 10 a.m. on a
foggy December morning, her labour began. But to Dr Harry
Grimshaw's alarm, the infant that at last emerged uttered no
wailing cry. Unable to breathe unaided he was, as if stricken
by the self-same virus, blue from lack of oxygen.

Grimshaw decided on drastic action. Calling for a pitcher of
icy water he plunged the child in. It worked. At once the baby
began to whimper indignantly.

William 'Billy' Clark passed his first night on earth beside
the family stove, wrapped in blankets; weak and afflicted with
colic, he was fed with diluted cow's milk every two hours of
his life until he was six months old. Yet against all the odds,

one mother's determination had cheated the pandemic of another victim.

In the gold-mining shanty-town of Westonia, West Australia, hardest hit of any in the 400 miles between Perth and Kalgoorlie, Mrs Elsie Marshall, a timber contractor's wife, knew she would lose her fifth child within days. Sited six miles from a railhead, Westonia's whitewashed canvas-built lean-tos formed as primitive a community as any on earth – and when a furniture-van ambulance carried her to the 'isolation hospital', the hessian-screened schoolhouse verandah, Elsie Marshall was resigned to the worst. From the first, only cases deemed fatal had been taken to the schoolhouse.

At first she had been conscious of the town band, intent upon its duty, marching importantly down the dusty main street each day, playing Handel's 'Dead March from Saul'. But slowly the band dwindled to a quartet, then a trio, until at last there was no more music. Every musician had succumbed.

By then, Mrs Marshall was too ill to be even aware of the 25 pounds of thrust that was needed to expel the baby from her womb. Time passed as in a dream, and her husband Jack, still on the danger list, was too ill even to know that his son had been born. It was three weeks before she awoke one morning to see a white-coated orderly standing in the doorway, holding a squalling underweight baby in roughly-fashioned swaddling clothes.

'Mine?' she asked faintly, unbelieving.

The orderly grinned. 'Yes – he's our mascot. Right from the Sunday he was born, there were no more deaths at all. So we've just had a mock christening ceremony.'

Mrs Marshall struggled to focus her thoughts. 'We always said if he was a boy we'd call him Paul.'

That, replied the smiling orderly, was up to her and her husband. But to the hospital's orderlies and nurses he would always be known by the name which they had just christened him, to them symbolising the end of the pandemic in Westonia: 'Fluey' Marshall.

* * *

In Washington, D.C., one doctor reached a conclusion so frightening it could scarcely be spoken aloud. Yet as a scientist his duty was to set down the facts in cold blood. As far back as 9 October, Major Victor Vaughan had calculated that in one week's time, ten people, daily passing the disease to ten others, could cumulatively infect a million people.

Since then, six million had died, and now, a more deadly manifestation than all the rest, the disease was striking at the yet unborn. As a statistician, Vaughan could but envisage a further logical step. It was an implication more chilling than any doctor had voiced until now.

In his firm slanting script, he wrote, 'If the epidemic continues its mathematical rate of acceleration, civilisation could easily have disappeared from the face of the earth within a matter of a few more weeks.'

As December dawned, it was too much for any man to comprehend. All at once, statistics had no more meaning. A million sick were reported in Java. The Punjab, in India's arid northwest, counted 250,000 deaths. In Barcelona, 1200 were dying every day.

With this realisation, a twilight calm fell upon the world. It was as if, with the knowledge that there was to be no respite, people faced death almost passively.

In Guatemala, where 43,000 were to die, one man's wry last words were: 'We die of the blessings of civilisation.' The Chinese, too, shrugged it off with a time-honoured proverb: 'After war comes plague.'

One Pathan tribesman brought his wife, dangerously ill with pneumonia, by donkey to India's Peshawar Medical Mission Hospital. At once the missionaries gave swift instructions: at the city gate he would find a stable to tether the donkey. Then, as his wife was critical, he should return to the hospital. A moment's cogitation, then the tribesman pointed out the economic priorities that times like these enforced.

His wife was in the missionary's care, he explained; moreover she was sick so nobody was likely to steal her. But the donkey was healthy; it was prudent to stay with the donkey.

Some faced death with caution. In Christchurch, New Zealand, solicitor Cranleigh Barton now spent almost all his days drawing up wills for nervous testators, his office floor 'one continuous puddle of disinfectant'. Others made their peace with life. In Tokyo, Count Hijikata Hisamoto, the only Minister granted permission to fall asleep in the Imperial presence after imbibing saké, died knowing that he enjoyed the Mikado's esteem to the end. No sooner had Emperor Taisho heard that he was sinking than he at once, to help Hijikata maintain face with his ancestors in the life to come, raised his Court status one degree, to Junior First Rank.

Some, knowing a worse fate awaited them, struggled to survive. Near Tengchow, China, foreign correspondent Josef Washington Hall, laid low in a rustic inn, literally willed himself to get better; most innkeepers, feeling a death in their house was unlucky, deposited sufferers on the temple steps, at the mercy of the pariah dogs. Shivering under a mosquito net in the jungle near Papua, New Guinea, Patrol Officer Wilfred Humphries had the same idea. Every man among his carriers, though ostensibly converted, had been a cannibal.

For others, it just wasn't their day. Asleep in the hospital commander's little lean-to at Camp Sherman, Chillicothe, Ohio, Major Carey McCord awoke with sudden disquiet: an old-fashioned hearse, its rear doors open and flapping had backed up almost against his army cot. As McCord arose, the engulfing black doors seemed suddenly 'like the wings of some evil spectre, beckoning me to enter'. Firmly, the Major declined – but 125 soldiers died that day.

Near Boissevain, Manitoba, a minister's wife, Flora Oke, had as strange a delusion as any. As sick as her own four children, Mrs Oke wanted nothing more from life but to close her eyes and rest – yet each time she did so a little old lady appeared. She was bent and ugly, leaning with difficulty on a cane, always approaching nearer to the bedside. Once she bent almost close enough to kiss Flora Oke. At once Flora opened her eyes – and the old woman disappeared.

Now it became a battle. Again Flora closed her eyes – and all at once the old woman was hovering again. With half her being, Flora wanted desperately to surrender to that embrace, which she knew well enough was the kiss of death. Then, though sleep was a drowsy torment, the thought of the children forced her yet again to open her eyes and keep them open: to stare the little old lady who was death out of countenance.

Some greeted death with ill-placed defiance. In Catania, Sicily, Donna Mattia, a wine-shop keeper, derisively saluted every truckload of coffins with a raised glass of Marsala and an earthly gesture, avowing, 'You won't get me – I drink wine.' But death claimed her sooner than any other in the street. Others awaited the last moment with dignity. At Bovalino, on the Ionian Sea, old 'Centoparole' (A Hundred Words), the hired man of the Celona family, so called for the fine yarns he spun for the children, rose shakily from his sick-bed to don his Sunday best: rusty black suit, watch-chain, black velours hat, stiff celluloid collar. Then in the silence he lay down and waited.

There were some who at the very end took more thought of others. Eighteen-year-old Gertrud Haefner, convinced she was dying in Stuttgart, left instructions she was to be buried in a paper shroud; Germany had suffered too much to waste precious material on a non-combatant. Police who broke into the Geneva house of Dr Kampagnian, an Armenian refugee, found written instructions as precise: to deliver his body to the Faculty of Medicine, for purposes of epidemic research.

At Naestved, Denmark, a young mortally sick Army captain sent word to Major Hage, chief of the garrison hospital: he had one last request to make. By now he was so near to death the Major had to bend close to hear his words: 'Try to keep me alive until the first of the month.'

Hage temporised. How could you, he thought, tell a man his life was numbered not in days but in hours? All at once, curiosity got the better of him. What special significance, he asked the Captain, did the first of the month hold for him?

'Then my mother will get her allowance,' whispered a widow's only son.

Through the gathering dusk, the neat white-clad form of Gustave-Henri-Jacques Julien was barely discernible. Framed against a back-drop of purple bougainvillaea, on the balcony of the Governor's palace, he seemed, to the distraught Hector MacQuarrie, a figure as remote from the tragedy engulfing Tahiti as some perfumed beruffed coxcomb from the court of Louis XVI. Try as he might, he could not seem to make the Governor hear or understand.

But the massive iron grilles of the front gate remained obstinately closed to the New Zealander. Never once since the epidemic began had Julien set foot outside the confines of his palace – and potentially-infected volunteers from Papeete's front line like MacQuarrie were barred from the Governor's presence.

It was in a vain attempt to rally the ineffectual Julien to his responsibilities that MacQuarrie had come to the palace gates to parley on this December evening.

'At least we could open the cinema halls, Your Excellency,' he called, 'and turn them into hospitals.'

Almost before he had finished speaking, the Governor had shaken his head. 'Impossible, my young friend,' he called back, in dismissal. 'I know this country. The natives hate hospitals. They would resist you.'

With this final interchange he was gone, retreating in haste to the safety of his shuttered room.

Though MacQuarrie had been too preoccupied, in the frantic days just past to keep pace with every aspect of the situation, he knew that from the outset the Governor had resisted all practical suggestions from every quarter.

No sooner had Consul Thomas Layton discovered Tahiti's radio communication was out than he had again been swift to act. Calling on the Governor, he guaranteed that if written authority were given him, he would ensure the transmission of an S.O.S. to New Zealand that very day. The British steamer

Salvor was in port and her radio operator was standing by. After much hedging and evasion, Julien gave his assent.

On 2 December, even a combined onslaught by a six-man pressure-group under Mayor Lucien Sigogne had failed to budge him. Above all, the Mayor urged a proclamation of martial law, enabling the gendarmes to break open padlocked shops and requisition scarce food supplies. Julien had dismissed this out of hand: such a measure 'would indicate a lack of calm'.

In truth, calm was now the one factor conspicuously absent in Papeete. Panic-stricken at the town's rising death-rate, boats were leaving the harbour on every tide, crammed with the sick, the well and the infected, carrying the disease to almost every one of the 120 inhabited islands that made up the Colony – from Raiatea, ninety miles north, to other groups almost 900 miles distant. Yet Julien had made no attempt to stem this exodus or impose a quarantine.

But why, Mayor Sigogne demanded, had not emergency aid been requested from America or Australia? A fast U.S. cruiser with medical personnel would be of sovereign help in slashing a death-rate which the Colonial Health Officer had reckoned as high as twenty per cent. Julien reassured him. The Associated Press representative, Alfred Rowland, had been authorised to cable his New York office in the Governor's name.

True, Julien had permitted Rowland to make a personal appeal – but at the same time expressly forbidding him to mention the Governor by name. A request by Consul Layton for the State Department to support Rowland's appeal met with another curt refusal. Armoured in stubborn pride, the Governor would allow no direct appeal to the United States Government.

'Our duty,' he wound up the meeting with meaningless rhetoric, 'lies in fighting the scourge without losing courage.'

For Hector MacQuarrie, staring wrathfully through the dusk after the Governor's retreating figure, this state of affairs was too appalling to contemplate. With Lovaina's death, Papeete had become a nightmare. The town's two undertakers and hearses could not cope with the work. The dead were buried in boxes, but the disease was claiming fifty people a day. It was impossible to make the boxes in time.

At first, working single-handed in the Rue Colette district, MacQuarrie had done his best. Yet he was painfully aware it was not enough. The district contained almost 500 patients. Time and again he would enter a straw-thatched *fare*, a one-storey communal dwelling, where ten people lay ill. To each man and woman he could give nothing but a small bottle of quinine tablets and advice. 'If you stay in bed, keep warm and take the medicine,' he counselled patiently, 'you will be well. But if you get up and bathe in the stream while you have fever, you will certainly die.'

The ritual never varied. Each man and woman promised solemnly to do his bidding. Next day he would find them slumped like sacks across the window sill while children poured cold water over their heads. At other times they were in the stream, face down, already dead. MacQuarrie was certain of just one thing. At this rate, 2000 in Papeete would die.

The Governor had said sea-burials were out of the question, for the fishermen would quit the reef – though the diamond-points of their lights had days ago flickered out, one by one. On this anguished night, the only lights in town were the headlamps of the death carts, three motor trucks, manned by drunken sailors from the tramp steamers, racing through the silent streets, legs and heads of hair dangling over the sides. Far beyond, on the hillside near Look-Out Point, the skyline trembled with dancing yellow flames: in a mass grave of blazing tar, the Mormon missionaries were disposing of the dead.

Now, in the darkness, MacQuarrie reached a sudden decision. It was Tina, the old masseuse who had saved his life, which clinched it for him. She had taken neighbours into her *fare* and nursed them, but that morning he had found her, alone and faltering, in a house nearby, trying to dress a corpse in its grave clothes to ensure it a happy passage to the land of spirits. '*Aita, pea-pea*, it doesn't matter, Tina,' MacQuarrie had consoled her, coaxing her back to her own *fare*, gravely aware of how sick she was.

MacQuarrie saw his chance. Tomorrow, whatever the Governor might say, he would open a hospital of his own. Somehow, with the help of friends, he would save Tina – and perhaps, with luck, fifty others from among the thousands who must die.

Although Hector MacQuarrie's first thought was for Tahiti's islanders, this spontaneous concern for mankind was now universal. Faced with the prospect of the world's eclipse, the people had achieved an outlook that knew no frontiers, a new maturity. Most could say, with England's seventeenth-century poet and divine, John Donne: 'Any man's death diminishes me, because I am involved in mankind.' One touch of sickness had made the whole world kin.

At first, understandably, community concerns had taken priority. The sudden onset of the pandemic, with that old perennial influenza, suddenly unmasked as the deadliest killer of all time, had been too stupendous to grasp. Negligence, greed, stupidity, had all played their part, as the people struggled to adjust – above all, well-meaning ineptitude. But now, with the realisation the pandemic's front line knew no demarcation, this attitude had changed. On 22 November, the Greek daily *Proodos* had summed up the abiding truth: 'Today all nations sneeze as one.'

The days of blaming one's next-door neighbour were past now. So, too, was undignified name-calling. No two nations had indulged in greater mutual recrimination than France and Spain, each charging the other had been first to spread the infection. But from December on, a five-man Spanish Medical Commission were welcome guests on French soil – working with the Pasteur Institute's Dr Emile Roux to exchange every available crumb of bacteriological and epidemiological data.

Everywhere there was the same spirit of cooperation. Already the American Red Cross had donated $125,000 to the stricken Swiss, and rushed doctors, nurses and medicines to Portugal.

From Rio de Janeiro, a Brazilian Medical Mission, sixteen-strong, had already reached France, though every man had been infected en route, and four of them had died. In Madrid, Ambassador Prince Max of Ratibor had offered the Ministry of the Interior the services of all those German surgeons from ships still interned in Spanish waters.

And the mood was contagious. In Berlin, bacteriologist August von Wassermann, famous for the determinant syphilis test that bore his name, set the keynote: 'For me there are no Germans, no Englishmen – only men who suffer and must be helped.' It was a sentiment one French prisoner-of-war, Private Robert Faucon, had come to appreciate above all. A twenty-one-year-old veteran of Verdun, working as a cowherd on a farm near Kassel, Germany, he owed his life to the local priest, Pastor Rabbe, who secured him a room in the village inn and nursed him back to health with his own hands. Now, as a farewell gift, he presented Faucon with a fine meerschaum pipe bearing the Kaiser's image.

'You'll surely get a kick out of burning the Kaiser,' the old priest chaffed him. 'As soon as you get back to France, send me one with Clemenceau.'

National concerns gave place to international: wherever the need was greatest, there a team was working. From Athens went a priority call to London's Scotland Yard, beseeching that a British police mission should set out for Greece to launch a crash course in elementary street hygiene. Surgeon Ruperto Borras, of Uruguay, in Paris for a conference, gave his time – and ultimately his life – to tend the sick in the city's poorest quarters. The Chief Medical Officer for Gambia, West Africa, had cut short a holiday to work for stricken diamond miners in Kimberley, and so, too, had the Principal Medical Officer for the Belgian Congo. As one New Zealand nurse on overseas service wrote: 'We are all one family, stricken and humbled, in the hands of an all-merciful God.'

Old grudges were forgotten. Between China and Japan there had been only centuries of distrust and enmity, but now, along the 300 miles of railroad between Harbin and Tsitsihar, Japanese military doctors, at the invitation of the Chinese, had become the region's doughtiest flu-fighters.

From Denmark sped a task-force of doctors and nurses to give aid to harder-hit Sweden; the Swedish Consul-General, not to be outdone, gave 100 beds to Copenhagen's Bispjeberg Hospital. And this chain of goodwill was unending. At first, Field-Marshal Sir Douglas Haig's British Expeditionary Force, still unscathed by flu, had undertaken to feed and medicate, for four crucial days, 700,000 French citizens who had returned to their villages on the Belgian border. Then, seeing that the hard-pressed civil authorities just couldn't cope, they rewrote the contract. For more than a month they scrounged fresh meat, white bread and hot milk for the flu-stricken of the Valenciennes area – providing more than five million meals and saving, by one estimate, 400,000 lives.

'France,' Georges Clemenceau wrote to Haig, 'owes you the salvation of a whole region.'

For some international Samaritans, it was harder going still. On Samoa, where more than 7000 islanders had died, a 44-strong Australian medical team under Surgeon Lieutenant Francis Temple Grey covered forty-five miles on foot through drenching rain forests to succour the stricken villages, with only a lone copra trader to act as interpreter, once stumbling for more than eight miles, the blood seeping from their boots, across a bed of solid lava.

Yet once more these were men fighting a battle which need never have been waged: on 30 October, eighteen days after the s.s. *Niagara* had brought the pandemic to New Zealand, Auckland's Harbour Board had taken no steps to check the s.s. *Talune*, with infected passengers aboard, sailing for Samoa. For Grey's party arriving one month later, it was as if a death ray had struck the island.

The warning was not unheeded. In almost identical terms, as nation after nation faced the implications of the disaster, a cry went up for the international liaison which until now had been so pitifully lacking. Urged Sir John Denniston, heading a commission appointed to probe into New Zealand's lamentable quarantine record: 'We strongly recommend that the Government enter into negotiations with other governments to establish and participate in an international bureau.'

'More particularly,' added Chairman Paul Cluver, whose South African commission had followed the same briefing, 'with the object of obtaining information in regard to epidemics.'

For the first time the men at the top were taking to heart the abiding lesson that the pandemic had brought home: no longer was any nation – or any man – an island standing alone.

CHAPTER TWELVE

'How Awful to Lose Six'
After 9 December 1918

Clad in his black soutane piped with red, with black buckle shoes, the stocky old Archbishop stood unflinching before the sentry's drawn bayonet outside Sydney's North Head Quarantine Station.

'Will you admit me?' he demanded.

'No,' the Sergeant of the Guard replied sternly.

'Is that absolute?' challenged Monsignor Michael Kelly, Roman Catholic Archbishop of Sydney.

'Absolute,' said the Sergeant flatly.

At this precise moment, a little after noon on Monday, 9 December, a vital religious principle was at stake. Outside the Quarantine Station's Darnley Road entrance, a grim-faced confrontation was in progress, watched agog by a fast-scribbling cohort of newsmen and their attendant photographers. Behind the Archbishop, a group of black-cassocked priests tensely awaited the next turn of events. Before him, barring his way, stood a determined tight-packed phalanx of soldiers and policemen.

No sudden caprice had prompted the sixty-eight-year-old Archbishop to arbitrarily challenge established authority. Nor could he deny that in three months Australia's rigid quarantine system had worked well: 80 vessels laid up, 10,000 people isolated for up to a week at a time, 1000 infected cases treated, island groups like the Solomons and New Hebrides preserved from all risk of infection. Yet everywhere in these hair's-breadth weeks, churchmen like Monsignor Kelly were conscious of the people's need for a true communion with God. Above all, a Catholic mortally sick had the right to die attended by a priest.

Six days earlier, in this crowded Quarantine Station where 1000 souls were now herded, Sister Annie Egan, a Catholic nurse, had died of pneumonia. For two days before her death, she had never stopped crying for a priest – yet all the efforts of the Reverend Father O'Gorman of St Mary's Cathedral, to gain admittance and hear her confession had been unavailing. A stone wall of regulations barred all access from the outside world.

Now, having wired every Australian diocese to enlist their support, the Archbishop had resorted to a time-honoured ruse: a full-scale confrontation, with every pressman in the city briefed in advance.

He had, Kelly told the assembled crowd, brought not only his portable altar but his sleeping kit. Now he was giving the authorities a chance to change their minds: he would abide by all regulations and remain in quarantine for months if need be, if they would accept him as resident chaplain. But still the police shook their heads stubbornly.

Knowing that he had made his point, the fighting Archbishop could not resist one last challenge as he climbed back into his carriage. 'If there were more like Nurse Egan calling for a priest now,' he told them, 'you would have to lay hands on me to keep me out.'

Already, Kelly guessed shrewdly, he had won. Within twenty-four hours, black banner headlines all over Australia had paid tribute to the Archbishop's lone stand – and Acting Minister for Customs Massey Greene had announced to the House of Representatives that 'following certain precautions' priests would be allowed to enter North Head Quarantine Station. Two days later, a duly-inoculated Padre, Father Peoples, took up his post as chaplain.

It was a timely gesture. Until now, as in Lynchburg, Virginia, most people had confined Sunday worship to their homes, armed with the prayer the Ministerial Union had composed for family use: 'Almighty God, hear, we beseech Thee, the cry of Thy helpless children, and take from among us the sickness with which our land is stricken.' Now, on the pandemic's ninety-eighth day, most felt the need for worship in public as never before.

All along, some ecclesiastics, like Cardinal French of Ontario, had steadfastly refused to close their churches. Others, like the Reverend John Houlihan of Deering, Maine, had complied until this moment. Now, though still abiding by the spirit of the regulations, Houlihan erected a simple altar in the doorway of a garage – and men and women, impelled by the need to seek strength from God, knelt silently in the snow.

Fighting men, too, felt that need. At Camp Fremont, California, a Lieutenant of the 12th Infantry Regiment wrote home that 'the soldiers have realised as never before that there is a chaplain'. It was the same as the churches now reopened in Richmond, Virginia. Impulsively a friend called on Mrs Barbara Trigg Brown, an officer's wife, and urged her: 'Let's go to church – I'm frightened.' Looking back now, Barbara Brown recalls: 'So in our hearts were we all.'

One city didn't wait for the ban to be lifted. Across the fifty-five square miles of Canada's largest city, Montreal, the great Bourdon of Notre Dame Church pealed forth the call to a different kind of worship. First, as Archbishop Bruchesi had instructed, the curé of every parish entered that silent sanctuary to celebrate mass on behalf of his absent congregation. Meanwhile, alert and expectant at home, the people waited.

What followed was something which those who witnessed it never forgot: a religious event unique in the city's history. From the church's main portal, heralded by the joyous clangour of a hand bell, and led by Archbishop Bruchesi himself, a small army of priests, clad in vestments of gold, followed by surpliced altar boys, set out by car and on foot all over Montreal to bring the Sacred Host to the very doors of the people – not borne in glittering monstrance as on Fête Dieu, but simply, as befitted a time of trouble, within the gold-veiled Ciborium.

As many knelt on the pavements, bearing lighted tapers in

their hands, to make their adoration, all over the city the cry
of bugles went up to prepare the people for their blessing.
Above it, wild and free, the pealing of the Bourdon filled the
winter sky. For some it struck a note they had all but forgotten
existed. It was the sound of hope.

'Oh God, I am very sorry.' To Hector MacQuarrie's ears,
the voice of the dying Frenchman was almost inaudible now,
yet somehow, amid the desperate rattling fight for breath, it
struggled to be heard. '... sorry for all the things that I have
done wrong ... please forgive me for Jesus Christ's sake ...'

He felt the man's eyes fixed on him imploringly, willing him
to stay. 'You must go now? That is sad.' And MacQuarrie, as
he had done so many times now, excused himself gently: 'Yes,
Monsieur, good night. There is much to do for many are sick.'
Then, with measured step, he crossed the floor to another
dying man.

In the little chamber he had christened 'the room of the
gateway', away from the main ward, MacQuarrie was alone
with two men. It was a pleasant brightly-lit room; a clean
island mat covered the floor, and the walls, at his instigation,
had been freshly whitewashed. Lace curtains draped the windows, and everywhere there were vases of crimson flamboyant
blossom. Yet for the New Zealander its whole concept was
symbolic of the problems besetting him in the days just past.
The men who occupied it would die before the night was out,
and both of them knew it. They had been carried here so that
their last moments of delirium should not disquiet those in the
main ward.

On Tuesday, 3 December, just as he had vowed, Hector
MacQuarrie had opened his emergency hospital. By then, he
noted wryly, Governor Julien had been past caring what anyone did. One more brief colloquy from iron-barred gate to
distant balcony had been enough. Feebly waving his assent to
MacQuarrie's plan, the Governor had again vanished from
sight.

Not for one moment had MacQuarrie hesitated as to his

choice of building. To him it was grimly appropriate that the site which had served so recently as the forcing-house of the infection should now be pressed into service to save perhaps fifty lives: the old military barracks on the coast road where the Governor had staged that disastrous victory banquet.

For MacQuarrie, there was bitter irony, too, that it was for old Tina he had conceived this hospital. Yet when he had gone in triumph to collect her she was at the point of death and would not come. '*Eriana*' (presently), was her unconvincing promise.

Yet by swift action, he knew, other lives could be saved. Along with the Associated Press's Alfred Rowland, who donated $5000 of his own money, Bjørn Kroepelein, a Swedish freelance photographer, and a handful of others, MacQuarrie next looted the store of beds the French garrison abandoned when departing for the front. Between them they had outfitted one large fifty-bed ward, and at once the New Zealander split them into shifts: three would nurse by day and two by night.

It was a titanic struggle from the first. Though the hospital was never short of patients, half were women – and for men under thirty, innocent of medicine, to care for twenty-five bedridden women was a near-impossible task. Despite all their efforts, there were deaths – which was why MacQuarrie had designed 'the room of the gateway'.

If it hadn't been for Renée it would have been easy to give up. She was a Tahitian café girl, one whom, though she stubbornly denied it, they had nursed back to health. Renée insisted she must convalesce, but MacQuarrie saw through her ruse. Within these crumbling walls, she had found, for the first time, a warmth and companionship absent from the dives of Papeete. But reluctantly MacQuarrie sent her packing. Her bed was needed.

Then, one afternoon, dozing from sheer exhaustion, Mac-Quarrie awoke to a vision of incredible loveliness: a copper-skinned Tahitian girl in a snowy-white linen head-dress, an ornate Red Cross adorning her brow. 'You don't know me?' she cried, gleeful at his perplexity. 'It's Renée!'

Such was her determination to stay, she had hastened to the store, bought soft muslin to bind round her head and red cotton to fashion a cross. If her days as a patient were over, Renée was now a nurse.

Shrewdly MacQuarrie guessed that in Papeete Renée's radiant appearance would draw many more volunteers. 'When you stop by the store,' he commanded her, 'get seven more outfits like that.'

And he was right. That same night, when eight breath-takingly lovely *vahines* from the cafés and brothels of Papeete reported for nursing duty, marked the turning-point. They flirted with the patients, they flirted with the volunteers, but they were kind and gentle and most who passed through Mac-Quarrie's makeshift hospital owed their lives to their care.

'You've got the eight worst "pretty ladies" in Tahiti as your nurses,' said one white visitor, shocked, but MacQuarrie was unrepentant. 'They're God's messengers none the less,' was his sober reply.

At such moments, he had known triumph – yet on nights like this, when he kept vigil beside the dying, he knew, by contrast, black despair. The urge to do more, to help so many others, jarred painfully with what he knew was the truth: there was no more any man could humanly do.

Now he knelt beside his second patient, an Australian schooner captain. His end was very near, and MacQuarrie, his head bowed, recited aloud the words of the Lord's Prayer. 'Be quick,' the skipper's eyes seemed to be saying. 'There's so little time.'

They shook hands. More confidently now, the Captain made a last request: a dying man's request was always honoured. 'Send Jim Smith to me,' he said, and MacQuarrie nodded quietly. Jim Smith and all his family had died days ago, but he said nothing of this. 'I'll try and get Jim for you, Captain,' he said.

Once more he glanced round the room. The light in the coconut-oil lamp, he saw, would outlive the spark of life in both these men. Then he passed into the tropical night.

Amid the scudding clouds, the full moon seemed to race across the sky; the air was heady with the scent of flamboyant blossom, and the gardenias that the islanders called *tiare Tahiti*. But soon, he thought, the blood-red flamboyants, the waxy-white gardenias would turn brown. They would fall and be trampled under foot on the moonlit sand, among the scuttling land crabs. This was the one sure truth: everything returned to earth.

A harsh strangled sound severed the darkness, barely audible above the rustling surf. Huddled against the crumbling wall of the hospital he had created, Hector MacQuarrie was weeping.

It was a time for tears. For untold numbers, on Tuesday, 11 December 1918 – the pandemic's one hundredth day – only one truth was now valid. Whatever the outcome for others, their own lives irrevocably had been turned upside down. Overnight, whole families had disintegrated.

Thousands were now orphans. Cape Town alone counted 2000, and in Stockholm, newspaper advertisements daily urged any family who could afford it that 500 children stood in crying need of adoption. For such as these, their sole hope was to find foster-parents as large-hearted as the Polish labourer in Cleveland, Ohio, who spoke up for his half-sister's children. Though his English was halting, he was fluent enough to tell Welfare Director Sherman Kingsley: 'Dem four kids can haf my roof till dey are tall like me.'

To many, all events from this time on were strangely unreal. For six-year-old Mary McCarthy and her brother, Kevin, kneeling in their pyjamas in a great-aunt's house in Minneapolis, the nightly prayer they uttered had small connection with the parents they had lost. 'Eternal rest grant unto them, O Lord, and let the perpetual light shine upon them,' their young voices recited, but in her mind's eye Mary saw only Tessa, her mother, with her husky singing voice, and Roy, her dashing father, who had planned those glorious backyard picnics and Easter egg hunts, and even drawn a gun on the conductor who tried to shunt his ailing family off the train.

It was the same for little Frances Cotter, in the manager's private apartment above the Bank of Nova Scotia in St Jacobs, Ontario. It was the first-ever Christmas Eve Santa Claus had not filled her stocking to the brim, so now, gently, her mother broke the news. All along, Santa Claus had been David Arthur Cotter, her father, who had died eight days earlier.

The irony was as bitter for Ada May Osman in Unley Bank, South Australia. Regulations decreed a yellow flag flew from the garden gate, signifying the house was quarantined while her husband Walter, aged forty-two, was dying from Spanish flu. But after ransacking the cellar, Mrs Osman found nothing to serve her purpose but a memento of last year's decorations: a yellow pennant, its red lettering proclaiming: A HAPPY CHRISTMAS.

Even now, the disease was striking as savagely as a headsman's axe. In Cheshunt, England, the Wilson family returned from their youngest daughter's funeral to find that trade union official Alfred Wilson had died in the hour they were absent from the house. Private William White, of Hoxton, East London, arrived home on leave without warning; he wanted to surprise his wife, Matilda. The surprise was White's alone: both Matilda and their fifteen-month-old daughter were already dying. Susanna Bourne, a Woolworth counter-hand, married her stoker husband, Thomas, in Dover, Kent; twenty-four hours later, in the same neat dark suit, he stood beside her grave. At the Campbell Funeral Church on Broadway, New York, a messenger tiptoeing up the aisle, abruptly halted the funeral of salesman John Jones. His wife had just died in King's County Hospital: a double service would be held the following day.

Some took the news with superhuman calm. On the Italian front, near Gorizia, Sergeant Cesaris Demel was escorting an officer's body to the cemetery when the cortège bogged down on a muddy road alongside a General's staff car. 'Who is this poor boy?' the General wanted to know. In truth, Demel had no idea, but he passed over the appropriate form authorising burial. Fifty-five years later, Demel still recalls how that senior officer 'turned to stone' as he looked for the last time on the body of his son.

For a few, stark tragedy, after weeks of agonising tension, was enough to unhinge the mind. In Haslev, Denmark, one doctor who lost his entire family just couldn't bring himself to countenance the facts of death. Neighbours suspecting something amiss entered the house to find as macabre a family group as existed anywhere in the world.

In his favourite armchair sat the doctor, smiling fixedly, as if to welcome guests he knew only just so well. Propped in other chairs, as rigid as waxworks yet all correctly attired in their Sunday best, were his wife and three young children – all of them dead.

'Albert, don't lie! I've got to know the worst!'

His voice impassioned, his eyes betraying his pain, Lieutenant Arthur Lapointe faced his old friend Albert Gagnon in the officers' quarters at Bramshott Camp. On this cold sparkling morning of 10 December, the young French-Canadian, after weeks of silent torment, knew that the man who stood before him had it in his power to resolve, in part at least, the uncertainties that had beset him.

In an unguarded moment, Gagnon had confessed to receiving a letter from home with news concerning Lapointe's family. Then, realising Lapointe himself was in the dark, he grew uneasy and evasive. 'But I've mislaid the letter,' he sidestepped Lapointe's request. 'I just can't seem to find it.'

But Lapointe would not be denied. Passionately he pleaded with Gagnon: whatever had happened to his family, he had to know. Uncertainty was worse than even the bitterest truth. 'Because of our old friendship,' he begged, 'let me see that letter.'

Gagnon hesitated. 'You will need all your courage,' he ventured, 'to stand the blow.' For answer, Lapointe, silently, extended his hand – then, as Gagnon produced the crumpled missive, he, in turn, knew hesitation. Had he the courage to read it, now it had come to the test. Slowly, he unfolded it.

It was worse than he could ever have imagined. Guillaume had gone, this much he had been prepared for, after his mother's letter, and Martine, too – so his dream had in truth been a terrible reality. But now Anselme, too, was dead.

Dimly he was aware Gagnon had taken a clean pocket-handkerchief to wipe away the tears coursing unchecked down his friend's cheeks. 'I was too proud,' Lapointe heard himself confess brokenly. 'I thought I'd return to see them all with an officer's rank badges. But Albert, believe me, I'm not proud any longer.'

Abruptly another officer entered the room. A native of the St Léandre district, he took in the situation at a glance. 'Poor comrade,' were his first compassionate words, 'how awful to lose six.'

For a moment Lapointe felt the room spin before his eyes. Then, as calmly as possible, he answered: 'Not six – I have lost two brothers and one sister.'

Palpably he saw the man hesitate. 'Oh, I see,' he said, after a moment's pause, 'then it must be another family I heard about.'

Yet he can't, Lapointe thought, hide the pity in his eyes. Now, as remorselessly as a cancer, the uncertainty would grow inside him until the very end.

Dr John Linson was baffled. Day after day, like every one of Surgeon-General Blue's Public Health Officers, he had sought to do his duty as a front-line flu fighter. Yet now it had become a near-impossible task. Overnight the Spanish Lady had become as elusive as a will o' the wisp.

Two months earlier, after reporting to the Division of Domestic Quarantine in Washington, D.C., Linson had sped hotfoot to Boston, Massachusetts, in response to Lieutenant-Governor Calvin Coolidge's urgent call for help. But in Boston, Linson had found four other P.H.S. officers already assigned to Health Commissioner Eugene Kelley. After interim work at that first open-air hospital on Brookline's Corey Hill, Linson had been sent on a priority mission to nearby Lawrence, where another tent hospital had sprung up.

Next, orders came to report on the organisation of every influenza clinic in Massachusetts – but as fast as Linson travelled the virus was a step ahead of him. In Boston it was then on the wane; it was days, too, since a case had been reported in Framingham. At this moment, Linson's orders changed yet again: move on to take charge in Providence, Rhode Island.

But once on the spot, it seemed almost as if evangelist Billy Sunday's prayers had been answered. Flu was a thing of the past in Providence. Instead, Linson was needed urgently 120 miles away in Hartford, Connecticut.

Yet in Hartford, the local health officials shook puzzled heads. 'Things have been pretty quiet here for a spell,' Linson was told. 'Our orders are for you to report back to Washington.'

All through the 300-mile journey Linson wondered. Had the pandemic now come full circle, to strike Washington with cyclone force? Once again, hopeful of playing his part to the full, Linson reported to the Division of Domestic Quarantine.

Now he received final orders: to report that very day to Assistant Surgeon General C. C. Pierce. At this moment, Linson knew his flu-fighting days were over. Surgeon-General Pierce headed a division newly created to deal with quite another sickness, one closely linked to war though rarely looming large in the nation's headlines: venereal disease.

A few blocks away, in the Butler Building, just as he had done every night for four months past, Surgeon-General Rupert Blue was studying the daily wires from health inspectors all over the United States. At first it wasn't easy for the burly Health Chief to take in the full impact of what he read. In a few cities – Boston, San Francisco – another sharp wave was inexplicably reported. Yet ever since 1 December, the requests for outside aid routed to his Wasington headquarters had been steadily diminishing. Now, comparable reports from cities far removed from the United States told the same story. Miraculously, Major Victor Vaughan's dire prophecy had not come to pass.

In New York, where the mortality rate ten weeks back had struck down sixty people in every thousand, less than eighteen deaths were now reported – and the same held good in Belfast, London, Berlin, Paris and Stockholm. Trade was resumed again in Cape Town and Rio de Janeiro, Rome and Madrid, and New Zealand had, on Christmas Eve, relaxed all restrictions.

On Tuesday 31 December 1918, as deep-toned clocks all over the world told the stroke of midnight and the passing of the Old Year, for most of civilisation, the Spanish Lady, as mysteriously as she had come, had vanished from the face of the earth.

The 120 days were over.

On New Year's Day, 1919, the people awoke to a world largely purged of its sickness. To be sure, some regions had still to experience the pandemic's full virulence for the first time. As late as 26 May 1919, the disease, re-christened 'Indian Flu', hit Bristol Bay, Alaska, with the fury of an Arctic blizzard – twelve days after claiming 15,000 lives on the tiny island of Mauritius.

But most of the world was free: to mourn their dead, to take up their lives anew, to count the cost of an unparalleled devastation.

It was a staggering total. More than 21 million had been wiped out – and by some counts the disease had affected fifty times that number. More than 540,000 Americans had died, 450,000 Russians, 375,000 Italians, 228,000 Britons, 225,000 Germans, but even these figures paled beside those of India: twelve-and-a-half million dead, four per cent of its population.

On Samoa, where 7500 had died, feeling now ran so high against the New Zealand administration for its wilful disregard of quarantine, that the Island's Chiefs formally petitioned King George V to annex them as a British Crown Colony.

In economic terms, the losses were incalculable. By New Year's Eve, 1918, the Prudential Insurance Company in Britain alone, had paid out £650,000 in eight weeks – while New York's Metropolitan Life had settled no less than 85,000 claims. As early as December, before the pandemic had even run its course, President Henry Moir of the Actuarial Society of America was to estimate that deaths in the United States alone represented an economic waste of ten million years.

Yet it was not all loss. No one agency had focussed a more merciless spotlight on prevailing conditions of housing and hygiene than the Spanish Lady – and from this time on, the war against poverty and contagious disease was to gather crucial momentum.

In Arizona, avowing 'there is no place in the State that is thoroughly safe from the health standpoint', Dr Orville Harry Brown, State Superintendent of Public Health, seized the chance to draft a whole new sanitary code: from now on it was mandatory for hotels, restaurants and drugstores to wash dishes in scalding water, furnish clean towels, maintain sterile toilets, and at all times be open to inspection. Within months, these same standards of elementary hygiene were being enforced for the first time in places as far apart as Cheyenne, Wyoming, and Calgary, Alberta – while other towns like Winnipeg and Vancouver laid down hard-and-fast rules on everything from wrapped bread to antiseptic sponges for bank-tellers.

Gone was the era in which public health had been narrowly limited to using the state's police force to enforce sanitation and control the spread of communicable disease. Instead, the emphasis was now on prevention and early detection – and health horizons would broaden to include chronic diseases, mental health, alcoholism, drug addiction and accident prevention.

Already, many cities like New York were instituting the first rudiments of an aftercare system – with social workers persuading flu sufferers to visit newly-opened health stations for periodic check-ups. As a result, many cases of neglect and

malnutrition were revealed for treatment that would otherwise have gone undetected; Cincinnati alone reported 200
bread-winners unable to return to work through post-influenzal
weakness or because their jobs had been filled. Other countries,
too, got the message: as a direct result of the pandemic, medical inspection for Italian schoolchildren became compulsory
from this time on.

The sights that most doctors and health-workers had witnessed would never be forgotten – as one Spanish volunteer
recalls, 'what I saw is engraved on my memory as if written
in letters of fire.' Now, in many centres, the public conscience,
profoundly stirred, was to demand – and get – sweeping action.
For Barcelona landlords, the provision of running water and
flush toilets became a duty. In Auckland, New Zealand, the
shocked revelations of M.P.s like Peter Fraser resulted in a
dramatic £250,000 slum clearance plan – the identical sum
voted by Cape Town's Council to rehouse those below the
poverty line. For Britain, the provision of 300,000 council-
owned houses for slum-dwellers became priority – and from
Montreal to Berlin, whole areas of decaying tenements were
ripped out and rebuilt.

Then, as now, no one of these problems admitted of easy
solution but some windows, once opened, can never be closed
again.

Of paramount urgency became the issue of centralisation
to co-ordinate the team work of epidemiologists, bacteriologists,
chemists and sanitary engineers. The time when a government
could stand comfortably aloof from a national crisis, passing
the buck to a local authority, was gone for ever. Even before
the pandemic was spent, Canada had announced the organisation of a Public Health Bureau, and others were swift to
follow. For Britain, a Ministry of Health to replace the old
Local Government Board, which equated public health with
the welfare of paupers, met at first with bitter reactionary
opposition. But by 1919, backed by such powerful sponsors as
Lady Rhondda, Lord Leverhulme and Major (later Lord)
Astor, it had become reality – with acute influenza-pneumonia

rated as a notifiable disease from this time on.

Soon South Africa, France and Australia – backed by the expert aid of the Rockefeller Foundation – had adopted this same system, and for many such fledgeling bodies, influenza was the first priority. For India's newly founded Medical Research Institute, the first task was to prepare 300,000 doses of serum in readiness for the next wave. Russia, too, had inaugurated its People's Commissariat of Health, with an influenza fighting fund of 245 million roubles.

Above all, the medical frontiers stayed down. Until now, independent research workers had attacked the influenza problem in small compact groups, like guerrilla fighters – independent of any central authority. But from January 1920 on, the League of Nations Health Organisation (now the World Health Organisation) ensured by a system of cables and weekly returns that flu fighters everywhere worked as an international team. From 1949 on, the World Influenza Centre of WHO, sited at Mill Hill, North London, would serve as the clearing-house of a world-wide alerting system linking 85 laboratories in 55 countries, keeping track of virus-mutations from Durban to Atlanta, Georgia.

Not until 1933 did an alert team of British researchers, headed by Professor Wilson Smith, succeed in artificially transmitting influenza to ferrets – and only in 1943 did the advent of the powerful electron microscope enable American researchers to espy the killer for the first time: a fluffy white virus resembling a miniature cotton boll, yet so minuscule that up to 30 million could be placed on the head of a pin. But whether this virus, christened Type A, was the death-dealing Spanish Lady will never be known for certain. Never was that virus seen by any human eye.

These were high-level concerns. For almost two billion people swept up by this cataclysm, their greatest concern, in the months to come, was in taking up the threads of a life they had counted as lost.

Many would suffer complications which endured for months, even a lifetime. Some remained stone-deaf for fully a year, following severe middle-ear infection. Others were so weak they hobbled like cripples, pausing for breath every hundred yards. All over the world, doctors noted, almost a third of those who had suffered an attack later came down with cardiac disorders, pulmonary tuberculosis or nephritis. At the Philadelphia Graduate Hospital, Dr Henry Davidson noted another distressing facet: the high proportion of young men who had early developed parkinsonism (chronic trembling paralysis), rarely known in patients under fifty.

For Keith Fairley, a Melbourne medical student in his final year, the aftermath of the flu was encephalitis, which for almost a year left his mind as blank as a slate. Each night throughout the term he sedulously read the first thirty pages of Sir William Osler's classic *The Principles and Practice of Medicine* – and next morning could not recall one word.

But more knew the supreme joy of coming alive to a world they could never take for granted again: after passing through the valley of the shadow, it was the little things that counted above all. Thus one man recalls the smell of black bitter coffee in a Milan barracks ... another the taste of an apple in a South Bend, Indiana, garden ... while a woman remembers a bowl of hot barley broth and Sydney Harbour sparkling in the sunlight. For kitchenmaid Inez Fagrell, in Uppsala, Sweden, who had lost all hope of ever hearing again, it was the sudden magic ticking of a wristwatch that filled her eyes with tears.

Many recall strange quirks of appetite that persisted for long afterwards. To Mrs Emily Bertino, in Jerome, Arizona, every morsel of food was as bitter as aloes for fully six months. Cadet Josef Krosh, convalescing in the German Naval Hospital at Kiel, could face nothing but crayfish; all cigarettes 'stank like burning bamboo'. In Bayreuth, all four members of the Zehender family developed an inexplicable craving for pickled cucumbers. After weeks of semi-starvation in Florence, South Carolina, Henry McKeithen finally pulled himself round with a plump partridge.

Few were as disillusioned as sixteen-year old Günther Trulsen in Rensburg, Germany. For six weeks, 'as ill as a kitten' and convinced he would die, he was sustained by thoughts of the get-well treat his parents had promised him: two fine Westphalian hams that hung secretly in the family chimney. Now, on Günther's first day of convalescence, his father ceremoniously lifted them from their hiding-place – to find both had been gnawed to the bone by vermin.

Almost everywhere, life was resuming its normal tenor – as if only the familiar daily round had power to banish past terrors. Back into the medicine cabinets went the salves and the eucalyptus, the camphor bottles and the rubbing alcohol. For a long time, frilly boudoir caps, to hide fallen hair, would be fashionable for women, but thousands, like the Reverend Maclaren Brydon, in Richmond, Virginia, found a homelier use for those medicated flu masks: to ward off the coal dust when he shook down the furnace in winter. In a million movie houses, the projectors whirred again; the Crawford Theatre, Beatrice, Nebraska, announced a gala reopening with 'That Great Dispeller of the Flu, Douglas Fairbanks, in "Mr Fix-It"'. No longer were calls routed to the emergency switch-board of Strawbridge and Clothier's Department Store, Philadelphia. Now the operators took orders for feather boas or the new one-piece shirt with collar attached for men.

Overnight the laws concerning public assemblies and over-crowding were swept away, though a few, through oversight, lingered on for half a century. Only in 1968 did Budapest's City Fathers repeal a flu ordinance forbidding more than five to stand in a tramcar – three years after Elko, Nevada, an-nulled the law compelling all persons to wear gauze masks on its streets.

For most, there was a fierce urge to rejoice. In Stockholm, Lehar's operettas played to packed houses. From the Portu-guese village of Paranhos da Beira, the sickness had vanished as mysteriously as the owls that heralded it – and now the candles and lanterns of a thanksgiving procession bathed that whole mountain amphitheatre in a sea of light. There was an urgent need to blot out the past. To one ship's navigator leaving Auckland Harbour, it seemed at first that Mount Eden was erupting like a giant volcano. Then, with a telescope, he identified it: a mammoth bonfire of mattresses from countless stricken households.

In a dozen languages, newspaper for-sale ads announced unrepeatable bargains: 'Mourning hat with crêpe veil, almost unused ... 10 dozen sleeve bands, various lengths.' At Toronto General Hospital, Nurse Gladys Brandt had daily proof that life was going on, despite all; the clothing storage room was choked out with the garments of deceased patients, and in every case she must phone relatives for permission to dispose of them. But many a husband, she recalls, replied: 'Oh, keep them – I've married again.'

Some could not forget. Never again would Martha Coulter, in Wellington, New Zealand, hear 'O God, Our Help In Ages Past', without breaking down; the line 'Time like an ever-rolling stream, bears all its sons away' recalled too poignantly those who had gone. And in Weser, Germany, church organist Günther Wäsche, deputising for the pastor at Sunday services, realised a nightmare task confronted him: to read from the pulpit a list of all those parishioners who had died.

As he read and the bells tolled, he saw the whole congregation was weeping. Doggedly, the tears streaming down his own face, Wäsche read on to the end.

For some, inevitably, the hard realities of daily life took precedence. To British Tommies, returning to 'the land fit for heroes to live in' that David Lloyd George had promised them, there was an important choice to be made: a civilian suit or a cash payment of fifty-two shillings and sixpence. For fifteen-year-old Sydney Durrance, a flu sufferer leaving Leicester Infirmary following an operation for empyema, things were tighter still. The doctors had told him to take it easy – but Durrance decided that by walking seven miles home he could save the two-and-threepence fare.

On the main street of Hälsingborg, Sweden, Mrs Hanna Forsberg had ventured forth for the first time since the loss of her eighteen-year-old son, Åke, when a neighbour shyly approached her. To Mrs Forsberg, her first request seemed to sum up the whole economic plight of the world as 1919 dawned.

'Hanna,' she asked, 'do you want a wreath for Åke – or would you rather have a loaf of white bread?'

In the murky twilight of the panelled courtroom in Belfast's Custody Court, there was a muted hush. Pale and composed in his neat dark suit, the foreman had returned the unanimous verdict of the eleven jurors ranged beside him: 'Guilty'. Now all eyes were focussed on the trial judge, Mr Justice Dodd, as he received the black cap.

The Judge spoke. His words were as chilling and ultimate as death itself.

'I do hereby adjudge that you, Nathaniel Osborne M'Connell, be taken from the bar of the court where you now stand to the place whence you came, His Majesty's Prison for the county city of Belfast, and that on Wednesday, 23 April, which shall be in the year of Our Lord, 1919, you be taken to the common place of execution within the walls of the prison in which you shall then be confined, and that you be then and there hanged by the neck until you are dead ... and may the Lord have mercy on your soul.'

'The prisoner,' noted the *Irish Telegraph*'s court reporter, 'was visibly moved.'

The s.s. *Newport* nudged slowly towards the dockside in Corinto, Nicaragua. Seamen were doubling to make fast the lines, and now the gangway was run up.

Impulsively Emilio Alvarez Lejarza grasped Dr A. E. Dilley by the hand. 'Thanks to you, my friend,' he said sincerely, 'it seems that we made it.' For answer, the surgeon smiled and shrugged. 'You were a lucky man,' he confided. 'To be honest, I didn't hold out much hope. As much as anything your wife's nursing pulled you through.'

Lejarza nodded soberly. Now, as he extended his arm to Juanita, he reflected that more than gallantry was involved.

After his fight for life, he was still as weak as a child: he would need his wife's support to descend the gangway at all. But this time without the need of rouge on his cheeks, for he was a man twice-blessed. Just as he had prayed he had come home to Nicaragua, but to live, not to die.

Arm in arm, oblivious to everyone but each other, Emilio and Juanita Alvarez went ashore.

Down the gangway of the s.s. *Salvor*, in Auckland, New Zealand, hefting his one battered suitcase, strode Hector Mac-Quarrie. On the dockside, the newsmen were clustered: the *Star*, the *Weekly News*, *The New Zealand Herald*. Would MacQuarrie please fill them in on conditions in Tahiti? Had he been there long? What was the death rate? Was the epidemic on the wane?

The scrupulous MacQuarrie did his best. The deaths must run into hundreds – more he didn't know. (In fact, the final estimate was 640 in Papeete alone – one-seventh of its population.) The epidemic had reached its peak on 10 December, one week after he had opened his emergency hospital. By 17 December, when MacQuarrie, at breaking-point, had handed over to Mayor Lucien Sigogne and boarded the *Salvor* for his native New Zealand, that hospital had cared for 175 patients, of whom only nine had died.

There were some details he did not give the newsmen. That Governor Gustave-Henri-Jacques Julien had not even informed the French Colonial Ministry of the disaster until 20 December was something the reporters would not learn from him. Nor did he add that every volunteer like himself had contemptuously refused a citation from the Governor – or that eighty leading citizens had petitioned Premier Georges Clemenceau, with ultimate success, for Julien's recall.

Next morning, curious as to how the reporters had handled his story, MacQuarrie scanned the papers over breakfast. He read of dairy shows, municipal squabbles, sale bargains – but found no mention of the sickness or Tahiti.

Already the pandemic belonged to history – and history, as

every news editor knew, had never been a Page One story.

In the living-room behind the hardware store at Ejstrup, the telephone rang shrilly. With an effort, Else Dahl reached over to answer it.

She was still weak and shaky, for just as Marius had prophesied she had contracted the Spanish flu. Worse, he and Kirsten had gone down with it, too – luckily without serious results for any of them. Even now she didn't for a moment regret doing her duty as she had seen it, though she wondered what Marius would have to say when he had fully recovered. But she thought that secretly he had been proud when the local paper wrote up her long battle – and expressed its regret that she had succumbed herself.

Now, it seemed, someone had taken that announcement too literally. From the capital an unknown sympathiser was enquiring in solemn tones: 'Can you tell me, please, when Mrs Dahl's funeral takes place? I would so much like to send a wreath.'

An irreverent sound echoed back up the wire to Copenhagen. Between puffs of the black cigar she now felt well enough to indulge in, Else Dahl was chuckling.

Ahead of Dr Juan Zamora, the passengers filing through the main exit of Madrid's Mediodia Station, terminal for the south, shuffled to an obedient halt. Puzzled, the young doctor frowned. The epidemic had long since passed from Algeciras. He had returned to the capital seeking a fresh assignment.

Now he saw the cause of the delay. At the head of the queue, two sanitary auxiliaries in white smocks were solemnly fumigating each passenger as they trooped past – as if even now they feared any relaxation would once more see the pandemic in their midst.

A moment, and it was his turn. Then the man who had valiantly fought the flu across 500 miles of Spain from Zaragoza to Algeciras, was drenched, like any tourist, in a blinding ignominious cloud of disinfectant.

For Charles Clapp, Junior, noisily drunk in a Greenwich Village speakeasy, the days following the pandemic were an unremitting blur fading insensibly into years. Ahead of him, though he stubbornly refused to acknowledge it, stretched sixteen years of moral disintegration.

His marriage to Margaret Macdonald, just after his twenty-first birthday in May 1919, was soon a cat-and-dog free-for-all of stormy quarrels and uneasy truces. Play-angel ... Wall Street bond salesman ... New York Stock Exchange member when the great crash came ... Clapp tried them all, but the back-drop to his high, wide and handsome living were the eight highballs that preluded dinner ... the sherry flips that stood in for breakfast ... the three-day benders and the agony of drying-out ... the sly concealment of liquor in safe hideaways in their Bedford Hills home. There were the speakeasy girls, too – so many he couldn't even remember their names.

Not until October 1935, when only an 'earthquake' – one part gin, one part Scotch, one part absinthe – had any power to stupefy him did a chance acquaintanceship with the Oxford Group (later Moral Rearmament) change not only Clapp's way of thinking but his whole mode of life. From this time on, at length reconciled with Margaret, he was never to take another drink.

But by then he was an obscure Connecticut real-estate broker, one year bankrupt. From that first bottle of White Rock in Ithaca, New York, he had piled up debts of $680,000.

It was probably the most costly flu cure in history.

Momentarily lifting her eyes from the hard stone floor, Lydia Phillips brushed a wisp of fair hair from her eyes. Then, once more dipping her brush in the bucket of sudsy water, she went on scrubbing. Never, it seemed, would the floors of Twist Street School Emergency Hospital be freed from their daily patina of grime. Yet by now her work as a volunteer had become a way of life. Of one thing, too, she was sure: in these last weeks she had come of age.

'Nurse,' a man's voice called, near at hand. Once, she thought, her sole aspiration was to be addressed like that, but Fate had decreed otherwise.

'Nurse!' came the voice again – harder now and more imperative. This time Lydia looked up. If a nurse was needed, perhaps she should go in search of one. But it was her the doctor was hailing – seemingly indifferent to her lowly status as a scrub girl.

'Nurse, it's you I'm talking to. Didn't you hear? Come with me, will you? – I need some help.'

Cheeks glowing, head held high, she followed joyfully in his wake. For Lydia Phillips, the battle was over, but that one word was her accolade.

Rigidly at attention on the parade ground at Andernach, Germany, John Lewis Barkley, newly promoted Corporal, was in a daze. Nobody had told him what was going on or why he was here. As far as he could see, the field was choked with top brass and doughboys, and there were bands, too, all of them playing. But automatically, as his name was called, he stepped forward. Bemused, he followed a captain's orders: to march with an assorted group of men, ranging from colonels to privates, to a chalk centre before the saluting base.

All at once, Barkley recognised the man standing on the raised platform before them. Never before had he seen him in the flesh, yet he knew him at once. It was 'Black Jack' himself – General John Pershing.

Still Barkley couldn't figure it out. The General was saying something about 'decorating as brave soldiers as the world had ever seen' – but even now he was none the wiser. Standing there with a bunch of brass, three divisions at ramrod attention behind him, he felt nothing but uneasy.

All at once Pershing stepped from the platform. Now he stood directly in front of Barkley. Salutes snapped like reflexes – then, stepping close, the General fumbled with the front of

Barkley's battle-blouse. At this moment, the doughboy from Holden almost yelled aloud. A pin had gone clean through the fabric into the flesh of his chest.

In a fog he felt Pershing pump his hand and say something about 'a fellow Missourian'. Conscious that he had been decorated, Barkley still didn't know why. Between 7 October 1918, and this morning, 17 March 1919, nobody had made any mention of his lone stand against the Germans at Cunel. Somehow the bout of Spanish flu, his warm encounter with that French family, had driven it clean from Barkley's own mind.

As Pershing passed from view along the line, Barkley squinted covertly down his nose. All he could see was a small blue ribbon with white stars, but now he knew. It was the highest award a soldier could attain: the Congressional Medal of Honour.

With a hiss of steam as harsh as an expiring breath, the train slid into Mont-Joli Station, Quebec Province. With pounding heart, Lieutenant Arthur Lapointe descended to the platform. Who, he wondered, would be here to meet him? But at 2 a.m. the station was silent and deserted. Perhaps the wire he sent ahead had not even arrived in time.

In the freezing silence, a door creaked. Framed against the lighted back-drop of the waiting-room, he saw his father and his brother, Alphonse. As they embraced fervently, the youngster saw the old man's face deeply lined, his moustache snow-white. But he could not bring himself to pose the question uppermost in his mind. Instead, he asked carefully, 'How is Mother?' 'She is well,' his father told him, 'and waiting for you at home.' Moments of guarded small-talk followed.

Suddenly Lapointe could bear the aching silence no longer. He blurted out what he had yearned to know for six months now: how were the others? For an instant, his father's face worked painfully. 'We did not tell you,' he said slowly, 'for we wanted to spare you all the sorrow we could. The epidemic carried off your three brothers and two sisters in nine days.'

Lapointe looked at Alphonse, finding no words. This was the

one brother left to him. The rumour had been true in all but one detail: he had lost not six but five. Was it for this, he thought, that he had returned? Many were sleeping for ever in France who would have been so happy to come home.

From the jetty, the Reverend Walter Perrett no longer recognised the terrain. Still visible beneath the snow were mounds and hummocks that had the shape of huts, yet each showed a black gaping hollow where the chimney flue had collapsed. All round him were scattered fragments of flint, broken knives and tools, a litter of punctured tins and shelves, lengths of rotted driftwood. Overnight, the village called Okak, where his long crusade had begun twenty-seven years earlier, had died.

Even now, on Tuesday, 4 March 1919, Perrett couldn't really grasp the implications. Not until 20 February had words of the havoc at Okak and Hebron reached him at Hopedale. All along, Perrett had consoled himself that if anything was amiss, the Reverend Andrew Asboe at Okak, or Bishop Albert Martin at Hebron would have sent a messenger by sledge. Now, on the shore of the frozen bay where Okak had stood, Asboe told him the stark truth. He had sent no sledge because no man had been able to walk.

The mission-barque *Harmony* was the unwitting culprit. Already, when it docked at Hebron, one sailor had shown signs of the sickness, and Captain Jackson had at once warned the Eskimos to keep clear of the crew's quarters. But neither at Hebron nor the next port of call, Okak, had the happy-go-lucky villagers paid any heed. Among 220 people at Hebron, only seventy now survived. From Okak's 266, no more than fifty-nine.

What the flu had begun, the dogs had ended. Crazed with hunger, they had smashed through windows, worried down doors, attacking those still alive as impartially as the dead. At Okak alone, Asboe, his rifle propped on a window-sill, had shot more than 100 of them. Then, with the thermometer still 30 below Fahrenheit, he and the storekeeper had began the

Herculean task of hacking a mass grave thirty-two feet wide and eight feet deep. In it they had laid all those Eskimos whom the dogs had not claimed first.

Little John, the pathfinder, and Big Josef, a king among hunters ... old Abia, who drove the sledge, and crippled Ernestina, who played the harmonium ... all those peace-loving men and women who in their neat white smocks had made part of Perrett's congregation, had gone. For ever etched on his mind's eye was the memory of them clustered in their huts while he read aloud from the Eskimo Bible, their huge smiles when 'Fader Karismas' doled out turnips to their children. Now all were part of the graveyard the Eskimos called 'God's Garden'.

In this moment, lost in thought beside the bay, the faith of the Christian soldier Perrett was momentarily shaken. He would recover it, to labour on for eighteen more years, but on this day, at first, the impact was too awful to bear. The work of twenty-seven years was undone in a night, as if he and Ellen had never set foot here. When next the cartographers went to work, Okak (latitude 75°40') would have vanished from the map. A man needed courage at such a time.

'All those fine men and women,' he said aloud, painfully. 'It's hard to accept that they've gone.'

Screened behind the Confessional grille in the Church of San Giorgio, the priest was no more than a disembodied voice. Yet instinctively Tersilla Vicenzotto sensed the compassion in his tones. No hint of frosty rebuke had greeted her first admission: that it was six years since she last confessed.

Now, after her halting *Confiteor*, she told her painful secret: on the day following Oscar's death she had cursed God by spitting in the face of San Antonio of Padua. In the years since then she had worked hard, back here in her hometown, Udine, struggling to bring up their daughters as Oscar would have wished, working by day in a furniture factory, by night as an usherette at the Teatro Puccini, pinching and scraping to make ends meet. Yet without Oscar, without faith, life was barren.

Nothing could bring Oscar back; she accepted that. Yet there could still be faith. And she believed that San Antonio himself had forgiven her and had willed this confession.

The priest paused, weighing his words thoughtfully. It seemed, he said, that this had been a moment of understandable desperation, though one thing must be made clear. It was not in his power to absolve her of her sin unless her mind was resolved never to repeat it. 'But it is, Father,' Tersilla whispered, meaning it with all her heart.

'Then,' replied the priest softly, 'I will ask God to give you absolution.'

In that instant, for one widow and mother, all the bitterness and rancour the world's most awesome plague had engendered fell away. In gratitude and humility, with love and with longing, Tersilla Vicenzotto once more embraced the God whom she had forsaken.

Epilogue

Perhaps the most puzzling factor about the Spanish Lady was her impermanence. On the face of it, the most appalling epidemic since the Middle Ages, which cost more than 21 million lives and in some way or other affected over one billion people – th'n half the world's population – should have imprinted itself indelibly on the public consciousness these fifty-six years past. Yet except to those who suffered it the Spanish Lady is now little more than a folk-memory – as remote from the conscious mind as the Black Death itself. Many readers under sixty can scarcely be aware that such a pandemic ever existed.

Even at the height of the slaughter, there was this same ambivalence. The disease took at least half a million American lives – ten times as many as the Germans took during the war – yet only in the hardest-hit cities did it ever win through to the newspapers' front pages. In those months of 1918, when the Allied troops were engaged in their last great push across the ruined countryside of France and Belgium, it was the crumbling of the Central European empires, the inexorable peace terms of Woodrow Wilson, that always took pride of place. To some medical men, at least, the fate of civilisation hung in the balance, for medicine could do little more than in the Middle Ages, when a red cross painted on the door of a stricken house, with the legend 'God have pity on us', was the sum total of medical knowledge. Yet no such stark facts were ever voiced by the world's headlines.

The Spanish Lady inspired no songs, no legends, no work of art. Even fundamental facts were meagre. To this day, no one can say with certainty where the disease began, where it ended, or even which virus was at fault. As one leading authority has summed it up: 'The resemblance to the disappearance of the Cheshire Cat in *Alice in Wonderland* is striking.' And to this day, too, flu remains one of the great medical imponderables: a disease which could, as recently as 1969, cost Britain's economy alone £150 million – and still escape the headlines. Yet, despite the sophistication of prophylactic techniques since 1918, few governments have shown themselves willing to take a positive lead in advocating mass vaccination.

To take but one example: in Britain alone, in 1967, the purely medical cost of influenza – drugs, doctors' time and hospital costs – amounted to £15 million. Yet the medical report which publicised this figure also estimated that if four out of five people had been vaccinated in that year, the total cost could have been cut to £9 million, and, more important by far, many hundreds of lives could have been saved.

But, just as in 1918, all too many authorities tend to regard the ravages of flu not as a challenge but as an uncomfortable truth, consistently to be ignored until too late. The late H. L. Mencken's commentary on the Spanish Lady, written as far back as 1956, sadly remains as true today: 'The epidemic is seldom mentioned, and most Americans have apparently forgotten it. This is not surprising. The human mind always tries to expunge the intolerable from memory, just as it tries to conceal it while current.'

Facts About the Flu

Few events in world history have attracted more speculation, folk-lore and often distorted legends – alongside informed medical comment – than the influenza pandemic of 1918-19. And while this is in no sense the definitive history of those 120 days when the fate of civilisation hung in the balance, here, nonetheless, is an attempt to answer some major queries concerning flu that have puzzled the world from that day until our own:

How many lives were lost?

Of necessity, this is only an estimate, since in many regions of Asia or Africa no death records exist or have ever existed. But a noted U.S. epidemiologist, Edwin Oakes Jordan (*Epidemic Influenza*, 1927), computed mortality by continents as follows: *North and Central America*, 1,075,685; *Latin America*, 327,250; *Europe*, 2,163,303; *Asia*, 15,757,363; *Australia and Oceania*, 965,245; *Africa and Madagascar*, 1,353,428. Total mortality: 21,642,274.

All told, over a billion people – more than half the world's population – are thought to have been attacked.

Which countries suffered most heavily?

Again, figures are approximate only, since for some countries, the totals are no more than estimates. In *North America*: United States (548,452), Mexico (300,000). In *Latin America*: Brazil (180,000). In *Europe*: Russia (450,000), Italy (375,000), Germany (225,330), United Kingdom (228,917), Spain (170,000), France (166,000), Scandinavia (37,154). In *Asia*: India (12,500,000), Japan (257,363). In *Australia and Oceania*: Netherlands East Indies (800,000), Philippines (93,686), South Sea Islands (50,000), Australia (13,320); New Zealand (6680). For *Africa*: Union of South Africa (139,471).

Heaviest death-rates per 100,000 of population are as follows:

India (4000); Madagascar (3500); Mexico (2300); South Africa (2280); New Zealand (2260), (this statistic representing Maoris only); Guatemala (2200); Netherlands East Indies (1600); Chile (1100); Italy (1060).

How did 1918 compare with past pandemics?

The only pandemics comparable in recorded history are the fifty-year Plague of Justinian, centring round Byzantium from A.D. 542, which reportedly slew 100 million people and the Black Death (1347-50), estimated to have slain 37 million in the east and 25 million Europeans. Again, such statistics should be treated with caution.

Which virus was responsible?

No one knows for certain – for not only was it invisible at the time, but apparently failed to survive. The proof: back in 1951, a medical team from the State University of Iowa, led by Dr Albert McKee, journeyed to Alaska to exhume the bodies of Eskimo victims preserved for thirty-three years within the earth's perma-frost line. In an endeavour to infect laboratory animals, lung sections packed in ice were returned to Iowa City – but in vain. No trace of the Spanish Lady had survived.

What of the infected swine theory?

On this question, medical men are still divided. From 1928 on, one American doctor, Dr Richard Shope of the Rockefeller Institute, dedicated an intensive research programme to investigating the theory Dr J. S. Koen had formulated, on 30 September 1918, at the National Swine Breeders' Show at Cedar Rapids, Iowa. Shope's ultimate conclusion: the fairly mild hog flu virus, acting in conjunction with the equally mild Pfeiffer bacillus – a process virologists call synergism, or working together – combined to produce a maverick killer that injured the human lungs beyond their capacity to recover.

Today, most influenza experts will at least agree that today's swine flu virus – Swine 'A' – may be a direct descendant of 1918's killer virus. As the late Sir Patrick Laidlaw, of Britain's National Institute for Medical Research put it: 'The virus of swine influenza is really the virus of the great pandemic of 1918 adapted to the pig.' And Dr Thomas Francis Jr, of the University of Michigan School of Public Health, Ann Arbor, has added: 'Evidence strongly supports the concept that a strain of virus similar antigenically to swine influenza virus was the prevalent one in 1918.'

But still unexplained, if this is true, is why the virus has retained its ability to affect pigs, yet lost its hold on man.

Then where did the virus go after 1918?

Again, scientists are uncertain. As Sir Christopher Andrewes, sole surviving member of the 1933 team which isolated Virus A, sees it: 'I can believe that the virus goes "underground", and perhaps does so all over the world ... that it can persist in an area without causing outbreaks ... but able to become active and epidemic when the time is ripe.' Recent research has shown, too, that an 'A' virus may survive in animal reservoirs – in pigs, horses, and in domesticated birds such as chickens, turkeys and ducks – though none of the strains recorded are identical with the human virus.

This rules out any question of humans being infected by animals – but not that an animal strain may combine with a human strain to produce a new virus lethal to man.

Which other viruses are involved?

Since 1933, three groups of virus – A, B, and C – have been identified. Group A viruses cause almost all epidemic and pandemic influenza – but within this one group over 1000 different strains are stored in the 'library', an outsize ice-locker at the World Influenza Centre's London headquarters, frozen at – 70°F.

Then, too, viruses change continually, not only after each epidemic but from area to area. A flu virus particle is a tiny blob of nucleic acid in a protein coat – but, chameleon-style, is for ever rearranging the proteins to become a new strain. Virus A, which Professor Wilson Smith's London team isolated in 1933, had, by 1947, become Virus A 1. Ten years later, in February 1957, came Virus A 2 – the famous 'Hong Kong Flu', which killed 23,000 Americans and 7000 Britons.

And Virus A2–Hong Kong–68 – 'Mao Flu' to the public – which struck with unparalleled virulence in the winter of that year was, in the words of the World Influenza Centre's Dr Geoffrey Schild, 'an unique and completely different virus', with almost no cross-relationship with former A2 viruses. Striking a path of devastation across the world, it claimed 20,000 American lives and over 9000 British. The economic cost to Britain alone was estimated at £150 million.

How does the World Health Organisation tackle the problem?

The crucial problem is identification. Through a world-wide alerting system of 85 laboratories in 55 countries, London's World Influenza Centre examines hundreds of strains èach year – seed virus flown in from abroad during the early stages of an outbreak, to be grown in live fertilised eggs. (The average consumption: 4000 eggs per week.) After candling, the eggs are chilled in cold vaults to kill the embryo, the virus drawn out, killed with formaldehyde, then concentrated to form a vaccine. By mid-January 1969, the peak of the 'Mao' epidemic, American pharmaceutical manufacturers alone had produced 20 million doses.

Then is inoculation the answer?

Only up to a point. Vaccine made from A2 virus in 1957 gave protection against other A2 viruses – but because the flu-bug is a quick-change artist would have given none at all against A2–Hong Kong–68. And since it takes up to five months to produce a new vaccine, a virus may travel round the world and infect millions before preventive action can be taken. As Professor Sir Charles Stuart-Harris, of the University of Sheffield, sums up: 'It is impossible to formulate a vaccine against pandemic virus with existing viruses until the antigenic (body-invading) constitution of the former is known.' Another inhibiting factor is laboratory capacity. For example, British laboratories can produce no more than 3 million doses a year – for a population of 52 million.

Recent developments have included the claim of the U.S. National Institutes of Health's Allergy and Infectious Diseases, in August 1972, to have perfected a vaccine which may control flu effectively for the first time: a combination of live if weakened viruses, administered by nasal spray, too sensitive to function in the high (98.6°F) temperature of the lungs but thriving in the nose and throat to produce crucial antibodies. Received with greater reserve was the February 1973 claim of the Pasteur Institute, Paris, to have developed a vaccine guaranteeing protection up to 1978. Comments Dr Schild: 'No one can ever say that senior strains in nature will be the same as in the laboratory.'

What about antibiotics?

If administered early enough, antibiotics are effective in curing most bacterial infection to which the flu virus makes man susceptible. But the staphylcoccus, for example, which causes one virulent form of pneumonia, has developed strains resistant to antibiotics. An increase of staphylcoccal pneumonia, otherwise rare, always occurs during a flu epidemic.

Who is most vulnerable?

Above all, the aged. A British Ministry of Health report showed that 33,000 more deaths than normally expected occurred during the 1957 outbreak – and 86,000 above average were reported from the United States. From these totals, in both instances, two out of three were among people over sixty-five. At risk, too, are sufferers from chronic heart, lung or kidney disease, diabetes and women in late pregnancy.

Who should be inoculated?

Health authorities recommend immunisation for (1) the very young and the very old – i.e. from three months to one year and persons over seventy years (2) Pregnant women (3) Persons in the age-group from five to twenty-five years (4) Persons with an occupational hazard, such as doctors, teachers, postmen and policemen (5) Those affected by the diseases listed above.

Can it happen again?

Given that the virus believed to have caused the pandemic still exists in pigs, most virologists answer yes. Says Professor Stuart-Harris: 'This threat makes the continual watch for new variants as necessary now as at any time in the past.' Sir Christopher Andrewes: 'It is still possible that a pandemic might return and kill its millions ... the variation of the virus is not yet fully understood.' Dr Geoffrey Schild: 'If a man tending turkeys in China picks up a flu strain from one, and another strain from a human contact, he can be the origin of a new strain – and a new pandemic.'

Since 1957, both major epidemics have stemmed from the Chinese mainland – where virologists, to date, have eschewed all contact with WHO. And Hong Kong, from where WHO linkmen first reported the viruses, is now but a jet-flight away from every major world capital – just over eighteen hours flying-time to New York, sixteen hours to London, fifteen and a half to Paris, twelve hours to Rome, fourteen to Madrid.

Thus, despite the vigilance of WHO, it is not inconceivable that a latterday Spanish Lady, harboured by an unsuspecting passenger, might one morning touch down at Kennedy, Heathrow, Orly or Leonardo da Vinci ... hitting the runway at a braking speed of 160 miles an hour ... checking through Passport Control ... passing all unsuspected through Health Control and Immigration ...

Acknowledgements

'As a world affair,' says Dr Carey P. McCord, 'the epidemic was the medical catastrophe of all time. Its like was never seen before or seen since. But for those who lived through it, that epidemic exists today.'

A survivor of those life-and-death days, Dr McCord speaks with authority. Now a veteran of the Institute of Industrial Medicine, Ann Arbor, Michigan, he recalled for me vividly the horror, the humanity, the determination, even the humour, of the days when, as a young Army Officer, he and his fellow medics battled the Spanish Lady at Camp Sherman, Chillicothe, Ohio.

Everyone who played a part in this book showed a similar spirit. Doctors, nurses, health workers and civilians everywhere in the world willingly gave of their time without stint, that this record of the 1918 pandemic was as complete as might be. All told, 1770 people helped with the compilation of this book. Over a period of years, they contributed hundreds of written accounts, many of which were supplemented by in-depth interviews. They furnished private diaries, contemporary letters, rare photographs, newspaper clippings and personal documentation. Their memories were further cross-checked with a multitude of contemporary sources: public health reports, medical treatises, hospital records, consular and diplomatic reports, war diaries, and the minutes of medical commissions.

The entire project would never have been possible without the help of forty-seven dedicated men and women, who made up my research team in twenty-nine countries. For months at a time they painstakingly investigated the epidemic at source, tracking down eye-witnesses, translating written accounts, combing archives and contemporary newspaper files, functioning as on-the-spot post-boxes. They provided such vital contacts and gems of research that I feel it only fair to name them in alphabetical order, by country. ARGENTINA (with URUGUAY): Dr Julio Chapper. AUSTRALIA: Tim Curnow. BRAZIL:

Dr Riccardo Olivo. CANADA: Kathleen Conrod, Marise Dutton, Ian McClymont. CHINA (with HONG KONG): Elizabeth Leslie. CZECHOSLOVAKIA: Pavel Szekely. DENMARK: Michael de la Cour, Grace Rembourn Fry. FRANCE: André Heintz. GERMANY: Brigid Allen, Eva Yeloff. GREECE: Stella Dimitracos. HUNGARY: John S Weissmann. ICELAND: Alwin Glendinning. INDIA: Indira Devi. ITALY: Marisa Beck, Donatella Ortona Ferrario, Maria Teresa Williams. JAPAN: Katsumi Iwamoto. MEXICO: Benito Gómez. NETHERLANDS: Elly Beintema. NEW ZEALAND: Chris Lamaison. NORWAY: Margareta Runqvist. PERU: Camilla Serro. POLAND: Lorraine and Leszet Toporowski. PORTUGAL: Anna Wysochi. SPAIN: Mariá Consolación, Fernández López. SWEDEN: Inga Forgan, Lisbeth Lindberg. UNION OF SOUTH AFRICA: Gill Garb, Sue Michel. UNION OF SOVIET SOCIALIST REPUBLICS: Margaret Duff. UNITED STATES OF AMERICA: Hildegard Anderson, Mildred Clarke, Jeanne McGrain. YUGOSLAVIA: Rosemary Edmonds. From first to last, these front-liners were back-stopped in a score of ways by Count Clemente Colonna (Spain), Hans Hermann Hagedorn (Germany), Erich Linder (Italy), Ilidio da Fonseca Matos (Portugal), Renata Schou Pedersen (Denmark), Dorothy Pemberton (South Africa), Lennart Sane (Sweden), and Nadia Stolt-Nielsen (Norway). None of their loyal and tenacious support will easily be forgotten.

Next I must thank the many officials who made it possible to research in their historical archives. In particular, at the U.S. National Archives and Records Service, I want to acknowledge the help of Edwin Flatequal, Director, General Archives Division, and Jerome Finster and Kenneth Hall, of the Industrial and Social Branch. Other archivists, too, spent long hours conducting research on my behalf, prodigal of time: Mrs Mary Aris (Caernarvonshire); W. H. Baker (Monmouthshire); W. T. Barnes (Carmarthenshire); E. J. Davis (Buckinghamshire); R. N. De Armand (Alaska State Historical Society); E. G. Earl (Isle of Wight); Michael Farrar (Cambridgeshire); P. William Filby and Mrs Nancy Boles (Maryland Historical Society); Joseph Ford (Owensboro Area Museum, Kentucky); Joseph G. Gamone (Kansas State Historical Society); Franklin M. Garrett (Atlanta, Ga. Historical Society); Norman Higson (East Riding); Mrs Arlene Hiu (Dept of Education, State of Hawaii); Margaret Holmes (Dorset); S. W. Horrall (Historian, Royal Canadian Mounted Police); Felix Hull (Kent); Mrs Mary G. Jewett (Georgia Historical Commission); Sheila MacPherson (Cumberland and Westmorland); John B. Mitchell (Symes-Eaton Museum, Hampton, Va.); W. E. Mizener and C. V. Carroll (Auxiliary Services Section, Manuscript Division, Public Archives of Canada); R. Sharpe-France (Lancashire); Sylvia J. Sherman (Maine State Archives); Ruby J. Shields (Manuscripts Division, Minnesota Historical Society); Joan Sinar

(Derbyshire); A. C. Spencer (Oregon Historical Society); Martha R. Stewart (Utah State Historical Society); John L. Vantine (State Historical Society of North Dakota); Alma Vaughan and Goldena Howard (State Historical Society of Missouri).

Many went far beyond anything I had a right to expect in an effort to put the pandemic in its correct medical perspective. Above all, I owe a special debt to Dr Geoffrey Schild, Director, World Influenza Centre, World Health Organisation, for his guidance and encouragement, but I am indebted, too, for valuable advice and clarification to Sir Christopher Andrewes and Professor Sir Charles Stuart-Harris. Sterling leads were furnished by Dr Susan Crawford and Dolores Huttner of the American Medical Association, Dr Edgar Thomson, Secretary, Australian Medical Association, and Dr A. D. Kelly, Canadian Medical Association, and I am grateful, among others, for the intriguing information they furnished, to Dr Giuseppe Agostoni, Dr Enrico Bedeschi, Dr Cesaris Demel, Dr H. Denny Donnell, Jr, Bureau of Communicable Diseases, Division of Health of Missouri, Dr Keith Fairley, Dr Arnold W. Fieber, Dept of Health and Hospitals, City of Boston, Dr E. Hilary Harries, Dr Rose Hu, Dr John Linson, Dr Lucien Montel, Dr Ernst Ottsen, Professor Eaver Pozderovic and Dr A. Wesselius-de-Casparis.

Inevitably, a heavy burden fell on many librarians and their staffs, and in this respect I should like to pay a special tribute to George C. Goossens and the staff of the British Museum Newspaper Library. Colindale, North London, who at the height of research were coping imperturbably with the requests of nineteen individual researchers in the course of a day. But of vital help, too, were the efforts made by Dr John Blake, Chief of the History of Medicine Division, National Library of Medicine, Bethesda, Maryland; Eric Gaskell, Wellcome Institute of the History of Medicine, London; Stanley Gillam, and the staff of the London Library; H. A. Izant, Chief Librarian, World Health Organisation, Geneva; Justine Johnson, of the Westchester Medical Centre Library, Valhalla, N.Y.; C. W. Schooling, Librarian for the Moravian Church in Great Britain and Ireland; Alva W. Stewart and Mrs Dortha H. Skelton, of the Earl Gregg Swem Library, College of William and Mary in Virginia, Williamsburg, Va.; Stanley Sutton and Mrs Valerie Weston of the India Office Library, London, and to C. R. H. Taylor, Janet Horncy and Jacqueline McAuliffe, of the Alexander Turnbull Library, Wellington, New Zealand. Nor should the patient help accorded by the staffs of the British Museum Reading Room, the Library for the College of Physicians and Surgeons, Columbia University, New York, and the Mount Vernon Public Library, Mount Vernon, N.Y. go unrecorded.

I am grateful, too, to some whom I never met for the trouble that they took in all corners of the globe, to narrow down facts or supply additional details; some of them, overnight, became my voluntary local experts on the subject, in particular Dr Emilio Alvarez, in Managua, Nicaragua, and Señor Jaime Gonzalez Parra in Bogotá, Colombia. But many vital leads would have been missed altogether had it not been for the generous aid of Mrs George H. Carroll, Mrs Lillian T. Collings, Julia J. Naylor, R. P. Patrick O'Reilly, Mrs Gabriel Politis, Fausta Segrè, of the Department of French and Italian, University of California, Santa Barbara, Susan Sherk, of the Department of Anthropology, Memorial University, St John's, Newfoundland, Mrs Charles J. Short, Chester B. Stevens, P. H. Townson and A. C. Van Gooyer.

But this book is based, above all, on the testimony of 1708 survivors, and to locate them without the help of more than a thousand newspapers who generously made public my appeal would have been an insuperable task. To mention only a handful by name seems almost invidious, but some entered so whole-heartedly into the project and gave such wide publicity to my quest, that success was assured from the first. It would be ungrateful indeed not to single out the help of Suzanne Burrell, *New Zealand Nursing Journal*; Rémy Daure, *Nice-Matin*; Colin Enderby, *Bank Notes*, Sydney; Margaret Hinkle, *Tipton (Ind) Daily Tribune*; Charles House, *Milwaukee Journal*; Ben Kent, *Messenger-Inquirer*, Owensboro, Ky; Edith P. Lewis, *Nursing Outlook*; Walter Lowe, *Greensburg Daily News*; Sten Lundgren, *VI*, Stockholm; Lillian Mackesy, *Appleton (Wis) Post-Courier*; R. L. Pennells, *British Legion Journal*; Benjamin Pogrund, *Rand Daily Mail;* Rachel Ramsey, Greencastle *(Ind) Banner-Graphic*; Nancy C. Reitz, *Johnstown (Pa.) Tribune-Democrat*; Ivan Sandrof, *Worcester (Mass) Evening Gazette*; Dan Valentine and Vickie Sorensen, *Salt Lake Tribune*. My heartfelt thanks, too, to good if unknown friends on the *Aberdeen Press and Journal, Bristol Evening Post, Cape Argus, Cape Times, Corriere della Sera, Fresno Bee, Leicester Evening Mercury, Oxford Mail, Stuttgarter Nachrichten*, and the *Yorkshire Evening Post*.

The survivors and their relatives whose testimony I was thus enabled to record for posterity are listed elsewhere in this book, but among them I owe an unequalled debt to Mrs John L. Barkley, Hector MacQuarrie, Miss Edna Perrett, Fru Else (Dahl) Ullerup, Mrs Lydia (Phillips) Van Gass, Signora Tersilla Nardini Vicenzotto, and Dr Juan Zamora.

Finally, how can I thank those who worked closest to me throughout? Without the help of my friends at *The Reader's Digest*, notably Fulton Cursler Jr, Walter Hunt, and Kenneth Wilson, none of this would have been possible. In London, Joan St George Saunders and her research team handled a multitude of global queries with unflurried calm. Streamlined secretarial help came just when it was needed from Simone Busch, Christine Garner, Leonora Marshall and Barbara Welzel.

Elly Beintema, Michael Freeman and J. W. C. Garner solved all my photographic problems. Jill Beck's final typescript was the usual miracle of precision. My agents in London and New York, Graham Watson and John Cushman, never lost faith in the project even in the darkest days. And I am everlastingly grateful to my publishers in those cities, Lord Hardinge of Penshurst and Herman Gollob, who waited so long and patiently for the finished book.

Without the help of those researchers who in moments of dire emergency crossed their designated 'frontiers', I should have been lost indeed. Brigid Allen, Margaret Duff, Elizabeth Leslie, Margareta Runqvist and Maria Teresa Williams, all at times made an enormous contribution to the final manuscript by tackling research and interviews in countries other than their own.

For the first nine months of the project I had the invaluable support of Maria Teresa Vasta, who oversaw every step of the research planning. Though ill-health temporarily forced her to put aside this burden, she resisted with the tenacity of a 1918 flu-fighter and once again took her place in the battle-line.

Lastly, to my wife, goes as ever my deepest gratitude. Apart from researching and handling a mountain of correspondence from the earth's four corners which grew weekly, even daily, more formidable, she typed and re-typed the final draft, kept the home running serenely, and was always there when I needed her most to offer her support, her advice and encouragement.

Bibliography

Newspapers and Periodicals

A.B.C., Madrid; *Aftenposten*, Oslo; *Aftonbladet*, Stockholm; *Alabama Journal*, Montgomery; *Albuquerque Journal*, N.M.; *Algemeen Handelsblad*, Amsterdam; *Alkotmány*, Budapest; *Allmänna Svenska Läkartidn*, Stockholm; *All the World*, London; *L'Alsace*, Besançon; *American City*, New York; *American Legion Magazine*, New York; *American Journal of Clinical Medicine*, Chicago; *American Journal of Medical Science*, Philadelphia; *American Journal of Nursing*, New York; *American Journal of Public Health*, Boston; *American Medical History*, Chicago; *American Review of Reviews*, New York; *Arbetet*, Malmo; *Archives of Internal Medicine*, Chicago, Ill.; *Archives Medicales Belges*, Brussels; *The Argus*, Melbourne; *Arizona Republic*, Phoenix; *Arkansas Democrat*, Little Rock; *Atlanta Journal*; *The Auckland Weekly News*; *Avanti!* Milan; *Az Est*, Budapest; *Az Ujság*, Budapest.

Baltimore Sun; *Barbados Standard; Barre-Montpelier Times-Argus*, Vt.; *La Bataille*, Paris; *Beaufort Courier*, Beaufort West, Cape Province; *The Beira News and East Coast Chronicle*, Mozambique; *Belfast Telegraph*; *Bergens Tidende*; *Berliner Morgenpost*; *Berlingske Tidende*, Copenhagen; *Bermuda Colonist and Weekly Daily News*, Hamilton, Bermuda; *Bismarck Tribune*, North Dakota, U.S.A.; *Bohemia*, Prague; *Bollettino dell'Istituto Storico Italiano dell'Arte Sanitaria*, Rome; *Bosnisa Posta*, Sarajevo; *Boston Globe*; *Boston Medical and Surgical Journal*; *The Brandon Weekly Sun*; *The Brantford Expositor*; *Bremer Bürger-Zeitung*, Bremen; *British Medical Journal*, London; *Budapesti Hirlap*; *The Bulawayo Chronicle*; *Bulletin of Historical Medicine*, Baltimore, Md.

The Calgary Daily Herald; *The Cape Argus*, Cape Town; *The Cape Times*, Cape Town; *Ceylon Independent*, Colombo; *Ceylon Morning*

Leader, Colombo; *Ceylon Observer*, Colombo; *Charleston Gazette*, W.Va.; *The Charlottetown Herald*, Prince Edward Is.; *Chemung Historical Journal*, Elmira, N.Y. *The Chicago Daily Tribune*; *China Medical Journal*, Shanghai; *The Civil and Military Gazette*, Lahore; *The Clarion*, Belize; *The Clarion-Ledger*, Jackson, Miss.; *Colonial and Provincial Reporter*, Freetown Sierra Leone; *Columbia-State*, S.C.; *Columbus Dispatch*, Ohio; *Corriere della Sera*, Milan; *Courant*, Hartford, Conn.; *La Croix*, Paris; *Cromos*, Bogotá.

Dagbladet, Oslo; *Dagens Nyheter*, Stockholm; *The Daily Chronicle*, Georgetown, Guyana; *The Daily Colonist*, Victoria, B.C.; *Daily Express*, London; *The Daily Gleaner*, Fredericton, New Brunswick; *The Daily Gleaner*, Kingston, Jamaica; *Daily Mail*, London; *The Daily Malta Chronicle*, Valletta; *Daily Telegraph*, London; *Denver Post*, Colo.; *La Dépêche*, Toulouse; *La Dépêche Marocaine*, Tangier; *Derevenskaya Kommuna*, Leningrad; *Des Moines Register*, Iowa; *Deutsche Warschauer Zeitung*, Warsaw; *Deutsches Volksblatt*, Vienna; *Le Devoir*, Montreal; *Diamond Fields Advertiser*, Kimberley; *Dispatch*, St Paul, Minn.; *Dresdner Nachrichten*; *Dublin Evening Mail*; *Düsseldorfer Nachrichten*; *Dziennik Poznanski*, Poznan.

The East African Standard, Mombasa; *The East London Daily Despatch*; *The East Rand Express*, Germiston; *The Eastern Province Herald*, Port Elizabeth; *L'Echo de Bulgarie*, Sofia; *L'Echo de Paris*; *Edinburgh Medical Journal*; *The Egyptian Mail*, Cairo; *English-American News*, Berlin; *The Englishman*, Calcutta; *The Evening Post*, Wellington, N.Z.; *The Evening Star*, Dunedin, N.Z.; *The Evening Telegram*, St John's, Newfoundland.

The Federalist, St Georges, Grenada; *Le Figaro*, Paris; *Fiji Times and Herald*, Suva; *Folkets Dagblad Politiken*, Stockholm; *La France Libre*, Paris; *Frankfurter Zeitung*.

Il Giornale d'Italia, Rome; *The Glasgow Medical Journal*; *The Globe*, Toronto; *Głos Narodu*, Cracow; *The Gold Coast Nation*, Cape Coast, Ghana; *Good Old Days*, Denver, Mass.

Hamburger Echo; *Hamburger Nachrichten*; *The Hamilton Spectator*, Ont.; *The Hawkes Bay Herald*, Napier, N.Z,; *Hilal*, Istanbul; *L'Homme Libre*, Paris; *Hospital Social Services Quarterly*, New York; *Hufvudstadsbladet*, Helsinki; *L'Humanité*, Paris.

Idaho Statesman, Boise; *Illinois State Journal*, Springfield; *L'Illustration*, Paris; *L'Independance Roumaine*, Bucharest; *The Independent*, New

York; *Independent-Record*, Helena, Mont.; *Indian Medical Gazette*, Calcutta; *Indianapolis Star*; *Industrial Arts Magazine*, Milwaukee, Wis.; *Industrial South Africa*, Cape Town; *Insurance*, Cape Town; *L'Intransigeant*, Paris; *Irish Telegraph*, Londonderry; *Isafold*, Reykjavik; *Izvestiya murmanskovo Kraevovo soveta rabochix*, Murmansk; *Izvestiya narodnovo kommissariyata zdravokhraneniya*, Moscow.

Jamaica Times, Kingston; *Japan Times*, Tokyo; *Japan Weekly Chronicle*, Kobe; *Jornal do Comércio*, Lisbon; *Jornal do Comércio*, Rio de Janeiro; *Le Journal*, Paris; *Journal*, Wilmington, Del.; *Le Journal de Genève*; *Journal-Lancet*, Minneapolis, Minn.; *Journal Officiel des Etablissements Français en l'Océanie*, Papeete; *Journal of Infectious Diseases*, Chicago; *Journal of Laboratory and Clinical Medicine*, St Louis, Mo.; *Journal of Occupational Medicine*, Pitman, N.J.; *Journal of the American Medical Association*, Chicago; *Journal of the Canadian Medical Association*, Toronto; *Journal of the Kansas Medical Society*, Topeka, Kansas; *Journal of the Medical Society of New Jersey*, Newark, N.J.; *Journal of the Royal Naval Medical Services*, London.

Kansas City Star, Kansas City, Mo.; *Kennebec Journal*, Augusta, Me.; *København*, Copenhagen; *Kölnische Volkszeitung*, Cologne; *Köningsberger Tageblatt*, Kaliningrad; *Konstanzer Zeitung*; *Krasnaya Gazeta*, Petrograd; *Kurjer Poznański*, Poznan.

The Labour World, Johannesburg; *The Lagos Weekly Record*; *The Lancet*, London; *Laval Médical*, Quebec; *Lexington Herald*, Ky.; *La Libre Parole*, Paris; *Lincoln Journal*, Nebr.; *The Livingstone Mail*, Zambia; *Los Angeles Times*; *L.S.D.*, Johannesburg; *Lyon Républicain*; *The Lyttelton Times*, Christchurch, N.Z.

The Madras Mail; *The Mafeking Mail*; *Magyar Hirlap*, Budapest; *The Malay Mail*, Kuala Lumpur; *The Malaya Tin and Rubber Journal*, Ipoh; *Manchester Guardian*; *Manitoba Free Press*, Winnipeg; *Le Matin*, Paris; *Medical Journal of Australia*, Sydney, N.S.W.; *Medical Journal of South Africa*, Cape Town; *Medical Press and Circular*, London; *The Medical Record*, New York; *Medicinhistorisk Årsbok*, Stockholm; *Medicinsk Forum*, Copenhagen; *Le Messenger d'Athènes*; *Miami Herald*; *Michigan State Journal*; *Military Medicine*, Washington, D.C.; *The Military Surgeon*, Washington, D.C.; *The Milwaukee Journal*; *The Missouri Historical Review*, Kansas City, Mo.; *Modern Hospital*, St Louis, Mo.; *Moghreb Al-Aksa*, Tangier; *Monitor and New Hampshire Patriot*, Concord, N.H.; *The Montreal Gazette*; *Morgenbladet*, Oslo; *The Morning Bulletin*, Edmonton, Alberta; *The Morning Chronicle*, Halifax, N.S.; *Munchener Post*, Munich.

La Nación, Buenos Aires; *Nationaltidende*, Copenhagen; *La Nazione*, Florence; *Nebraska Medical Journal*, Lincoln; *Népsava*, Budapest; *Neues Pester Journal*, Budapest; *Nevada Appeal*, Carson City; *The New Orleans Times-Picayune*; *The New York Medical Journal*; *The New York Statistician*; *The New York Times*; *The New Zealand Herald*, Auckland; *New Zealand Medical Journal*, Dunedin; *The New Zealand Times*, Wellington; *Nieuwe Rotterdamsche Courant*; *The North Carolina Medical Journal*, Raleigh; *North China Herald*, Shanghai; *Le Nouvelliste de Lyon*; *Nowa Riforma*, Cracow; *The Nyasaland Times*, Blantyre, Malawi.

L'Oeuvre, Paris; *The Oklahoman*; *The Oregon Historical Quarterly*, Portland, Oreg.; *Oregon Statesman*, Salem; *Otago Daily Times*, Dunedin, N.Z.; *The Otago Witness*, Dunedin, N.Z.; *The Ottawa Evening Citizen*; *The Overland Monthly*, San Francisco; *The Oxford Mail*.

The Papuan Courier Weekly, Port Moresby; *Patris*, Athens; *The Penang Gazette*; *Pester Lloyd*, Budapest; *Pesti Hirlap*, Budapest; *Le Petit Journal*, Paris; *Le Petit Marseillais*; *Le Petit Parisien*; *La Petite Gironde*, Bordeaux; *Philadelphia Bulletin*; *The Pictorial*, Durban; *Pierre Capital-Journal*, S.D.; *The Pioneer*; *The Pittsburgh Gazette*; *The Polynesian Gazette*, Levuka, Fiji; *Il Popolo D'Italia*, Milan; *Le Populaire*, Paris; *The Port of Spain Gazette*; *The Practitioner*, London; *Pravda*, Moscow and Petrograd; *La Prensa*, Buenos Aires; *The Press*, Christchurch, N.Z.; *Proodos*, Athens; *Providence Journal*, R.I.

The Quebec Telegraph.

Raleigh News and Observer, N.C.; *Rand Daily Mail*, Johannesburg; *Il Resto del Carlino*, Bologna; *Revista de la Sociedad Venezolana de la Medicina*, Caracas; *Revue Médicale de la Suisse Romande*, Geneva; *The Rhodesia Herald*, Salisbury; *Richmond Times-Dispatch*, Richmond, Va.; *Riforma Medicina*, Naples; *The River Plate Observer*, Buenos Aires.

The St Louis Post-Dispatch, St Louis, Mo.; *The Salt Lake Tribune*, Salt Lake City, Utah; *The San Francisco Chronicle*; *The Sarawak Gazette*, Kuching; *Science*, New York; *Scientific American*, New York; *The Scotsman*, Edinburgh; *Scribner's Magazine*, New York; *Seattle Post-Intelligencer*; *O Seculo*, Lisbon; *Severnaya Kommuna*, Petrograd; *Sierra Leone Weekly News*; *The Singapore Free Press*; *Social-Demokraten*, Stockholm; *El Sol*, Madrid; *South African Fruit Grower*, Johannesburg; *The South African Lady's Pictorial*, Cape Town; *South African Mining and Engineering Record*, Johannesburg; *The South*

China Morning Post, Hong Kong; *La Stampa,* Turin; *The Star,* Auckland, N.Z.; *The Statesman,* Austin, Tex.; *The Statesman,* Calcutta; *The Straits Echo,* Georgetown, Malaya; *The Straits Times,* Singapore; *Sudhoffs Archiv für Geschichte der Medizin,* Leipzig; *The Survey,* New York; *Svenska Dagbladet,* Stockholm; *Svenska tidningen,* Helsinki.

Der Tag, Berlin; *De Telegraaf,* Amsterdam; *Le Temps,* Paris; *Tenessean,* Nashville; *Tidens Tegn,* Oslo; *Tideskrift for den norske laegeforening,* Oslo; *The Timaru Herald,* Timaru, N.Z.; *The Times,* Kingstown, St Vincent; *The Times,* London; *Times of Ceylon,* Colombo; *Times of India,* Bombay; *The Times of Malaya,* Ipoh; *Today's Health,* Chicago; *Tondernsche Zeitung,* Tondern, Denmark; *Topeka Journal*; *Transactions of the Medical Society of the State of New York*; *Transactions of the Royal Society of Medicine,* London; *La Tribune Congolaise,* Antwerp; *The Trinidad Guardian,* Port of Spain.

The Uganda Herald, Kampala.

Vancouver Daily Province; *Vercherniye izvestiya,* Moscow; *Virginia Medical Monthly,* Richmond, Va.; *De Volkstem,* Pretoria.

The Waimate Times, Waimate, N.Z.; *The Wanganui Herald,* Wanganui, N.Z.; *The Washington Post*; *Weekly Rangoon Times and Overland Summary*; *The West Australian,* Perth; *Wyoming State-Tribune,* Cheyenne.

The Yale Review, New Haven, Conn.; *The Yorkshire Post,* Leeds.

Za Narod, Shenkursk; *Znamiya Trudovoi Kommuni,* Moscow; *The Zululand Times,* Eshowe.

Printed Sources

Ackerknecht, Dr Edwin H., *History and Geography of the Most Important Diseases* (New York: Hafner Publishing Co., 1955).

Adam, H. Pearl, *Paris Sees it through: a Diary, 1914-19* (London: Hodder and Stoughton, 1919).

Aldrich, Mildred, *When Johnny comes marching home* (Boston: Small Maynard, 1919).

Alexander, Frederick W., *Twenty Years working of the Electrolytic Disinfectant Plant of Poplar* (Poplar: Public Health Office, 1923).

Allen, F. L., *Only Yesterday* (New York: Harper & Bros., 1931).

Alport, A. Cecil, *The Lighter Side of the War* (London: Hutchinson, 1932).

Arbeiten aus dem Kaiserlichen Gesundheitsamte, vol. 53 (Berlin: Julius Springer, 1922).

Baker, Ray Stannard, *Woodrow Wilson, Life and Letters*, vol. VIII (New York: Doubleday Doran, 1939).

Baker, Sarah, J., *Fighting for Life* (London: Robert Hale, 1940).

Balfour, Andrew, and Scott, Henry H., *Health Problems and the Empire* (London: Collins, 1925).

Banov, Dr Leon, *As I Recall* (Columbia, S.C.: R. L. Bryan Co., 1970).

Barkley, John Lewis, *No Hard Feelings* (New York: Cosmopolitan Book Co., 1930).

Baron, A. L., *Man against Germs* (New York: E. P. Dutton, 1957).

Bayly, Hugh Wansey, *Triple Challenge* (London: Hutchinson, 1935).

Bean, C. E. W., *The Australian Imperial Force in France, 1918*, vol. VI (Sydney: Angus & Robertson, 1942).

Bennett, F. O., *Hospital on the Avon* (Christchurch, N.Z.: North Canterbury Hospital Board, 1962).

Benwell, Harry, *History of the Yankee Division* (Boston: Cornhill, 1919).

Berger, Maurice, *Germany after the Armistice* (New York: Putnam, 1920).

Bishop, R. W. S., *My Moorland Patients* (London: John Murray, 1922).

Blenkinsop, Maj.-Gen. Sir L. J. and Rainey, Lt.-Col. J. W., *History of the Great War – Veterinary Services* (London: H.M.S.O., 1925).

Bourne, Geoffrey, *We met at Barts* (London: Frederick Muller, 1963).

Bowen, Louise de Koven, *Growing up With a City* (New York: Macmillan, 1926).

Bowerbank, Sir Fred, *A Doctor's Story* (Wellington, N.Z.: The Wingfield Press, 1958).

Boylston, Helen Dore, *Sister* (New York: Ives Washburn, 1927).

Bridges, Philippa, *A Walk-about in Australia* (London: Hodder & Stoughton, 1925).

Bull, William P., *From Medicine man to Medical man* (Toronto: Parkins-Bull Foundation, 1934).

Burman, Jose, *Disaster struck South Africa* (Cape Town: C. Struik (Pty), Ltd, 1971).

Burnet, Sir Francis and Clark, Ellen, *Influenza* (Melbourne: Macmillan, 1942).

Burr, Dr C. B. (ed.), *Medical History of Michigan*, vol. 1 (Minneapolis: Bruce Publishing Co., 1930).

Burton, Alfred, *The First Ten Years of the Heart of Africa Mission* (London: Heart of Africa Mission, 1920).

Byam, William, *The Road to Harley Street* (London: Geoffrey Bles, 1963).

Cameron, Charlotte, *A Cheechako in Alaska and the Yukon* (London: T. Fisher Unwin, 1920).

Casson, Stanley, *Steady Drummer* (London: G. Bell and Sons, 1935).

Cavina, Giovanni, *L'influenza epidemica attraverso i secoli* (Rome: Possi, 1959).

Charteris, Brig.-Gen. John, *At G.H.Q.* (London: Cassell, 1931).

Chierici, Aldo, *Italiani e Arabi in Libia* (Rome: Editrice M. Garra, 1919).

Clapp, Charles, Jr., *The Big Bender* (New York: Harper & Bros., 1938).

Clarkson, Grosvenor, B., *Industrial America in the World War* (Boston: Houghton Mifflin, 1923).

Close, Upton, *In the Land of the laughing Buddha* (New York: Putnam, 1934).

Cocks, E. M. Somers, *A Friend in need* (Christchurch, N.Z.: Nurse Maude District Nursing Association, 1950).

Coffman, Edward T., *The war to end all wars* (New York: Oxford U.P., 1968).

Collins, Joseph, *Italy re-visited* (London: T. Fisher Unwin, 1920).

Collis, Robert, *The Silver Fleece* (London: Thomas Nelson, 1936).

Colony of Fiji, The, 1874-1931 (Suva: J. J. McHugh, 1931).

Cook, J. Gordon, *Virus in the Cell* (New York: Dial Press, 1957).

Cooksey, J. J. and McLeish, A., *Religion and Civilisation in West Africa* (London: World Dominion Press, 1931).

Coolidge, Calvin, *Autobiography* (New York: Cosmopolitan Book Co., 1929).

Cooper, Page, *The Bellevue Story* (New York: Crowell, 1948).

Corday, Michel, *The Paris Front* (New York: E. P. Dutton, 1934).

Cormack, Annie, *Chinese Birthday, Wedding, Funeral and Other Customs* (Peking: China Booksellers Ltd, 1922).

Counsell, H. E., *37, The Broad* (London: Robert Hale, 1943).

Cross, Arthur J., *Twenty Years in Lambaland* (London: Marshall Bros, 1925).

Crosthwait, William L. and Fischer, Ernest G., *The Last Stitch* (Philadelphia: J. B. Lippincott, 1956).

Cummins, S. L. (ed.), *Studies of Influenza in Hospitals of the British Armies in France, 1918* (London: Medical Research Committee, 1919).

Cumpston, Dr J. H. L. and McCallum, Dr Frank, *Public Health Services in Australia* (Geneva: League of Nations, 1926).

Cunningham, John T., *Newark* (Newark: New Jersey Historical Society, 1966).

Cushing, Harvey, *From a Surgeon's Journal* (London: Constable, 1936).

Davis, Michael M. Jr, *Immigrant Health and the Community* (New York: Harper Bros, 1921).

De Debrovits, Dr Alexander, *Public Health Services in Hungary* (Geneva: League of Nations, 1925).

De Gooyer, A. C., *De Spaanse griep van '18* (Amsterdam: Philips-Duphar, 1968).

De Vibraye, Count Tony, *Carnet de Route d'un Cavalier* (Paris: privately printed, 1939).

Delaunay, Paul, *Paysages de Guerre* (Paris: Librairie Amédée Legrand, 1921).

Del Mar, Frances, *A Year among the Maoris* (London: Ernest Benn, 1924).

Dock, Lavinia, *History of American Red Cross Nursing* (New York: Macmillan, 1922).

Dos Passos, John, *Mr Wilson's War* (New York: Doubleday, 1963).

Drew, Lieut. H. T. B., *The War Effort of New Zealand* (Auckland, N.Z.: Whitcombe & Tombs, 1923).

Dublin, Dr Louis, *Twenty-five years of Health Progress* (New York: Metropolitan Life Insurance Co., 1937).

Edmonds, Brig.-Gen., Sir James and Davies, Maj.-Gen. H. R., *History of the Great War: Military Operations, Italy, 1915-19* (London: H.M.S.O., 1949).

Eisenmenger, Anna, *Blockade, 1914-24* (London: Constable, 1932).

An Englishwoman, *From a Russian Diary* (London: John Murray, 1921).

Enriquez, Colin, *A Burmese Arcady* (London: Seeley Service Co., 1923).

Etherton, Lt.-Col. Percy, *In the Heart of Asia* (London: Constable, 1925).

Fairbrother, R. W., *Handbook of Filterable Viruses* (London: William Heinemann, 1934).

Falls, Capt., Cyril, *History of the Great War: Egypt and Palestine*, pt. II (London: H.M.S.O., 1930). *History of the Great War: Military Operations, Macedonia* (London: H.M.S.O., 1935).

Farwell, George, *Last Days in Paradise* (London: Gollancz, 1964).

Fedden, Marguerite, *From an Abbeville Window* (Bristol: J. W. Arrowsmith, 1922).

Fine, Joseph, *Filterable Virus Diseases in Man* (Edinburgh: E. & S. Livingstone, 1932).

Fletcher, Maisie, *The Bright Countenance* (London: Hodder & Stoughton, 1965).

Fokeer, A. F., *The Spanish Influenza in Mauritius* (Port Louis: Mauritius Indian Times, 1931).

Forbes-White, F. A. C., *Checkmate* (London: George Harrap, 1927).

Franck, Harry R., *Vagabonding through changing Germany* (New York: Harper & Bros, 1920).

Frey, Dr Gottfried, *Public Health Services in Germany* (Geneva: League of Nations, 1924).

Frost, W. H., *The Papers of Wade Hampton Frost* (New York: Commonwealth Fund, 1941).

Frothingham, Thomas G., *The American Reinforcement in the World War* (Garden City, N.Y.: Doubleday Page, 1927).

Garland, Joseph E., *To Meet these Wants* (Providence, R.I.: Rhode Island Hospital, 1963).

Garrett, Franklin M., *Atlanta and Environs*, vol. II (Athens, Georgia: University of Georgia Press, 1969).

Gibson, John, *Physician to the World* (Durham, N.C.: Duke U.P., 1950).

Gifford, Edward Winslow, *Tongan Society* (Honolulu: Bernice P. Bishop Museum, 1929).

Glemser, Bernard, *The Last Safari* (London: Bodley Head, 1970).

Godsell, Philip, *Arctic Trader* (New York: G. P. Putnam, 1934).

Gogarty, Rev. H. A., *In the Land of the Kikuyus* (Dublin: M. H. Gill & Son Ltd, 1920).

Golosmanoff, Dr Ivan, *The Public Health Services of Bulgaria* (Geneva: League of Nations, 1926).

Gordon, Doris, *Backblocks Baby-Doctor* (London: Faber & Faber, 1955).

Gosse, Philip, *Memoirs of a Camp Follower* (London: Longmans Green, 1934).

Gram, Dr H. M., *The Public Health Services in Norway* (Geneva: League of Nations, 1927).

Graves, Charles, *Invasion by Virus* (London: Icon Books, 1969).

Graves, Robert and Hodge, Alan, *The Long Week-End* (London: Faber & Faber, 1940).

Grayland, Eugene C., *New Zealand Disasters* (Wellington, N.Z.: A. H. and A. W. Reed, 1957).

Greenwood, Alfred, *The Public Health Administration of Yugoslavia* (Maidstone: W. P. Dickinson, 1925).

Gullett, H. S., *The Imperial Australian Force in Sinai and Palestine* (Sydney: Angus & Robertson, 1923).

Gunn, Clement B., *Leaves from the Life of a Country Doctor* (Edinburgh: The Moray Press, 1935).

Hackett, J. D., *Health Maintenance in Industry* (Chicago: A. W. Shaw Co., 1925).

Haldane, Elizabeth S., *The British Nurse in Peace and War* (London: John Murray, 1923).

Hall, Grace, *No Time to Die* (Cape Town: Howard Timmins (Pty), Ltd, 1959).

Hare, Ronald, *Pomp and Pestilence* (New York: The Philosophical Library, 1955).

Harley Street Doctor, *A Doctor's Diary* (London: Hutchinson, 1925).

Headlam, Lt.-Col. Cuthbert, *History of the Guards' Division in the Great War* (London: John Murray, 1924).

Heagerty, John J., *Four Centuries of Medical History in Canada*, vol. 1 (Toronto: Macmillan, 1928).

Health Organisation in Denmark (Geneva: League of Nations, 1924).

Health Organisation in Japan (Geneva: League of Nations, 1925).

Heiser, Victor, *A Doctor's Odyssey* (London: Jonathan Cape, 1936).

Henrikson, Viktor, *A Doctor's Story* (London: Michael Joseph, 1959).

Henschen, Folke, *The History and Geography of Diseases*, trans. Joan Tate (New York: Delacorte Press, 1966).

Herman, Leon, *A Surgeon thinks it Over* (Philadelphia: University of Pennsylvania Press, 1962).

Herrick, James B., *Memories of Eighty Years* (Chicago: University of Chicago Press, 1949).

Hirsch, Dr August, *Geographical and Historical Pathology*, vol. I (London: The New Sydenham Society, 1883).

Hoehling, A. A., *The Great Epidemic* (Boston: Little Brown, 1961).

Holden, Frank, *War Memories* (Athens, Georgia: Athens Book Co., 1922).

Holmgren, Israel, *Mitt liv*, vol. II (Stockholm: Natur och Kultur, 1959).

Hooper, H. D., *Africa in the Making* (London: United Council for Missionary Education, 1922).

Hoover, Herbert, *Memoirs*, vol. I, *The Years of Adventure* (New York: Macmillan, 1951).

Hope, E. W., *Industrial Hygiene and Medicine* (London: Baillière, Tindall & Cox, 1923).

Howard, William Travis, Jr, *Public Health Administration and the Natural History of Disease in Maryland, 1797-1920* (Washington, D.C.: Carnegie Institution, 1924).

Huber, Michel, *La Population de la France pendant la Guerre* (Paris: Les Presses Universitaires de France, 1931).

Humphries, Wilfred, *Patrolling in Papua* (London: T. Fisher Unwin, 1923).

Hutson, Rev. James, *Chinese Life in the Tibetan Foothills* (Shanghai: Far Eastern Geographical Settlement, 1921).

Hutton, Samuel K., *A Shepherd of the Snows* (London: Hodder & Stoughton, 1936).

——, *Health Conditions and Disease Incidence among the Eskimos of Labrador* (Poole, Dorset: J. Looker, 1925).

—— and Binney, George A., *The Eskimo Book of Knowledge* (London: Hudson's Bay Company, 1931).

Ingle, Dwight, *A Dozen Doctors* (Chicago: University of Chicago Press, 1963).

Inglis, Theodora, *New Lanterns in Old China* (New York: Fleming H. Revell Co., 1923).

Ireland, Maj.-Gen. M. W., *The Medical Department of the United States Army in the World War* (15 vols) (Washington: Government Printing Office, 1923-7).

James, A. T. S., *Twenty-Five Years of the L.M.S.* (London: London Missionary Society, 1923).

Jitta, Dr N. M. J., *Public Health Services in the Netherlands* (Geneva: League of Nations, 1924).

Keable, Robert, *Tahiti: Isle of Dreams* (London: Hutchinson, 1925).
Keesing, Felix, *Modern Samoa* (London: Allen & Unwin, 1934).
Kernodle, Portia, *The Red Cross Nurse in Action* (New York: Harper Bros, 1949).
Kincaid, C. A., *Forty Years a Public Servant* (Edinburgh: William Blackwood, 1934).

Lamb, Dr Albert, *The Presbyterian Hospital and the Columbia-Presbyterian Medical Center, 1868-1943* (New York: Columbia University Press, 1955).
Lambie, Mary, *My Story* (Christchurch, N.Z.: N. M. Peryer, 1956).
Langdon, Robert, *Island of Love* (London: Cassell, 1959).
Lapointe, Arthur, *Soldier of Quebec* (Montreal: Editions Edouard Garard, 1931).
Lee, Roger I., *Health and Disease: Their determining factors* (Boston: Little Brown, 1920).
Lethbridge, Alan, *Germany as it is Today* (London: Eveleigh Nash, 1921).
Livingstone, W. P., *Laws of Livingstonia* (London: Hodder & Stoughton, 1921).
London, Charmian, *The New Hawaii* (London: Mills & Boon, 1923).
Lucas, Sir Charles, *The Empire at War*, vols III, IV and V (Oxford: O.U.P., 1921-4).
Ludendorff, Gen. Erich, *My War Memories* (London: Hutchinson, 1919).

McCarthy, Mary, *Memories of a Catholic Girlhood* (London: Heinemann, 1953).
Macartney, William, *Fifty Years a Country Doctor* (London: Geoffrey Bles, 1938).
McCoy, Donald, *Calvin Coolidge: the Quiet President* (New York: Macmillan, 1967).
MacDonald, David, *Twenty Years in Tibet* (London: Seeley Service & Co., 1932).
Mackie, Alexander, *Memories of a Scotch Doctor* (Aberdeen: privately printed, 1949).
MacPherson, Maj.-Gen. Sir W. G., *History of the Great War: Medical Services, General History*, vol. III (London: H.M.S.O., 1924).
MacQuarrie, Hector, *Tahiti Days* (New York: George Doran Co., 1921),
Magnuson, Paul, *Ring the Night Bell* (London: William Heinemann, 1961).

Mann, A. J., *The Salonica Front* (London: A. & C. Black, 1920).

Manson, Cecil and Celia, *Dr Agnes Bennett* (London: Michael Joseph, 1960).

March, Gen. Payton, *The Nation at War* (Garden City, N.Y.: Doubleday Doran, 1932).

Marshall, Max, *Crusader Undaunted* (New York: Macmillan, 1958).

May, Earl Chapin and Oursler, Will, *The Prudential* (Garden City, N.Y.: Doubleday, 1950).

Mess, Henry A., *Industrial Tyneside* (London: Ernest Benn, 1928).

Mignon, Henri, *La service de santé pendant la guerre*, 4 vols (Paris: Masson, 1926).

Millard, Shirley, *I saw them die* (London: George Harrap, 1936).

Mr Punch's History of the Great War (London: Cassell, 1920).

Moberley, Brig.-Gen. F. J., *History of the Great War: the campaign in Mesopotamia, 1914-18*, vol. IV (London: H.M.S.O., 1927).

Monti, Achille, *La Malaria, l'ittero infettivo, l'influenza* (Milan: Hoepli, 1921).

Moore, Harry H., *Public Health in the United States* (New York: Harper Bros, 1923).

Moorshead, R. Fletcher, *The Way of the Doctor* (London: The Carey Press, 1926).

Mortara, Giorgio, *La salute pubblica in Italia durante e dopo la guerra* (Bari: Laterza, 1925).

Mowrer, Edgar, *Triumph and Turmoil* (New York: Weybright & Tulley, 1968).

Namora, Fernando Goncalves, *Retalhos da Vida de um Médico* (Lisbon: Guimâraes Editores, 1954).

Nathan, Manfred, *South Africa from within* (London: John Murray, 1926).

Nevinson, H. W., *Last Changes: Last Chances* (London: Nisbet, 1928).

Newman, George, *Report on the Pandemic of Influenza, 1918-19* (London: H.M.S.O., 1920).

Nichols, Henry J., *Carriers in Infectious Diseases* (Baltimore: Williams & Wilkins Co., 1922).

Oakenfull, J. C., *Brazil, Past, Present and Future* (London: John Bale, Sons & Danielson Ltd, 1919).

O'Brien, Frederick, *Mystic Isles of the South Seas* (New York: The Century Co., 1920).

——, *Atolls of the Sun* (New York: The Century Co., 1921).

Oliver, Wade, *The Man who lived for Tomorrow* (New York: E. P. Dutton, 1941).

Owen, H. Collinson, *Salonica and After* (London: Hodder & Stoughton, 1919).

Oxford and Asquith, Earl H. H. A., *Letters to a Friend* (London: Geoffrey Bles, 1933).

Palmer, Alan, *The Gardeners of Salonika* (London: André Deutsch, 1965).
Palmer, Frederick, *Newton D. Baker: America at War*, 2 vols (New York: Dodd Mead, 1931).
Pamietnik bezrobotynch, 2nd ed. (Warsaw: Panstowe Wydawnictwo Ekonomiczne, 1967).
Pantazzi, Ethel Greening, *Roumania in Light and Shadow* (London: T. Fisher Unwin, 1921).
Parry, Robert Hughes, *Under the Cherry Tree* (Llandysul: The Comerian Press, 1969).
Parsons, Robert P., *Trail to Light* (Indianapolis: Bobbs-Merrill, 1943).
Patterson, Lt.-Col. J. H., *With the Judaeans in the Palestine Campaign* (London: Hutchinson, 1922).
Paul, Dr Hugh, *The Control of Communicable Diseases* (London: Harvey & Blythe, 1952).
Peel, Mrs C. S., *How we lived then* (New York: Dodd Mead, 1929).
Pelc, Dr Hynek J., *Organisation of the Public Health Services in Czechoslovakia* (Geneva: League of Nations, 1924).
Pemberton, John, *Will Pickles of Wensleydale* (London: Geoffrey Bles, 1970).
Pershing, Gen. John J., *My Experiences in the World War* (New York: F. A. Stokes Co., 1931).
Pitt, Barrie, *1918: The Last Act* (London: Cassell, 1962).
Platt, Kate, *The Home and Health in India* (London: Baillière, Tindall & Cox, 1925).
Portman, Lionel, *Three Asses in Bolivia* (London: Grant Richards, 1922).
Pottle, Frederick, *Stretchers!* (New Haven: Yale U.P., 1929).
Power, Harold, *Bush Doctor* (London: Robert Hale, 1970).
Preston, Lt.-Col. the Hon. R. M. P., *The Desert Mounted Corps* (London: Constable, 1921).
Prévost, Jean, *Dix-huitième année* (Paris: Gallimard, 1929).
Pritchett, V. S., *A Cab at the Door* (London: Chatto & Windus, 1968).
Prokl, K. and Kowalczewski, Dr J., ed., *Polskie prawo sanitarne* (Warsaw: Lekarski Instytut Naukowo-Wydawniczy, 1946).
Ptaschkina, Nelly, *Diary*, trans. Pauline De Chary (London: Jonathan Cape, 1923).
The Public Health Services in New Zealand (Geneva: League of Nations, 1928).

Quinto, Gian Bino, *Appunti di un ragazzo genovese di tanti anni fa* (Genoa: Pagano, 1970).

Rey, Charles E., *Unconquered Abyssinia* (London: Seeley Service & Co., 1923).
Rice, Thurman, *A Textbook of Bacteriology* (Philadelphia: W. B. Saunders Co., 1942).
Riddell, Lord, *War Diary* (London: Ivor Nicholson & Watson, 1933).
Robb, Douglas, *Medical Odyssey* (Auckland, N.Z.: William Collins, 1967).
Rogers, Fred B. and Sayre, A. R., *The Healing Art* (Trenton, N.J.: Medical Society of New Jersey, 1966).
Rondthaler, Bishop Edward, *Memorabilia of Fifty Years* (Raleigh, N.C.: Edwards & Broughton Co., 1928).
Rorie, David, *A Medico's Luck in the War* (Aberdeen: Milne & Hutchinson, 1929).
Ross, Leyland and Grobin, Allen, *This Democratic Roosevelt* (New York: E. P. Dutton, 1932).
Rowe, N. A., *Samoa under the Sailing Gods* (London: G. P. Putnam, 1930).
Rudin, Harry, *Armistice 1918* (New Haven: Yale U.P., 1944).

Sams, Lt.-Col. H. A., *The Post Office of India in the Great War* (Bombay: The Times Press, 1922).
Sandes, Major Edward, *In Kut and Captivity with the Sixth Indian Division* (London: John Murray, 1919).
Sandilands, Lt.-Col. H. R., *The 23rd Division* (Edinburgh: William Blackwood, 1925).
Sauerbruch, Fernand, *A Surgeon's Life* (London: André Deutsch, 1953).
Schofield, Alfred, *Behind the Brass Plate* (London: Sampson Low and Marston, 1928).
Schroetter, Dr Hermann, *Public Health Services in Austria* (Geneva: League of Nations, 1923).
Scott, Ernest, *Australia during the War* (Sydney: Angus & Robertson, 1936).
Sen, Rajendra Kumara, *A Treatise on Influenza with Special Reference to the Pandemic of 1919* (North Lakhimpur, Assam: privately printed, 1923).
Shipley, Arthur E., *The Voyage of a Vice-Chancellor* (Cambridge: C.U.P., 1919).
Slosson, Preston, *The Great Crusade and After* (New York: Macmillan, 1930).
Smith, Lesley, *Four Years out of Life* (London: Philip Allan, 1931).
Snell, Sidney, H., *A Doctor at Work and Play* (London: John Bale,

Sons & Curnow, 1937).

Sonnenberg, Max, *The Way I saw it* (Cape Town: Howard Timmins (Pty) Ltd, 1957).

Spagnol, Tito, *Memoriette marziali e veneree* (Milan: Mario Spagnol, 1970).

Speakman, Marie, *Memories* (Wilmington, Del.: The Greenwood Bookshop, 1937).

Stamp, Winifred, *Doctor Himself* (London: Hamish Hamilton, 1949).

Starr, John, *Hospital City* (New York: Crown, 1957).

Stroebel, Heinrich, *The German Revolution and After*, trans. H. J. Stenning (London: Jarrolds, 1921).

Stuck, Hudson, A., *A Winter Circuit of our Arctic Coast* (London: T. Werner Laurie, 1919).

Sullivan, Mark, *Our Times*, vol. v (New York: Scribner, 1972).

Sutherland, Halliday, *A Time to Keep* (London: Geoffrey Bles, 1935).

Swann, Herbert, *Home on the Neva* (London: Victor Gollancz, 1968).

Sydney Morning Herald and Its Record of Australian Life (Sydney: John Fairfax & Sons, 1931).

Tailhade, Laurent, *Reflets de Paris, 1918-19* (Paris: Jean Fort, 1921).

Tales from the African Jungle (London: Church Missionary Society, 1924).

Tamagawa, Kathleen, *Holy Prayers in a Horse's Ear* (New York: Ray Long & Richard R. Smith, 1932).

Tarrassevitch, Lev, *Epidemics in Russia since 1914* (Geneva: League of Nations, 1922).

Tayler, Henrietta, *A Scottish Nurse at Work* (London: The Bodley Head, 1920).

Taylor, Emerson Gifford, *New England in France, 1917-19* (Boston: Houghton Mifflin, 1920).

Taylor, Harry P., *A Shetland Parish Doctor* (Lerwick, Shetland: J. & J. Manson, *Shetland News* Office, 1948).

Teichman, Eric, *Travels of a Consular Officer in North-West China* (Cambridge: C.U.P., 1921).

Teichman, Capt. Oskar, *The Diary of a Yeomanry M.O.* (London: T. Fisher Unwin, 1921).

Thalmann, Dr Hans, *Die Grippeepidemie 1918-19 in Zürich* (Zürich: Juris Druch Verlag, 1968).

Top, Dr Franklin H., ed., *The History of American Epidemiology* (St Louis: C. V. Mosby Co., 1952).

Vaughan, Victor C., *Epidemiology and Public Health* (St Louis: C. V. Mosby Co., 1922).

——, *A Doctor's Memories* (Indianapolis: Bobbs-Merrill, 1926).

Wald, Lilian D., *Windows on Henry Street* (Boston: Little Brown, 1941).

Warner, Jack (with Dean Jennings), *My First 100 Years in Hollywood* (New York: Doubleday, 1964).

Wauchope, Gladys, *The Story of a Woman Physician* (Bristol: John Wright & Sons, 1963).

Weinthal, Leo, *The Story of the Cape-Cairo Railway, 1887-1922* (London: Pioneer Publishing Co., 1923-6).

Westman, Stefan, *A Surgeon's Story* (London: William Kimber, 1962).

Weymouth, Anthony, *Who'd Be a Doctor?* (London: Rich & Cowan, 1937).

Whitshed, Juliet De Key, *Come to the Cookhouse Door*, (London: Herbert Joseph, 1932).

Williams, Greer, *Virus Hunters* (London: Hutchinson, 1960).

Williams, Richard and Dorothy, *Family Doctor* (London: Peter Davies, 1954).

Williams, T. G., *The Main Currents of Social and Industrial Change in England, 1870-1924* (London: Pitman, 1925).

Williams, William Carlos, *Autobiography* (London: MacGibbon & Kee, 1968).

Willinsky, Abraham, *A Doctor's Memoirs* (Toronto: Macmillan, 1960).

Wilson, Dorothy Clarke, *Dr Ida* (London: Hodder & Stoughton, 1960).

Wilson, Dorothy Clarke, *Ten Fingers for God* (London: Hodder & Stoughton, 1965).

Wilson, Rev. G. H., *A Missionary in Nyasaland* (London: Universities Mission to Central Africa, 1920).

Wilson, R. McNair, *Doctor's Progress* (London.: Eyre & Spottiswoode, 1938).

Winslow, Charles, *The Conquest of Epidemic Disease* (Princeton, N.J.: Princeton U. P., 1943).

Withington, Alfreda, *Mine Eyes Have Seen* (London: Robert Hale, 1945).

Woodward, Ernest, *Short Journey* (London: Faber & Faber, 1942).

Woolley, C. L., *From Kastamuni to Kedos* (Oxford: Basil Blackwell, 1921).

Wratislaw, Albert, *A Consul in the East* (Edinburgh: William Blackwood, 1924).

Zhdanov, V. M., Soloviev, V. D. and Epshtein, F. G., *Uchenie o grippe* (Moscow: Medgiz, 1958).

Zinsser, H. A. W., *A Textbook of Bacteriology* (Philadelphia: G. Appleton Co., 1922).

Manuscript Sources

Alaska Packer's Association: Reports on the 1919 Influenza Epidemic at Kvichak, Naknek and Nushagak Stations, Bristol Bay. (Courtesy R. N. De Armand, State of Alaska Historical Library, Juneau.)

Balanguer, Spain: 'Libro Verde', Minutes of the Town Council concerning La Gripe. (Courtesy Mayor and Council of Balanguer.)

Barton, Cranleigh H. Journal of the District Solicitor to the Public Trust Office, Christchurch, N.Z. (Courtesy Cranleigh H. Barton.)

Bedeschi, Lieut. Enrico. Diary of Lager E. Josefstadt, Bohemia, 1917-18. (Courtesy Dr Enrico Bedeschi.)

Brydon, Anne P. A War Diary for 1918: Richmond, Va. (Courtesy Miss Anne Brydon.)

Burcalow, Benson. Letter of 13 Oct 1918: Monroe, Wis. (Courtesy Mrs Burnett Painter.)

Coleman, Mary H. Diary, 1918-19: Williamsburg, Va. (Courtesy Dr Janet Kimbrough.)

Crichton, Agnes. Letter from St Andrews, Scotland, 19 Dec 1918. (Courtesy James J. Ward.)

Dann, Pte. Reuben. Extracts from a Diary, 1st Ox. and Bucks Light Infantry, 1918: Bangalore, India. (Courtesy Reuben Dann.)

Davies, William. Narrative Account of the Spanish Influenza at Sea Point, Cape Town. (Courtesy Mrs Mavis L. Davies.)

Diamond, A. I. Fiji and the Spanish Influenza Epidemic: an unpublished study. (Courtesy Chief Archivist, Crown Colony of Hong Kong.)

Gordon, Rev. Henry. A Winter Diary of Labrador, 1918-19. (Courtesy Provincial Archives, Colonial Building, St John's, Newfoundland.)

India, Government of. Proceedings of the Department of Education (Sanitary), October 1918, vol. 10364. (Courtesy Commonwealth Relations Office (India Office), London.)

Klemming, Lieut. Nils. Letter from Boden, 24 September 1918. (Courtesy

War Archives, Stockholm, Sweden.)

Lavender, Dr Charles. Letters, 1918-19: Marthasville, Mo. (Courtesy Mrs Melissa Larson.)

Longmont, Colo. City Council Minutes, 1918. (Courtesy P. K. Spangler.)

Lorenz, Cpl. Frank. Private Diary, 1918-19: Supply Co. 310, Q.M.C. (Courtesy Mrs Dorothe L. Wright.)

McPeck, Lieut. Howard R. Letters from Camp Perry, Toledo, Ohio, 1918. (Courtesy Mr and Mrs Howard McPeck Jr.)

Myrick, Pfc. Donald. Letters from Camp Kearny, San Diego, Calif. (Courtesy the late Mrs Charlotte Myrick.)

North Canterbury Hospital Board, Christchurch, N.Z. Official Board Minutes, 23 Dec 1918, and 26 Feb 1919. (Courtesy Mr D. Horne, Acting Chief Executive.)

Norway, Ministry of Foreign Affairs. Correspondence with Embassies and Consulates Concerning the Spanish Influenza Epidemic. (Courtesy Chief Archivist, Norwegian Ministry of Foreign Affairs.)

Olsen, Pte. Archie. Letter from Camp Grant, Rockford, Ill., 8 Oct 1918. (Courtesy Minnesota Historical Society.)

Paddon, Dr Henry. A Diary of North-West River. (Courtesy Dr Tony Paddon.)

Perrett, Rev. Walter. Letters from Labrador, 1892 etc. (Courtesy Miss Edna Perrett.)

Ress, Laura. Family letters from Fairview, N.J. (Courtesy Mrs Charles J. Short.)

Rossiter, Rev. Ernest. Missionary Experiences in Tahiti, unpublished MSS. (Courtesy Church of Jesus Christ of Latter Day Saints, Salt Lake City, Utah.)

Royal North West Mounted Police. Correspondence concerning Spanish Influenza, 1918-19: RG 18, vols 565, 567, 568, 1003; RG 91, vol. 67. (Courtesy Auxiliary Services Section, MSS Division, Public Archives of Canada, Ottawa.)

Samoa, Western. Reports of Consul Mason Mitchell to Secretary of State, Washington: 29 Nov, 3, 7, 10 Dec 1918; 20 Jan 1919. (Courtesy Dept. of State Records, U.S. National Archives, Washington, D.C.)

South Africa. Missionary Reports for 1918-19. (Courtesy Society for the Propagation of the Gospel in Foreign Parts, London.)

Tahiti. Reports of Consul Thomas Layton to Secretary of State, Washington, 10 Dec 1918 to 16 Jan 1919. (Courtesy U.S. National Archives, Washington, D.C.)

Treves, Nurse Silvia. Diary of Camp Hospital 0110, Marsan, Italy. (Courtesy Sra. Silvia Vidale.)

Unknown Soldier: a private diary of 157 F.A. Brigade, Jan-Apr 1919 (Courtesy Maryland Historical Society.)

U.S. Public Health Service, Records of: correspondence with Commerce

Dept, Labor Dept, and Children's Bureau. (Courtesy Industrial and Social Branch, Civil Archives Division, U.S. National Archives, Washington, D.C.)

Vicenzotto, Oscar and Tersilla. Letters from Padua–Pisa, 1918. (Courtesy Sra Tersilla Vicenzotto.)

Young, L/Cpl. George. Diary, 33rd M. G. Battalion, 1918-19. (Courtesy G. S. Young.)

The Survivors

The 1708 senior citizens listed below have an unique distinction in common: all of them survived the third greatest pandemic mankind has ever known. Between them, they provided the hard core of facts on which this book is based. While some furnished contemporary letters or specially written accounts, many patiently submitted themselves to a series of in-depth interviews. To avoid confusion, the ranks, and, in many cases, the names given, are those which then pertained, followed by the location in which he or she experienced those nightmare days.

Aarseth, Sverre. Oslo, Norway.
Aas, Dina. Trondheim, Norway.
Aasmyr, Martin. Neverdal, Norway.
Abate, Wanda. Ascoli Piceno, Italy.
Abell, Ella. Evansville, Ind., U.S.A.
Abraham, Frieda. Cuxhaven, Germany.
Adair, Bessie. La Fayette, Ind., U.S.A.
Agazzi, Alberto. Bergamo, Italy.
Agostini, 2nd Lieut. Giuseppe. 53rd Infantry Regiment, Monte Roccolo, Italy.
Aguirre, Tomás. Bilbao, Spain.
Akesson, Nurse Gunhild. Samariterhemmet Hospital, Uppsala, Sweden.
Alberini, Gino. Cadelbosco Sopra, Italy.
Alexander, Betty. Bruny Is., Tasmania.
Allen, Horace. Swadlincote, England.
Allmeroth, Margaret. St Louis, Mo., U.S.A.
Almond, Dora. Roanoke, Va., U.S.A.
Altstatt, Helen, St Louis, Mo., U.S.A.
Alvarez, Ramon. Tampico, Mexico.
Ambrosetti, Gina. Varese, Italy.
Ames, Robert. San Bernardino, Calif., U.S.A.

Ammentorp, Agnes. Naestved, Denmark.
Amorth, Giuseppina. Modena, Italy.
Amundsen, Thea. Lillehammer, Norway.
Andersen, Johanne. Holstebro, Denmark.
Andersen, Karoline. Astrup, Denmark.
Andersen, Knut. Storslott, Norway.
Andersen, Yrsa. Sundholm, Denmark.
Anderson, Alberta. Fond du Lac, Wis., U.S.A.
Andersson, Eivor. Stockholm, Sweden.
Andersson, Karl. Mellanbäck, Sweden.
Andersson, Nurse Naëmi. Gothenburg Maternity Hospital, Sweden.
Andersson, Pte. Nils. 124 Infantry Regiment, Ljungbyhed, Sweden.
Andrews, Harry. Florence, Colo., U.S.A.
Andrews, James. Temuka, N.Z.
Andries, Tess. Many, La., U.S.A.
Ankermann, Sophy. Greifenburg, Germany.
Appolis, Fred. Claremont, Cape Town, S. Africa.
Aragonés Fas, Magin. Monastery of Cervera, Lérida, Spain.
Archambault, Rev. George E. Providence, R.I., U.S.A.
Von Arnim, Kathe. Elisabeth Hospital, Berlin, Germany.
Arsenault, Anne. Halifax, N.S., Canada.
Arthur, George. Ayr, Scotland.
Asboe, Rev. Andrew. Okak, Labrador, Canada.
Ashby, Helen. Tulsa, Okla., U.S.A.
Ashby, Marcella. Salt Lake City, Utah, U.S.A.
Ashley, Lenorah. Huddersfield, England.
Atkinson, Janet. Ings, England.
Aurelius, Bengt. Halmstad, Sweden.
Axelby, Gertrude. Northfield, Conn., U.S.A.
Baccarani, Cesare. Ancona, Italy.
Bacchelli, Iolanda. Bologna, Italy.
Bådshaug, Tor. Vestre Gausdal, Norway.
Bailey, J. W. Palmerston North, N.Z.
Baker, Driver Albert. Army Road Construction Coy, Amiens, France.
Baker, Elizabeth, Providence, R.I., U.S.A.
Baker, Ruth. Clovis, N.M., U.S.A.
Balbirnie, David. Dundee, Scotland.
Baldwin, Douglas. Coaticook, Quebec.
Balieu, Eva. Charleroi. Pa., U.S.A.
Ball, Angelina. Tomahawk, Wis., U.S.A.
Balliana. Pte. Pietro. 1/2 Infantry Regt, King's Brigade, Florence, Italy.
Barata, Antonia dos Santos. Obidos, Portugal.
Barden, Augusta. Cachoeira do Sul, Brazil.
Bardot, Denise. Algiers.

Barion, Vito. Pariole di Canaro, Italy.
Barker, J. Maxwell. Whakatane, N.Z.
Barlee, Herb. Conyong, N.S.W., Australia.
Barns, Elizabeth. Joliet, Ill., U.S.A.
Barontini, Renzo. Piombino, Italy.
Barr, David. Christchurch, N.Z.
Barrow, C. J. Wallasey, England.
Barrows, Edward Fletcher. Brattleboro. Vt., U.S.A.
Bartoloni, Edmond. Marseilles, France.
Barton, Cranleigh. Christchurch, N.Z.
Basset, Charles. Paris, France.
Bassi, Ugo. Fojano della Chiana, Italy.
Baudrand, Georges. Lyons, France.
Bauer, Hilde. Pirna, Germany.
Baumgardt, Albert. Malmesbury, C.P., S. Africa.
Baur, Elinor. St Louis, Mo., U.S.A.
Bauschelt, Nath. Port Washington, Wis., U.S.A.
Bayes, Gladys. Poplar (East London), England.
Bayford, Sarah. Bristol, England.
Beal, Everett. Hinton, Okla., U.S.A.
Beard, Edith. Kalkfontein South, S.W. Africa.
Beard, Florence. Kalkfontein South, S.W. Africa.
Beardsmore, George. Dunedin, N.Z.
Beatson, Muriel. Owhango, N.Z.
Beauchamp, Ethel. Anakiwa, N.Z.
Beaumont, Arthur. Leicester, England.
Bebbington, Aircraftman Frederick. Blandford Camp, Dorset, England.
Beckmayer, Elisabeth. Hamburg, Germany.
Bedeschi, Lieut. Enrico. Lager E, Josefstadt Prison Camp, Czechoslovakia.
Bedford, Douglas. Masterton, N.Z.
Bednarz, Rozalia. Wilkes-Barre, Pa., U.S.A.
Beet, L. G. Kimberley, C.P., S. Africa.
Behrend, Nurse Grace. Columbia Hospital, Milwaukee, Wis., U.S.A.
Beintema, Pte. Jelle. Leeuwarden, Holland.
Bekken, Marius. Arneberg, Norway.
Belcher, Horace. Bristol, England.
Bell, Dorothy. Logan, Ohio, U.S.A.
Bellingan, Violet. Port Elizabeth, C.P., S. Africa.
Beltrami, Albino. Darzo, Italy.
Bender, Barbara. Sanger, Calif., U.S.A.
Bengtsson, Anna. Brödhult, Sweden.
Bennett, Jack. Rotorua, N.Z.

Benning, Pauline. Cape Town, C.P., S. Africa.
Benöhr, Marie. Brussels, Belgium.
Berg, Regina. Rakkestad, Norway.
Berg, Nurse Thea. Tomahawk, Wis., U.S.A.
Bergeret, Jeanne. Citeaux, France.
Bergman, Dr Rolf. Uppsala, Sweden.
Berlin, Herbert. Rosewood. Queensl., Australia.
Bermel, Peter. Nickernich, Germany.
Bernardi, Capt. Guglielmo. 11th Heavy Field Artillery Regt, Villorba, Italy.
Berndt, Lutzi. Jassow, Germany.
Bernet, Eugène. Preméry, France.
Bertin, Ottavio. Pontelongo, Italy.
Bertino, Emily. Jerome, Calif., U.S.A.
Beugnot, Alice. Nevers, France.
Biggi, Antonietta. Milan, Italy.
Bishop, Eva. Melton Mowbray, England.
Bishop, Pfc. Frederick. Camp Custer, Battle Creek, Mich., U.S.A.
Bishop, Mary. Portneuf, P.Q., Canada.
Bjarke, Harald. Bjarkøy, Norway.
Björk, Karl. Gothenburg, Sweden.
Björklund, Anna. Forsa, Sweden.
Björnstaedt, Olof. Porsgrunn, Norway.
Blackwell, Phyllis. Remuera, N.Z.
Blackwell, Sylvester. Hobson Bay, N.Z.
Blades, Dorothy. Victor, Colo., U.S.A.
Blanchfield, Ivy. Auckland, N.Z.
Blanton, Natalia. Augusta, Mich., U.S.A.
Blogg, Grace. Melbourne, Vic., Australia.
Boath, Betty. Berkhamsted, England.
Bocchi, Sofia. Rome, Italy.
Boffi, Paolo. Montichiari, Italy.
Boger, Oistein. Oslo, Norway.
Bogost, Ben. Milwaukee, Wis., U.S.A.
Boizot, Georges. Luc-sur-Mer, France.
Bollen, Harold. Port Elizabeth, C.P., S. Africa.
Booth, C. Leslie. Montreal, P.Q., Canada.
Booth, Russell. Cranston, R.I., U.S.A.
Borchert, Mathilde. Göttingen, Germany.
Boscarelli, Silvia. Milan, Italy.
Bosson, Adele. Charleroi, Pa., U.S.A.
Boulanger, Gilberte. Toul, France.
Boursse, Loekie. Amsterdam, Holland.
Bouse, Erika. Wolfenbüttel, Germany.

Bouvier, Louis. Marcillé, France.
Boverhof, Albert. Academic Hospital, Groningen, Holland.
Bowden, C. F. Kempsey, N.S.W., Australia.
Bowden, Pte. Anne. W.A.A.C., Parkhurst (I. of W.), England.
Bowen, Kathleen. Cambridge, England.
Bowler, D. R. Goulburn, N.S.W., Australia.
Bowles, Helen. Richmond, Va., U.S.A.
Bowman, Charles. Richmond, Va., U.S.A.
Bowman, Major Frederick, C.A.M.C. No. 2 Stationary Hospital, Abbe-
  ville, France.
Bowring, Edgar. Coventry, England.
Boyd, Evelyn. Winnipeg, Man., Canada.
Brace, C. A. Dargaville, N.Z.
Brandel, Nurse Kate. Military Hospital No. III, Brussels, Belgium.
Brandstätt, Luise. Stuttgart, Germany.
Brandstetter, Georg. Stuttgart, Germany.
Brandt, Probationer Nurse Gladys. Toronto General Hospital, Canada.
Brännlund, Ottilia. Högsjö, Sweden.
Bravo, Rodríguez. Mexico City.
Brayley, Pte Jack. H.M.A.S. *Encounter*, Savau, Samoa.
Brazão, Didio Pereira. Rio Maior, Portugal.
Brealey, Mary. Carlton Women's Hospital, Vic., Australia.
Breda, Fiorina. Pozzo di Codroipo, Italy.
Breiel, Harold. Chillicothe, Ohio, U.S.A.
Brentin, John. Bessemer, Pa., U.S.A.
Brereton, V. C. Pilgrim's Rest, Tvl., S. Africa.
Breuning, Anna. Dagersheim, Germany.
Brewer, Percy. Perth, W. Australia.
Briggs, Catherine. Wingham, N.S.W., Australia.
Briggs, Mae. Beloit College, Beloit, Wis., U.S.A.
Brill, Pharmacist's Mate Ernest, U.S.N. Great Lakes Naval Training
  Station.
Brinkley, Roy. Max Meadows, Va., U.S.A.
Brittingham, Edna. Hampton, Va., U.S.A.
Brizi, Medical Orderly Angelo. *Quarto*, Taranto Naval Base, Italy.
Broersma, Sjouke. Groningen, Holland.
Brown, Alice. Adrian, Mich., U.S.A.
Brown, Barbara. Richmond, Va., U.S.A.
Brown, Beatrice. Waiki, N.Z.
Brown, Bella. Chipman, N.B., Canada.
Brown, Charlie. Auckland, N.Z.
Brown, Florence. Witney, England.
Brown, Harvey. Williams, Calif., U.S.A.
Brown, Winifred. Southampton, England.

Browning, Walter. Richmond, Va., U.S.A.

Brownlee, Fannie. Tulsa, Okla., U.S.A.

Von Bruenchenhein, Eugene. Chicago Heights, Ill., U.S.A.

Brugman, Jacoba. Apeldoorn, Holland.

Brundu, Salvatore. Benetutti, Sardinia.

Brunken, Pfc. John. 3rd Training Regiment, Camp Pike, Little Rock, Ark., U.S.A.

Bruse, Göta. Kiruna, Sweden.

Bryan, Willard. Fisher, La., U.S.A.

Bryant, Mary. Sydney, N.S.W., Australia.

Brydon, Anne. Richmond, Va., U.S.A.

Buchan, Elsie. Fraserburgh, Scotland.

Budd, Alice. Camaru, N.Z.

Budd, Evelyn. Prescott, Ariz., U.S.A.

Buehrer, Amalia. Milwaukee, Wis., U.S.A.

Buitenhuis, Gerrit. Arnhem, Holland.

Buker, Raymond. Kings, Ill., U.S.A.

Bullock, Francis. Doncaster, England.

Bulmer, W. J. Kimberley, C.P., S. Africa.

Burcalow, Marcia. Monroe, Wis., U.S.A.

Burdette, Amy. Foxwarren, Man., Canada.

Burgel, Jan Isaak. Nijmegen, Holland.

Burke, Henry. Brisbane, Queensl., Australia.

Burns, Nurse Rose. St Kilda Emergency Hospital, Melbourne, Vic., Australia.

Burt, Gunner Dermot. Royal Garrison Artillery, Brighton, England.

Burton, Bertha. Madison Heights, Va., U.S.A.

Burton, Kathleen. Taranaki, N.Z.

Bushell, Molly. Kohimarama, N.Z.

Busse, Pte Hans. 6th Signals Unit, Breslau, Germany.

Butler, J. C. Kimberley, C.P., S. Africa.

Buttenschoen, Dorothea. Schierensee, Germany.

Buyers, William. Aberdeen, Scotland.

Byerly, Margaret. Quincy, Ill., U.S.A.

Bylund, Ester. Sundborn, Sweden.

Byrne, E. J. Lytton Quarantine Station, Brisbane, Queensl., Australia.

Cabrera, Vicente Ortega. Badajoz, Spain.

Cahill, Irene. Rawdon, P.Q., Canada.

Caldwell, Ivy. Lebanon, Ind., U.S.A.

Callaghan, Signalman Harold, R.A.N., R.M.A.S. *Encounter*, Suva–Tonga Is–Sydney, N.S.W., Australia.

Callaway, Jessie. No. 8 (Aust.) General Military Hospital, Fremantle, W. Australia.

Calzavara, Rina. Milan, Italy.

Cambridge, Garnet. Penrith, N.S.W., Australia.
Campbell, Alice. Janesville, Wis., U.S.A.
Campbell, Esther. Lyttelton, N.Z.
Caraffini, Igino. Citerno, Italy.
Carissimi, Carlotta. Bergamo, Italy.
Carlene, James. Dunedin, N.Z.
Carlson, Lolita. Hanford, Calif., U.S.A.
Carnebo, Astrid. Alvsjö, Sweden.
Carr, Mae. Winnipeg, Man., Canada.
Carter, Nellie. Brandywine, Va., U.S.A.
Carulli, Marcella. Milan, Italy.
Carver, Agnes. Bingham, Utah, U.S.A.
Cassin, Miriam. Auckland, N.Z.
Castagnetti, Mario. Milan, Italy.
Castellaneta, Lieut. Giovanni. Malpensa Airfield, Italy.
Castelli, Enrico. Mantua, Italy.
Cavigioli, Capt. Riccardo. 5th Bersaglieri Regt, Pojana Maggiore, Italy.
Cazzola, Umberto. Bologna, Italy.
Ceccarelli, Luigia. Forlimpopoli, Italy.
Celada, Maria. Milan, Italy.
Celona, Rodolfo. Bovalino, Italy.
Cenci, Giulio. Rome, Italy.
Cerretelli, Lieut. Berto. 3rd Army Heavy Artillery, Santa Bona, Italy.
Cerro, Ambrosia. Buenos Aires, Argentina.
Cerveny, Lena. Leopolis, Wis., U.S.A.
Chamberlain, Naomi. Susquehanna Valley, Pa., U.S.A.
Chambers, Violet. Hastings Emergency Hospital, N.Z.
Chan, Flora. Locke, Calif., U.S.A.
Chand, Ram. Delhi, India.
Chapman, Gladys. Redlands Girls School, Neutral Bay, N.S.W.
Chapman, Pte. Samuel. 33rd Battalion, R.A.I.F.. Citorne, France/
  Sydney, N.S.W., Australia.
Chapuis, Jeanne. Dijon, France.
Chareyre, Marie. Cavaillon, France.
Charlet, Léon. Michel-Levy Military Hospital, Marseilles, France.
Chenery, Nell. Dalgety & Co., Sydney, N.S.W., Australia.
Chevalier, Josephine. Cotterets, France.
Chiggiato, Arturo. Venice, Italy.
Childers, Edna. Sand Hill, Mo., U.S.A.
Childers, Robert. Sand Hill, Mo., U.S.A.
Christensen, Neil. Brandon General Hospital, Man., Canada.
Chudoba, Anne. Camp Grant, Rockford, Ill., U.S.A.
Cignolini, 2nd Lieut. Pietro. 232nd Infantry Brigade, Fiesso d'Arco,
  Italy.

Clark, Eleanor. London, Ohio, U.S.A.
Clark, Emily. Johannesburg Isolation Hospital, Tvl., S. Africa.
Clarke, Mildred. Alameda, Calif., U.S.A.
Claussen, Nurse Gudrun. Wolston Park Mental Hospital, Sandgate, Queensl., Australia.
Cleaver, David. Rhondda Valley, Wales.
Cleland, Elsie. Hopewell, Va., U.S.A.
Clements, Helen. Madison, Ind., U.S.A.
Clère, Felix. Chalon-sur-Sâone, France.
Cliteur, Suzanna Johanna. Haarlem, Holland.
Clough, Ruth. Manchester, N.H., U.S.A.
Cochrane, Donalda. Qu'Apelle, Sask., Canada.
Cocker, Nurse Winifred. Carr House Isolation Hospital, Doncaster, England.
Coetzer, Catherine. Blaney, C.P., S. Africa.
Coffey, Lena. Christiansburg, Va., U.S.A.
Colborn, Jerrene. Bishop, Calif., U.S.A.
Coleman, Catherine. Woonsocket, R.I., U.S.A.
Coleman, Janet. Richmond, Va., U.S.A.
Colombo, Elda. Milan, Italy.
Comfort, James E. St Louis, Mo., U.S.A.
Conlan, L. R. Charleville, Queensl., Australia.
Conover, Nurse Elva. Rockford Hospital, Rockford, Ill., U.S.A.
Cook, Opal. Lamar, Colo., U.S.A.
Cooper, Douglas. Masterton, N.Z.
Cooper, Sgt F. W. Police H.Q., Lichtenburg, Tvl., S. Africa.
Cooper, Dr Janet. Melbourne Homeopathic Hospital, Vic., Australia.
Cooper, Joy. Avondale, N.Z.
Cooper, Larimore. Sparta, Tenn., U.S.A.
Copland, Watt. Gore, N.Z.
Copping, Bertram. Pentonville (North London), England.
Coppini, Adolfo. Vienna, Austria.
Corbett, Irene. Cape Flats, C.P., S. Africa.
Cordingley, Fred. Blair Athol, Queensl., Australia.
Correia, Renato. Paradela de Mirandela, Portugal.
Cortes, Concha Moragon. Zaragoza, Spain.
Cortese, Dino. Diamondville, Wyo., U.S.A.
Costello, Jack. Boulder, W. Australia.
Coulter, Martha. Wellington, N.Z.
Courtenay, Nurse Mary. Guy's Hospital, London, England.
Couson, Frank. Ballarat, Vic., Australia.
Cox, L. Machell. Long Eaton, England.
Cox, Rifleman Sidney. 8th Rifle Brigade, Lazarett 4, Rastatt, Baden, Germany.

Cragg, Georgina. Gerald, Sask., Canada.
Craig, Rita. Hartford, Conn., U.S.A.
Crawford, Irma. Eldon, Iowa, U.S.A.
Cremer, Leone. Freeport, Ill., U.S.A.
Cresci, Alfonso. Lezze, Italy.
Crescimanno, Vittorio. Palermo, Sicily.
Crespi, Lieut. Pier Paolo. 2nd Army, Borgotaro, Italy.
Cretara, Emilia. Rome, Italy.
Crichley, Lilian. Blackpool, England.
Criner, Ann. Butler, Pa., U.S.A.
Crispin, Buller. Waimate, N.Z.
Crowley, Theresa. Davenport, Iowa, U.S.A.
Culleton, James. Fresno, Calif., U.S.A.
Cullum, Bob. Prince of Wales Hospital, Randwick, Sydney, N.S.W.
Cummings, Nell. Rockford, Ill., U.S.A.
Cunha, Mario. Belo Horizonte, Brazil.
Currey, Winifred. Mowbray, Cape Town, S. Africa.
Curtis, Helen. Elm Grove, W. Va., U.S.A.
Curtis, J. H. Southall, England.
Cuzzoni, Maria Rosa. Mortara, Italy.
Da Cunha, Ciro Vieira. Rio de Janeiro, Brazil.
Dahl, Else. Ejstrup, Denmark.
Dahl, Hans. Oslo, Norway.
Dahlgren, Hildur. Högen, Sweden.
Dahm, Rosa. Koblenz, Germany.
Dainty, Winifred. Birmingham, England.
Dale, Emma. Bury St Edmunds, England.
Dalle Donne, Marshal Cesare. H.Q. XXX Armoured Corps, Monte Grappa, Italy.
Damon, Lily Belle. Dickens, Iowa, U.S.A.
Danford, Cpl. Asa. 81st Field Artillery, Camp Mills, N.Y., U.S.A.
Dann, Pte. Reuben. 1st Oxfordshire & Bucks Light Infantry, Bangalore, India.
Danvers, Pte. Joseph. 2/2 North Midland Field Ambulance Coy, Cambrai, France.
D'Arrigo, Domenico. Messina, Sicily.
Dart, Ruth. Montreal, P.Q., Canada.
Daur, Elisabeth. Stuttgart, Germany.
Davey, Beatrice. Wilkes-Barre, Pa., U.S.A.
Davids, Sydney G. Grand Hotel, Grahamstown, C.P., S. Africa.
Davidson, Elizabeth. Dundee, Scotland.
Davidson, Stuart. Uitenhage, C.P., S. Africa.
Davies, William. Pretoria, Tvl., S. Africa.
Davis, Bertha. Lake Charles, La., U.S.A.

Davis, Kathleen. Gardner's Siding, N.Z.
Davis, Ruby. Fort Dodge, Iowa, U.S.A.
Davison, Ella. Richmond, Va., U.S.A.
Davoren, Rachel. Blockhouse Bay, N.Z.
Dawbarn, Gwen. Eunice High School, Bloemfontein, O.F.S., S. Africa.
Dawe, Mildred. Elizabeth, Ill., U.S.A.
Dazzi, Gino. Rio de Janeiro, Brazil.
De Araujo, Belmiro. Porto, Portugal.
Dean, Marie. Spartanburg, S.C., U.S.A.
Death, Edna. Hawera, N.Z.
Deeks, Walter. Claremont, Cape Town, S. Africa.
De Freitas, Constantino. Rio de Janeiro, Brazil.
Degenne, Nurse Sardin. Hospital Claude-Bernard, Paris, France.
De Giampietro, Candido. Cavalese, Italy.
De Jong, Pieterje. Hallum, Holland.
Delanchie, James. Johannesburg, Tvl, S. Africa.
Del Monaco, Maria. Palmanova, Italy.
Delost, Antoinette. Neuilly-le-Réal, France.
De Mange, Eleanor. Berkeley, Calif., U.S.A.
Demel, Sgt Cesaris. 79th Surgical Ambulance Coy, Pradamano, Italy.
Deming, Clarissa. Waterbury, Conn., U.S.A.
Denham, Hannah. Dundee, Scotland.
Dennett, Laurence. Grahamstown, C.P., S. Africa.
Denny, Ruth. Melbourne, Vic., Australia.
De Oliveira, Antonia Ambrosio. Agua Limpa, Brazil.
De Paoli, Lieut. Mario. 58th Infantry Regt, Monte Grappa, Italy.
Deperraz, Léa. Marseilles, France.
Desjardins, Albert. Montreal, P.Q., Canada.
Diaz, Alonso. Mexico City, Mexico.
Diebels, Josiena. Oss, Holland.
Dieblich, Margarete. Brey, Germany.
Dilks, Edith. Market Harborough, England.
Dinsdale, Nurse Laurie. Infectious Diseases Hospital, Fairfield, Vic.,
    Australia.
Ditmas, Edith. Oxford, England.
Dixon, George. Hamilton, N.Z.
Dobrindt, Harry. Louth, Ont., Canada.
Dolceacqua, Anna. New York, N.Y., U.S.A.
Dolge, Henry. City of Milwaukee Health Dept, Wis., U.S.A.
Doll, Lena. Las Vegas, N.M., U.S.A.
Dolve, Arne. Vossevangen, Norway.
Domas, Seaman 1st Class Lemuel. U.S.N.R., s.s. *Eastland*, Lake Michi-
    gan, U.S.A.
Doran, Gordon. Woomelang, Vic., Australia.

Downman, Esther. Comet, Queensl., Australia.
Dray, Violet. Dunedin, N.Z.
Drewett, Christina. Auckland, N.Z.
Driscoll, Ruby. Portland, Oreg., U.S.A.
Drummond, Catharine. Cessnock, N.S.W., Australia.
Dubois, Roger. Collège Louis Léard, Falaise, France.
Duff, Arthur. Kiukiang, China.
Dunbar, Police-Constable Jack. Eden, N.S.W., Australia.
Dunn, Hazel. Valentine, Nebr., U.S.A.
Durmeir, Paulina. Waiuku, N.Z.
Durrance, Sydney. Leicester, England.
Duryea, Alta. St Louis, Mo., U.S.A.
Dymek, Karl. Üsküb, Albania.
Dymond, Carman. Melfort, Sask., Canada.
Eade, Arch. Sydney, N.S.W., Australia.
Earnshaw, Ivy. Christchurch, N.Z.
Eaton, W. F. Foxworth Hospital, Liverpool, England.
Ebeltoft, Nora. Arendal, Norway.
Eddleton, Juliet. Richmond, Va., U.S.A.
Eddy, Florence. Brantford, Ont., Canada.
Edey, Sister Mayme. Old Base Hospital, Toronto, Ont., Canada.
Edlund, Gösta. Stockholm, Sweden.
Edlund, Mary. Vreta Kloster, Sweden.
Edvardsen, Erling. Tromsø, Norway.
Edwards, Henry. Waverley, N.S.W., Australia.
Edwards, Hilda. Huddersfield, England.
Edwards, Lillian. St Marylebone (West London), England.
Edwards, W. J. Savanne, Ont., Canada.
Ekenborg, Conrad. Södra Salberga, Sweden.
Ekman, Einar. Grythyttan, Sweden.
Elliott, J. Colin. Auckland. N.Z.
Ellis, Ernestine. Montreal, P.Q., Canada.
Els, Marthinus. Bedford Cape, C.P., S. Africa.
Elson, Barbara. Pretoria, Tvl, S. Africa.
Eltoft, Mikal. Nordiland, Norway.
Emery, Ike. Korumburra, Vic., Australia.
Endersby, Doris. York, W. Australia.
Enestrom, Gudrun. Håkanstorp, Sweden.
Engels, Julia. Philadelphia, Pa., U.S.A.
Engkvist, Greta. Stockholm, Sweden.
Ericson, Valborg. Stockholm, Sweden.
Eriksson, Aina. Norn, Sweden.
Erikksson, Nils. Vilhelmina, Sweden.
Estment, Winifred. Port Elizabeth, C.P., S. Africa.

Eustace, Gunner Charles. S.A. Heavy Artillery, Potchefstroom, Tvl, S. Africa.

Everitt, Annie. Björneborg, Sweden.

Evins, Lewis. Wilburton, Okla., U.S.A.

Fagrell, Inez. Uppsala, Sweden.

Fairley, Keith. Wirth's Park Emergency Hospital, Melbourne, Vic., Australia.

Fangio, Aminta. Montevideo, Uruguay.

Fanning, William. Huntsville, Ala., U.S.A.

Faraudo, Giuseppe. Turin, Italy.

Farid, Mohammed. Cairo, U.A.R.

Farmer, J. C. Adelaide, S. Australia.

Faucon, Pte. Robert. 416th Infantry Regt, Bauerbach, Germany.

Feddersen, Nurse Martha. Lutheran Hospital, St Louis, Mo., U.S.A.

Felici, Adriano. Spoleto, Italy.

Felicori, Fausto. Bologna, Italy.

Fenske, Agnes. Platte Centre, Neb., U.S.A.

Ferdon, Joanna. Georgetown, S.C., U.S.A.

Ferguson, Isabella. Perth, Scotland.

Ferguson, Nellie. Lynchburg, Va., U.S.A.

Ferguson, Steward William. R.M.S. *Niagara*: Vancouver–Honolulu–Auckland–Sydney.

Fermo, Palmira. Fiume, Italy.

Ferrara, Josephine. Morgantown, W. Va., U.S.A.

Ferrari, Mario. Montesiro, Italy.

Ferreira, Gunner Percy. S.A. Field Artillery, Robert Heights, Pretoria, Tvl, S. Africa.

Ferretti, Vittore. Milan, Italy.

Ferris, Nurse Margaret. Victoria General Hospital, Halifax, N.S.

Finch, William. South Shields, England.

Fish, George. Deputy Mayor, Dordrecht, C.P., S. Africa.

Fissore, Giuseppina. Turin, Italy.

Flack, Frances. Gympie, Queensl., Australia.

Flanders, Jean. Cork, Ireland.

Flanery, Rena. Everett, Wash., U.S.A.

Fleming, Jessie. Titiroa, N.Z.

Fletcher, Kathleen. Evans Head, N.S.W., Australia.

Fleur, Catherine. Pertuis, France.

Flores, Luis Puga. Montanchez, Spain.

Florry, Rosaline. H.Q., G.P.O., London, England.

Flynn, Beatrice. Blenheim–Wellington–Rotorua–Auckland–Nelson, N.Z.

Flyvholm, Mette Marie. Thyborøn, Denmark.

Fontana, Maria. Milan, Italy.

Foppiano, Sgt. Pier Lorenzo. No. 325 Field Hospital, Malga Sunio, Italy.

Ford, Dorothy. Bowling Green, Ky, U.S.A.
Forfod, Elide. Trondheim, Norway.
Forman, Madeleine. Cape Town, C.P., S. Africa.
Forster, Florence. Camp Hancock, Pa., U.S.A.
Forsyth, Wilfred. Virden, Man., Canada.
Fosli, Anna. Maalselv, Norway.
Fosli, Rönning. Maalselv, Norway.
Foster, Dorothy. Cape Town, S. Africa.
Foster, Gertrude. Vancouver, B.C., Canada.
Foster, Mary. Derby, England.
Foster, Muriel. Cape Town, S. Africa.
Foster, Vera. Johannesburg, Tvl, S. Africa.
Fouche, Germina. Pretoria, Tvl, S. Africa.
Fournier, Pierre Claude. Paris, France.
Fournier, Alphonse. Belledune, N.B., Canada.
Frankel, James. Montreal, P.Q., Canada.
Frazier, Thelma. Fayette, Iowa, U.S.A.
Fredette, Yvette. Central Falls, R.I., U.S.A.
Fredriksson, Karin. Gothenburg, Sweden.
Freeburn, Mary. Lindsay, Ont., Canada.
French, Dorothy. Burgh Heath, England.
Frewer, Pte. Frederick. London Scottish Regiment, New Malden, England.
Friekel, Thekla. Eich, Germany.
Friskman, Lillian. Vallejo, Calif., U.S.A.
Frizni, Elena. Mirano, Italy.
Frost, Sister Jenny. Huntingdon County Hospital, England.
Fry, Robert. Adelaide, S. Australia.
Frye, Arthur. Dunedin, N.Z.
Fulton, Truman. Fredericktown, Mo., U.S.A.
Furbee, Margaret. Mannington, W. Va., U.S.A.
Furtado, Joâo Maria. Ceará-Mirim, Brazil.
Fussell, Gladys. Bristol, England.
Gadchaux, Maria. St Nicholas de Port, France.
Gafforio, Tullio. Portici, Italy.
Galloway, Alex. Perth, Scotland.
Garcia, Domingo. Buenos Aires, Argentina.
Garcia, S. Arce. Echevarrí, Spain.
Gard, Ruth. Berhampore, N.Z.
Gardiner, Henry. Tylerstown, Rhondda, Wales.
Garrett, Ellen. Cublington, England.
Garrett, Margot. Auckland, N.Z.
Garthe, John. Risör, Norway.
Gavaudan, Pte. Ferréol. 216th Infantry Regt, Lyons, France.
Gay, Rita. Genoa, Italy.

Geldenhuys, Myrtle. Willowmore, C.P., S. Africa.
Gelli, Giuseppina. Leona, Italy.
Gentry, Minnie. South Bend, Ind., U.S.A.
Genuel, Renée. Pierrecourt, France.
George, Doris. New Plymouth, N.Z.
Gregerson, Maude. Pemberton, Minn., U.S.A.
Ghosh, Provash Chandra. Calcutta, India.
Gibson, Jessie. Wellington, N.Z./Sydney, N.S.W., Australia.
Gieseke, Val. Bethlehem, Pa., U.S.A.
Gilmer, Mary. Eccles, N. Va., U.S.A.
Ginnetti, Rosa. Waupaca, Wis., U.S.A.
Giobbi, Cesara. Como, Italy.
Giovannini, Ebe. La Spezia, Italy.
Gisbert, Pascual. Alicante, Spain.
Glavine, Jane. Fortune Harbor, NF.
Gleason, Edna. Flagstaff, Ariz., U.S.A.
Gledcole, Nurse Violet. Pahiatua Hospital, N.Z.
Gleeson, Margaret. Seddonville, N.Z.
Gnutti, Lucia. Reggiolo, Italy.
Goble, Elton. Victorville, Calif., U.S.A.
Godbe, Hampton. Salt Lake City, Utah, U.S.A.
Goedhart, Cornelia. Oosterbeek, Holland.
Goering, S. C. Barcelona, Spain.
Goldshtein, Nathan. Jerusalem, Palestine.
Gollner, Stella. Milwaukee, Wis., U.S.A.
Goodwin, Gordon. Narrabri, N.S.W., Australia.
Goostrey, Stan. Sandgate, Queensl., Australia.
Gordon, J. Roy. Milford Station, N.S., Canada.
Gordon-Huntly, Yvonne. Durban Ladies' College, Natal, S. Africa.
Goring, Edith. Bloemfontein, O.F.S., S. Africa.
Görlt, Gertrude. Aus, S.W. Africa.
Gorsich, Marie. Joliet, Ill., U.S.A.
Gould, Margaret. Burford, Ont., Canada.
Graham, Alexander. South Shields, England.
Graham, Pfc. Charles, U.S.M.C., Camp Dodge, Des Moines, Iowa, U.S.A.
Graham, Nurse Lucy. Boulder/Kalgoorlie, W. Australia.
Graham, Martha. Sumter, S.C., U.S.A.
Grant, Christie. Amatikulu, Zululand.
Grant, Elizabeth. Sydney, N.S.W., Australia.
Grant, Richard. Berwick, Vic., Australia.
Granvogel, Elizabeth. Milwaukee, Wis., U.S.A.
Grassi, Gino. Leghorn, Italy.
Gray, Helen. Port Elizabeth, C.P., S. Africa.

Gray, Jean. Roanoke, Va., U.S.A.
Gray, Nurse Mary. Whangarei Hospital, N.Z.
Gray, Nellie. Wellington, N.Z.
Grayson, Avalyn. Gorgas, Ala., U.S.A.
Green, Elsie. Albany, W. Australia.
Green, Sgt. Fred. No. 27 Squadron, R.A.F., Beauvais, France.
Green, Robert. Wollongong, N.S.W., Australia.
Green, Rose. Auburn, N.Y., U.S.A.
Green, Ruby. Ring River, W. Australia.
Greene, Nell. Richmond, Va., U.S.A.
Greer, Jean. Blanco, near George, C.P., S. Africa.
Greuel, Katrin. Parz-Elsdorf, Germany.
Grezler, Claudio. Trento, Italy.
Grice, Harold. Elkhorn, Wis., U.S.A.
Grieve, Lloyd. Waiuku, N.Z.
Griffin, Trooper Charles. Anzac Mounted Division, *Ullamroa*, Woodman's Point, W. Australia.
Griffiths, Nellie. Auckland, N.Z.
Grosfils, Gisela. Brussels, Belgium.
Groves, Alice. Perth, W. Australia.
Groves, Steward Richard, s.s. *Nestor*, Liverpool–New York.
Grubb, Norman. Limerick, Pa., U.S.A.
Grzegorz, Marie. Kishnau, Germany.
Guareschi, Lieut. Antonio. Vesio Camp Hospital, Italy.
Gudgeon, Eva. Carnforth, England.
Gulino, Pietro. Caltagirone, Sicily.
Gunston, Officer-Cadet C. A. No. 11 Officer Cadet Battalion, Pirbright, England.
Gunter, Eva. Harrow, England.
Gustafsson, Anna. Nossebro, Sweden.
Gustavsson, Alice. Södermanland, Sweden.
Haack, Hans. Charleville, France.
Habeck, Edgar. Milwaukee, Wis., U.S.A.
Haddock, Chauncey. Plymouth, Ind., U.S.A.
Haddock, Maybelle. Plymouth, Ind., U.S.A.
Haefner, Gertrud. Stuttgart, Germany.
Haite, Vera. Auckland, N.Z.
Haldorsen, Otto. Havøysund, Norway.
Halford, W. H. C. Kalgoorlie, W. Australia.
Hall, Edna. Clinton, Ill., U.S.A.
Hamilton, Nurse Ethel. Winnipeg, Man., Canada.
Hammer, Pauline. Koblenz, Germany.
Hammond, Cushla. Waikumete, N.Z.
Hammond, Elmer. Akron, Ohio, U.S.A.

Hammond, Lucia. Bloomsburg State Normal School, Pa., U.S.A.
Hanhart, Carlos. La Paz, Bolivia.
Hankinson, J. H. Cape Town, C.P., S. Africa.
Hansen, Julie. Søllested, Denmark.
Hanson, Gladys. Coventry, England.
Hanssen, Günther. Schwerin, Germany.
Hards, Effie. Donkerkvek, C.P., S. Africa.
Hardwick, Eveline. Holmfirth, England.
Hardy, Sgt. George. Canterbury Mounted Rifles, Anzac Mounted Division, Jericho, Palestine.
Harnell, Rut. Julita, Sweden.
Harrison, Evelyn. Dunedin, N.Z.
Harrison, Mabel. Huddersfield, England.
Harrison, Ruth. Wadena, Sask., Canada.
Harsant, Florence. Tanoa, N.Z.
Hart, Ethel. Conway, C.P., S. Africa.
Hart, Raymond. New Britain, Conn., U.S.A.
Hartman, Howard. Perth Modern School, W. Australia.
Hasanbegovic, Semso. Sadici, Bosnia.
Haselden, Alice. Auckland, N.Z.
Hassenfeldt, Jessie. Hamilton, Ont., Canada.
Haugland, Bjarne. Brekke, Norway.
Haugsted, Ingeborg. Svendborg, Denmark.
Haw, Ethel. Fish Hoek, C.P., S. Africa.
Hawes, Evander. Rumford, R.I., U.S.A.
Hay, Annie. Lumsden, Scotland.
Hayden, Edith. East Brunswick, Vic., Australia.
Hayton, Margaret. Cockermouth, England.
Hazell, Daisy. Reigate, England.
Head, Alfred. Sandy Bay, Hobart, Tasmania.
Head, Nita. Flemington, Mo., U.S.A.
Headley, Florence. Sunderland, England.
Hecktor, Luise. Hanau, Germany.
Hector, Janie. Edinburgh, Scotland.
Hedrick, Luise. Gross-Queren, Germany.
Heenan, Pte Eric. H.M.A.T. *Boonah*, Sydney–Durban–Fremantle.
Hegardt, Dr Gunnar. Uddevalla Provisional Hospital, Sweden.
Hegert, Oscar. Milwaukee, Wis., U.S.A.
Heinrich, Pauline. South Bend, Ind., U.S.A.
Heiser, Serena. Milwaukee, Wis., U.S.A.
Hellens, C.P.O. John. R.N. H.M.S. *Royal Sovereign*, Rosyth, Scotland.
Hellesø, Arnt. Rørvik, Norway.
Hellström, Ingrid. Västerås, Sweden.
Hemus, Ethel. Okotoks, Alta., Canada.

Henderson, Leonard. Davenport, N.Z.
Henderson, Prudence. Wanganui, N.Z.
Henneky, Pieter. Krabbedijke, Zeeland.
Hennichs, Rut. Stockholm, Sweden.
Henriksen, Louise. Gedser, Denmark.
Henry, Mary. Annan, Scotland.
Hernya, Emilia. Sydney, N.S.W., Australia.
Herrero, Pedro. Bilbao, Spain.
Heymans, Gideon. Paul Roux, O.F.S., S. Africa.
Hickey, Kathleen. Blair Athol, Queensl., Australia.
Hidalgo, Rodolfo. Cordoba, Argentina.
Higgins, Agnes. Danvers, Mass., U.S.A.
Hijink, Jan Hendrik. Winterswijk/Utrecht, Holland.
Hill, Adeline. Birmingham, England.
Hill, Eva. Otago Medical School, N.Z.
Hillmann, Irma. Göttingen, Germany.
Hirstfield, Arthur. Middletown, Ohio, U.S.A.
Hirva, Jaakko. Helsinki, Finland.
Hobbs, Albert. Orange, N.S.W., Australia.
Hoddinatt, Milleah. Charlottesville, Pa., U.S.A.
Hodgins, Nurse Bertha. New Haven Hospital, New Haven, Conn.,
    U.S.A.
Hodgson, Jane. Alston, England.
Hogan, Nurse Ina. West Maitland, N.S.W., Australia.
Hogben, Julius. Thames, N.Z.
Hogg, Elsie. Balclutha, N.Z.
Hogg, Cpl. H. A., N.Z. Field Artillery, s.s. *Tahiti*, Sierra Leone.
Hognestad, Ingebjörg Maria. Bryne, Norway.
Hogstad, Eli. Trondheim, Norway.
Holland, Edith. Winton, N.Z.
Holloway, Leslie E. Cape Town, S. Africa.
Hollows, Pte. Alfred. N.Z.M.C., Victoria Hall Emergency Hospital,
    Wellington, N.Z.
Holman, Eva. Wellington, N.Z.
Holmberg, Nobel. Minnedosa, Man., Canada.
Holzer, Erna. Elbing, Germany.
Hong, Guan. Penang, Malaya.
Hood, Robert G. York County, N.B., Canada.
Hooker, Elsie. Christchurch, N.Z.
Hooper, Pte. Louis. S.A.T.C., Lafayette, La., U.S.A.
Hopkins, Frances. Providence, R.I., U.S.A.
Hormann, Greta. Bremen, Germany.
Horn, Emil. Bloemfontein, O.F.S., S. Africa.
Hornabrook, Jean. Adelaide, S. Australia.

Horne, Emily. Harewood, N.Z.
Horringa, Gerarda. The Hague, Holland.
Hornung, Luise. Stuttgart, Germany.
Houghton, Hazel. Sydney, N.S.W., Australia.
Houlton, Alice. Calgary, Alta., Canada.
Howe, Lillian. Sheffield, Tasmania.
Howell, Elizabeth. Dover, Del., U.S.A.
Howell, Vera. Hawera, N.Z.
Howes, Minnie. Durban, Natal, S. Africa.
Hunt, Frances. Tekuiti, N.Z.
Hunt, Mildred. Des Moines, Iowa, U.S.A.
Hunter, Leslie. Coromandel, N.Z.
Hunter, Pte. Thomas. 7th Bn Northumberland Fusiliers, 149th Brigade, 50th Division.
Hurd, Dorothy. Port Elizabeth, C.P., S. Africa.
Husdell, Mavis. Port Adelaide, S. Australia.
Hutcheson, Inez. Waverley, Kans.
Hutchinson, Doris. Dunedin, N.Z.
Hutchinson, Frank. Wellington Fever Hospital, N.Z.
Hutton, Frances Belle. Lewistown, Ill., U.S.A.
Ibbott, W. G. Melbourne, Vic., Australia.
Ingram, Faith. Auckland, N.Z.
Insausti, Isabel. Madrid, Spain.
Ives, Carroll Sanborn. Sherbrooke, P.Q., Canada.
Jack, Dorothy. New Deer, Scotland.
Jackson, Emma. Southampton, England.
Jacobs, Ethel. Beaver Dam, Wis., U.S.A.
Jacobsen, Peder. Uløybukt, Norway.
Jacobson, Cyril. Brisbane, Queensl., Australia.
Jacovelli, Espedito. Massafra, Italy.
Jago, Maurice. St Buryan, England.
James, Grace. San Diego, Calif., U.S.A.
Jansson, Agnes. Sävare, Sweden.
Jansson, Erik. Asarna, Sweden.
Jaraczewski, Esther. Milwaukee, Wis., U.S.A.
Jeanmaire, Louise. Connoy, France.
Jearey, Pte. H. N. 1st Queen's Royal West Surrey Regt, Namur, France.
Jellison, Harrison. Bladworth, Sask., Canada.
Jenkins, David. Leicester, England.
Jensen, Karl Henrik. Gudmandrup, Denmark.
Jenssen, Arthur. Herjangsholmen, Norway.
Jessup, Josephine. Frazier, Mont., U.S.A.
Johannison, Helga. Stockholm, Sweden.
Johansen, Sylvia, Trondheim, Norway.

Johansson, Erik. Enköping, Sweden.
Johansson, Pte. Hjalmar. 9th Coy, Västmanland Regiment, Västerås, Sweden.
Johansson, Linnea. Frändefors, Sweden.
Johns, Beatrice. Portsmouth, Va., U.S.A.
Johnsen, Harriet. Stavanger, Norway.
Johnsen, Sigvald. Brastad, Norway.
Johnson, Bernice. Melvin Hill, N.C., U.S.A.
Johnson, Elizabeth. Goodman, Wis., U.S.A.
Johnson, Ellen. Coventry, England.
Johnson, Elsie. Rockford, Ill., U.S.A.
Johnson, Jenny. South Shields, England.
Johnson, Lillie. Modesto, Calif., U.S.A.
Johnson, Linnea. Rockford, Ill., U.S.A.
Johnson, Nurse Myrtle. Augustana School of Nursing, Chicago, Ill., U.S.A.
Johnston, Sister Jean. Seacliff Mental Hospital, Auckland, N.Z.
Johnston, Vida Anne. Aberdeen, Scotland.
Johnstone, Janet. Auckland, N.Z.
Jones, Dorothy. Aylesbury, England.
Jones, Nurse Gwen. Camp Sherman, Chillicothe, Ohio.
Jones, Gwendoline. Hobianga, N.Z.
Jones, Lena. Lawrenceville, Va., U.S.A.
Jones, Pte. Leonard. 51st Bn. Royal Sussex Regt, Connaught Hospital, Aldershot, England.
Jones, Lorraine. Cache Junction, Utah, U.S.A.
Jones, Scout Ted. 3rd Green & Sea Point Scout Troop, Three Anchor Bay, C.P., S. Africa.
Jonger, Elisabeth. Arnhem, Holland.
Jönsson, Agnes. Malmö, Sweden.
Jonsson, Berndt. Broddetorp, Sweden.
Jonsson, Gösta. Glimåkra, Sweden.
Jönsson, Jenny. Råå, Sweden.
Jonsson, Margit. Hälsingborg, Sweden.
Jordan, Sue. Edenton, N.C., U.S.A.
Jörgensen, Anna. Tusenaes, Denmark.
Joy, Elsie. Penge (South London), England.
Kachelhoffer, Mauritz. Kimberley, C.P., S. Africa.
Kapadia, Chunilal. Bombay, India.
Kapfer, Ruth. Baring, Mo., U.S.A.
Karlsson, Dagny. Östersund, Sweden.
Kaske, Rose. Rib Lake, Wis., U.S.A.
Kaul, Ruth. Syracuse, N.Y., U.S.A.
Kauter, Josef. Mittelheim, Germany.

Kawasaki, Kyoshi. Kobe, Japan.
Kay, Harold. Manaia Taranaki, N.Z.
Keefer, Erlyne. Beaver Dam, Wis., U.S.A.
Kegel, Mathilda. Milwaukee, Wis., U.S.A.
Keightley, L. M. Kimberley, C.P., S. Africa.
Kelly, Doreen. Brisbane, Queensl., Australia.
Kent, Pte. Ada. W.A.C., Wisconsin Avenue Emergency Hospital, Milwaukee, Wis., U.S.A.
Kern, Mary. West Allis, Wis., U.S.A.
Kernan, Charles. Rural Retreat, Va., U.S.A.
Kerr, Claire. Nabiac, N.S.W., Australia.
Kettlewell, Pte. Charles. No. 11 C.C.S., Rouen, France.
Kilmer, Kathryn. North Liberty, Ind., U.S.A.
Kim, Jongshik, Seoul, Korea.
Kinard, Lois. Crystal Springs, Miss., U.S.A.
King, Francis. Willesden (North London), England.
King, Guy. Bulls, N.Z.
Kinley, Alice. Rockford, Ill., U.S.A.
Kirkpatrick, Floreta. Rushville, Ind., U.S.A.
Kish, Nurse Mabel. Cochran, Calif., U.S.A.
Klein, Bertha. Queens, N.Y.
Kleinschmidt, Regina. Merrill, Wis., U.S.A.
Klink, Kirsten. Fredericia, Denmark.
Klinke, Madeline. Riverside, Ill., U.S.A.
Kloosterhuis, Bougien. Markstede, Holland.
Klos, Geerling. Enschede, Holland.
Knepel, Florence. Leeds, England.
Knivestøen, Olaug. Skotselv, Norway.
Knorr, Elvira. Woodhaven, L.I., U.S.A.
Knowles, W. T. Wellington. N.Z.
Koch, Anja. Euskirchen, Germany.
König, Ottilie. Stuttgart, Germany.
Kosoric, Miko. Gorazde, Yugoslavia.
Krause, Minnie. Genesee, Wis., U.S.A.
Krautkremer, Mary. Hankinson, North Dakota, U.S.A.
Kriel, Fredrica. Cape Town, C.P., S. Africa.
Kristiansson, Herman, Kall, Sweden.
Kristoffersen, Andrea. Porsgrunn, Norway.
Krona, Pte August. 16-1 Infantry, Vänersborg, Sweden.
Krosh, Naval Cadet Josef. First Shipyard Division, Kiel, Germany.
Kruise, Wiert. Lethe, Holland.
Kühn, Margarethe. Sorau, Germany.
Kusenberg, Paul. Samsun, Turkey.
Kuskopf, Margaret. Brisbane, Queensl., Australia.

Kvarn, Einar. Ytterøy, Norway.
Kvikne, Martha. Sogn, Norway.
Labriola, John. Bethlehem, Pa., U.S.A.
Ladd, Lillie. Central, Ark., U.S.A.
Ladd, Sarah Belle. Norfolk, Va., U.S.A.
Ladwein, Hans. Pachten, Germany.
Lafond, Germaine. Fontain-sur-Saône, France.
La Gioia, Franco. Gravina di Puglia, Italy.
Lai, Cpl. Virgilio. 7th Artillery Regt, Marostica, Italy.
Laidlaw, W. G. High River, Alta., Canada.
Lange, Linga. Rockford. Ill., U.S.A.
Lani, Thelma. Elko, Nev., U.S.A.
Laperche, Marie Aline. Ochamps, Belgium.
Lappin, Dr Lazur. Villiersdorp, C.P., S. Africa.
Larsen, Karl. Nykøbing, Denmark.
Larsen, Mandrup. Bergen, Norway.
Larsen, Nurse Marie. Bispebjerg Hospital, Copenhagen, Denmark.
Larsen, Olga. Thy, Denmark.
Larsson, Pte. Carl. 1-17 Infantry, Uddevalla, Sweden.
Latham, Pte. Arch. H.M.A.T. *Boonah*: Sydney–Durban–Fremantle.
Lathwell, Lyn. Collie, W. Australia.
Latini, Angela. Este, Italy.
Lawrence, Effie. Shreveport, La., U.S.A.
Lawson, Fireman John. Auckland Central Railway Station, N.Z.
Learoyd, Philip. Rossall School, Fleetwood, England.
Leaver, Laurence. Laddonia, Mo., U.S.A.
Lebetkin, George. Hartford, Conn., U.S.A.
Lee, Elsie. Milan. Mich., U.S.A.
Lee, Flavia. Indianapolis, Ind., U.S.A.
Lee, Melva. Stratford Normal School, Ont., Canada.
Lehrer, Bettie. Pittsburgh, Pa., U.S.A.
Leide, Gunnar. Uddevalla, Sweden.
Leiffer, C. L. Green Point Rapids, B.C., Canada.
Lemaire, Charles. Cambrai, France.
Lemonnier, Marie. Pleurtuit, France.
Lende, Anna. Naerbø, Norway.
Leonard, Eugenie. Pueblo, Colo., U.S.A.
Le Person, Jeanne. Quimperlé, France.
Leppin, William. Grand Island, Nebr., U.S.A.
Le Roux, Kate. Woodstock, C.P., S. Africa.
Leschuitta, Elena. Sottoselva di Palmanova, Italy.
Leslie, Gladys. Winsley, England.
Levi, Haim. Jerusalem, Palestine.
Levinsohn, Jack. Ulster Farm, Grahamstown, C.P., S. Africa.

Levy, Graham. Waikamete, N.Z.

Lewis, Driver Charles. No. 3 Transport Corps, SASCO, The Castle, Cape Town, S. Africa.

Lewis, Marjorie. Colorado Agricultural College, Fort Collins, Colo., U.S.A.

Lewis, Nurse Una. Moore Park Emergency Hospital, Sydney, N.S.W., Australia.

Lewis, Vinetta Irene. Kokstad, C.P., S. Africa.

Lian, Sing. Ipoh, Malaya.

Libretti, Emma. Ferrara, Italy.

Liersch, Hattie. Kendall. Wis., U.S.A.

Lignell, Anna. Östersund, Sweden.

Liker, Edward. Saratoga Springs, N.Y., U.S.A.

Lindgren, Nelson. East Providence. R.I.

Lindstöl, Pte Toralf. Odderöen, Norway.

Lindstöl, Pte. Toralf. Odderöen, Norway.

Von Linsingen, Beatrice. Queenstown, C.P., S. Africa.

Linson, Dr John H. U.S. Public Health Service: Washington, D.C./ Boston, Brookline, Lawrence, Mass./Providence, R.I./Hartford, Conn., U.S.A.

Littler, Alex. Blackburn, England.

Ljunggren, Pte. Rolf, HQ Göta Life Guards, Stockholm, Sweden.

Llopis, Estela. Tarragona, Spain.

Locuoco, Captain Ettore. *San Giorgio*, Pola, Yugoslavia.

Lode, Kirsten. Naerbø, Norway.

Löf, Anna. Vänersborg, Sweden.

Lohrer, Else. Stuttgart, Germany.

Loida, Isabelle. Fornfelt, Mo., U.S.A.

Long, Edna. Bloomfield, N.B., Canada.

Lorenz, Cpl Frank. Supply Co 310, QMC, Vannes, France.

Loureiro, Francisco Henriques. Paranhos de Beira, Portugal.

Lowe, Lal. Hamilton, N.S.W., Australia.

Lowes, H.P. Health and Home Affairs Dept., Brisbane, Queensl., Australia.

Lubbi, Pte. Jan Jacobus. Harskamp Military Barracks, Holland.

Lucchesi, Frank. Richmond, Va., U.S.A.

Lucia, Sgt. Bernardo. 12th Sanitary Corps, Hospital della Maddalena, Messina, Sicily.

Lumsden, Nurse Alice. Collegiate Annexe Auxiliary Hospital, Brandon, Man., Canada.

Lund, Märta. Karlstad, Sweden.

Lundberg, Henning. Umeå, Sweden.

Lupinetti, Donatangelo. Castilenti, Italy.

Lutz, Ronald. Cedar Hill, Mo., U.S.A.

Lynn, Norval. Welland, Ont., Canada.

Lyons, Doris. Adelaide, S. Australia.

McCord, Major Carey P., M.C. Camp Sherman, Chillicothe, Ohio, U.S.A.

McCoy, Robert. Brown University, Providence, R.I., U.S.A.

MacCracken, F. H. Wellford, S.C., U.S.A.

McCullough, Jane. Leetsdale, Pa., U.S.A.

McCutcheon, Margaret. Lumsden, N.Z.

McDiarmid, Trooper Samuel. 6th Black Watch, Halifax, England.

McDonald, Clara. Bow (East London), England.

MacDonald, Donald. Auckland, N.Z.

McDonald, Nurse Flora. Brisbane Emergency Hospital, Queensl., Australia.

McDonald, Nurse Josephine, St. Vincent's Hospital, Norfolk, Va., U.S.A.

MacDonald, W. E. Timaru, N.Z.

MacDowell, Nurse Eula. Brockville General Hospital, Ont., Canada.

McFadyen, Nurse Jessie. Ballarat Base Hospital, Vic., Australia.

McGarth, Loretta. Freeport, Ill., U.S.A.

McGarth, Mary. Pawtucket, R.I., U.S.A.

McGeckie, Nell. Auckland, N.Z.

McGehan, Jetta. Bethlehem, Pa., U.S.A.

McGregor, Donalda. Chesley, Ont., Canada.

McGregor, Doris. Palmerston, N.Z.

McGruddy, Nurse Frances. Wanganui Hospital, N.Z.

Machado, Fernando. Coimbra. Portugal.

Machell, Sarah. Kendal, England.

Macias, Antonio Gonzales. Cadiz, Spain.

McIndoe, Amy. Clinton, N.Z.

McIntosh, Pte. Charles. 44th Bn. A.I.F., Sutton Viney, England/Cannington, W. Australia.

McIntyre, Florence. Durban, Natal, S. Africa.

McJoliet, Nurse Elizabeth. St Joseph's Hospital, St Paul, Minn., U.S.A.

McKay, Frances. Millwood, Va., U.S.A.

McKeithen, Mae. Florence, S.C., U.S.A.

MacKenzie, Pte. Kenneth. 12th Nelson Regt, Le Tréport, France.

MacKinnon, Iain. Aberdeen, Scotland.

McLay, Jock. Glenhaughton Station, Queensl., Australia.

McLean, Edith. Aberdeen, Scotland.

McLellan, Mary. Oklahoma City, Okla., U.S.A.

McLennan, Tom. Auckland, N.Z.

McLeod, Pte. George. 53rd Y.S. Bn, The Gordon Highlanders, Dundee, Scotland.

McLeod, Norman. Assistant Scoutmaster, Somerset West, C.P., S. Africa.

McMeniman, Caroline Veronica. Wallangarra, Queensl., Australia.

McMeur, Jean. Chefoo, North China.
McMillan, Nona. Elk River, Minn., U.S.A.
McMorris, Cevilla. Lyons, Nebr., U.S.A.
McMorris, Etta Mae. Tulsa, Okla., U.S.A.
McNamara, Marie. Westonia, W. Australia.
McNamara, Nurse Mary. Trinity Hospital, Milwaukee, Wis., U.S.A.
McNaught, Martha. Moorseville, Ind., U.S.A.
MacNeish, Ellen. Chicago, Ill., U.S.A.
Macomber, Ethel. American Red Cross, Le Mans, France.
McQuarrie, Clara. Heward, Sask., Canada.
MacQuarrie, Hector. Taunoa, Tahiti.
McQuilkin, Laura. Empire Hotel, Auckland, N.Z.
McRae, Milton. Rib Lake, Wis., U.S.A.
Maderna, Angelo. Milan, Italy.
Madsen, Dr Paul. Tasing, Denmark.
Maechtel, Maria. Heidelberg, Germany.
Maldonado, Miguel Sánchez. Málaga, Spain.
Malone, Emily. Bristol, England.
Maloney, Cornelius. Waterbury, Conn., U.S.A.
Malval, Gunner André. 30th Field Artillery Regt, St Julien-du-Saults, France.
Malvardi, Giovanna. Turin, Italy.
Manganelli, Enzo. Sassofortino, Italy.
Manna, Anne. Providence, R.I., U.S.A.
Mansour, Ibrahim Youssef. Cairo, U.A.R.
Mänsson, Ragnar. Stora Kopinge, Sweden.
Manzi, Pte. Massimo. 21st Artillery Regt, Mestre, Italy.
Manzionna, Michele. Capurso, Italy.
Marcellini, Cesare. Gazzuolo, Italy.
Von Marchtaler, Anneliese. Obernkirchen, Germany.
Mareth, Kathryn. Gray's Lake, Ill., U.S.A.
Marin, Naval Cadet Nicholas Torices. Arsenal of La Carraca, Cádiz, Spain.
Marks, Mary. St John, N.B., Canada.
Marlia, Anita. Milan, Italy.
Marshall, Elsie. Westonia, W. Australia.
Marsham, F. B. Huntley Preparatory School, Marton, N.Z.
Martin, Doris. Stepney (East London), England.
Martin, Grace. Taumarunui, N.Z.
Martin, Pte. John A. 37th Engineers, U.S.E.F., Allerey, France.
Martin, Joseph. Huntly, N.Z.
Martin, Mary. Quebec, P.Q., Canada.
Martin, Severiano. Gredos (Sierra), Spain.
Martinelli, Alfredo. Semogo, Italy.

Martinotti, Pte Giuseppe. Venaria Airfield, Italy.
Maryburn, Doris, Hastings, England.
Mason, Lucy. Auckland, N.Z.
Mastrorilli, Faustino. Monte Corno, Italy.
Mathewes, Christopher. Charleston, S.C., U.S.A.
Mathiesen, Hilbert. Townsville, N. Queensl., Australia.
Mathisen, Nils. Porsanger, Norway.
Mattson, Rupert. Blenheim, N.Z.
Maurel, Jeanne. Lunéville, France.
Maurizi, Giorgio. Bologna, Italy.
May, Arlene. Bates College, Lewiston, Me., U.S.A.
Mayes, R. J. York, W. Australia.
Mays, Joan Selwyn. Auckland, N.Z.
Mazzaglia, Antonio. Catania, Sicily.
Meehan, Sister Maisie. North Terrace Isolation Hospital, Adelaide, S. Australia.
Mejrli, Anna. Balsfjord, Norway.
Melani, Umberto. Milan, Italy.
Melck, Mary. Wynberg Girls' High School, C.P., S. Africa.
Mendes, Francisco. Porto, Portugal.
Mendis, Seraphina. Fresno, Calif., U.S.A.
Meng, Rudolf. Felt Mills, N.Y., U.S.A.
Menner, Freda. Northcote South, Queensl., Australia.
Menzer, Anthony. Hamilton, Ohio, U.S.A.
Menzer, Yvonne. Parey St Césaire, France.
Merlet, Kathleen. Featherston, N.Z.
Merlin, Assistant Superintendent Florence. Elyria Memorial Hospital, Ohio/Brook's Cubicle Hospital, Boston, Mass., U.S.A.
Merrill, Hazel. Omaha, Nebr., U.S.A.
Merrillees, Barbara. Roma, Queensl., Australia.
Merriman, Florence. Chiloquoia, Oreg., U.S.A.
Meroni, Pte. Aldo. 62nd Infantry Regt, Calestano, Italy.
Messina, Giuseppe. Catania, Sicily.
Messinger, Eva. Rockford, Ill., U.S.A.
Metcalf, Mary. Erlanger, Ky., U.S.A.
Metheny, Jennie. Delaplaine, Ark., U.S.A.
Mayers, Alice. Boulder City, W. Australia.
Micard, René. St Nicholas de Port, France.
Michael, Nurse Sarah. Winnipeg General Hospital, Man., U.S.A.
Middleton, Doris. Buninyong, Vic., Australia.
Milbauer, Rivie. Bronx. N.Y.
Milburn, Dr Henry Hall. Vancouver, B.C., Canada
Miles, Margaret. Keiskamma Hoek, C.P., S. Africa.
Millen, Eileen. Thames, N.Z.

Miller, Betsy. Blackpool, England.
Milne, Trooper William. 4/5th Black Watch, Brussels, Belgium.
Miranda, Elpidio Salas. Grecia, Costa Rica.
Mitoyo, Shizuo. Tokyo, Japan.
Mittendorf, Else. Schwerte an der Ruhr, Germany.
Mocke, E. J. Bothaville, O.F.S., S. Africa.
Mohr, Claudia. Plainview, Nebr., U.S.A.
Molina, Vicente. Nogales, Mexico.
Møller, Nurse Margit. Stavenger/Naerbø, Norway.
Momigliano, Lieut. Mario. 139th Sapper Engineering Coy, Val Giudi-
     caria, Italy.
Mondini, Giovanni. Bologna, Italy.
Montag, Lillian. Pittsburgh, Pa., U.S.A.
Montel, Capt. Lucien. 12th Bn. Chasseurs Alpins, Monts-en-Ternois,
     France.
Montenegro, Juan. Montevideo, Uruguay.
Moore, Elizabeth. Mahana, N.Z.
Moore, Mary. City Doctors' Receiving Office, Los Angeles, Calif., U.S.A.
Moquet, Marie Luce. Langon, France.
Mørch, Gunner Johannes. Kristiansholm Castle Battery, Klampenborg,
     Denmark.
Morelli, Carmine. Naples, Italy.
Morena, Antonio Serra. Vialdran, Spain.
Morgan, Irene. Miami University, Oxford, Ohio, U.S.A.
Morgan, Irene. Providence, R.I., U.S.A.
Morgan, Peg. Park City, Utah, U.S.A.
Morgan, T. V. Charleroi, Pa., U.S.A.
Morier, Gunner Lucien. 120th Heavy Artillery Regt, Cussy-les-Forges,
     France.
Morris, Ethel. Hell Hole, S.C., U.S.A.
Morris, Marion. Uitenhage, C.P., S. Africa.
Morrish, Stanley. Avondale, N.Z.
Morrison, Donald. Kyogle, N.S.W., Australia.
Morsilli, Peter. Providence, R.I., U.S.A.
Moses, Margaret. South Ohio, N.S., Canada.
Mostert, Ralie. Grootfontein Farm, Paarl, C.P., S. Africa.
Motwani, Satram. Bombay, India.
Moulton, Ward Attendant Gladys. Keswick Military Hospital, Adelaide,
     S. Australia.
Mulholland, Pte. Fitzgerald. 8th Bn. A.I.F., H.M.H.T. *Orantes*,
     Albany, W. Australia.
Mulholland, T. H. Auckland, N.Z.
Mullen, Helen. Scranton, Pa., U.S.A.
Muller, 2nd Lieut. Rodolfo. 24th Photo-Electric Coy, Crone, Italy.

Mullins, John. Etty, Ky., U.S.A.

Mullins, C. G. St Andrews Preparatory School, Grahamstown, C.P., S. Africa.

Munro, Elizabeth. Glen of Foulis, Scotland.

Munro, Mary. Kilmarnock, Scotland.

Murphy, Anna. Pittsburgh, Pa., U.S.A.

Murphy, Edward. Quebec, P.Q., Canada.

Murphy, R. V. Fall River, Mass., U.S.A.

Murray, H. B. Dubbo, N.S.W., Australia.

Mustoe, Florence. Belmont, Kan., U.S.A.

Mutch, Anne. Auckland, N.Z.

Myers, John. Christchurch, N.Z.

Myers, Mattie. Alicia, Ark., U.S.A.

Myles, Amelia. Moundsville, W.Va., U.S.A.

Myrick, Charlotte, Hubbard Woods, Ill., U.S.A.

Nadebaum, R. Henry. Milang, S. Australia.

Najfa, Zejnilagic. Blasanica, Bosnia.

Nakamura. Tetsu. Tokyo, Japan.

Nash, Pte. Mary. W.A.A.C. Bushley Hall O.T.C. Camp, Watford, England.

Nattermann, Käthe. Mayen, Germany.

Nava, Livio. Milan, Italy.

Naylor, Julia. Clifton Hill, Mo., U.S.A.

Needham, Barbara. Pittsburgh, Pa., U.S.A.

Nel, Police Constable D. J. Durban, Natal, S. Africa.

Nepean, Lidia. Sydney, N.S.W., Australia.

Nestor, Mary. Koo Wee Rup, Vic., Australia.

New, Sgt. Maurice. 1st Bn. Hampshire Regt, Belfast, N. Ireland.

New, Violet. Ashburton, N.Z.

Newell, Eric. King's School, Canterbury, England.

Newman, Burgess. Owaka, N.Z.

Newton, Alan. Bloemfontein, O.F.S., S. Africa.

Ney, Darcy. Warwick, Queensl., Australia.

Nichols, Artia. Skiatook, Okla., U.S.A.

Niemann, Ruth. Zuoz, Switzerland.

Nienaber, Maria. Vrede, O.F.S., S. Africa.

Nikolic, Zarko. Gorazde, Yugoslavia.

Nilssen, Ole. Trondheim, Norway.

Nilsson, Carl. Ränneslöv, Sweden.

Nilsson, Elon, Malmslätt, Sweden.

Nilsson, Esther. Fryserum, Sweden.

Nilsson, Mia. Katslöse, Sweden.

Nilsson, Pte. Oscar. HQ., Heavy Artillery Regt, Stockholm, Sweden.

Nissinen, Lilv. Helsinki, Finland.
Noll, William. Wein, Mo., U.S.A.
Nordberg, Eva. Gothenburg, Sweden.
Norman, Kathleen, Winchester, N.Z.
Norris, Gladys. Qumbu, C.P., S. Africa.
Norstad, Ole. Drammen, Norway.
Northover, Joseph. Auckland, N.Z.
Nott, Dorothy. Elgin, Nebr., U.S.A.
Nowland, Isabelle. Muswellbrook, N.S.W., Australia.
Nuthall, Gladys. Christchurch, N.Z.
Nyberg, Hilda. Arnö Island, Sweden.
Nye, Clare. Westonia, W. Australia.
Nyheim, Oluf. Bjerkvik, Norway.
Oddy, Martha. Leeds, England.
Oke, Bessie. Boissevain, Man., Canada.
Oldford, Beatrice. Bonavista Bay, NF.
Oliphant, Nurse Isa. 4th Scottish Military Hospital, Glasgow, Scotland.
Oliver, Cpl. Charles, R.A.F. *City of Marseilles*: Newcastle, England/
    Murmansk, Russia.
Oliver, Ruby. San Francisco, Calif., U.S.A.
Olivetti, Gemma. Rome, Italy.
Olsen, Petra. Halstad, Norway.
Olsson, Signe. Gothenburg, Sweden.
O'Neale, Harry. Featherston, N.Z.
O'Neall, Eleanor. Greenville, S.C., U.S.A.
Oreno, Carmela. Trabia, Sicily.
Orsi, Giuseppina. Spinetta Marengo, Italy.
Osborn, Roma. Cedar City, Utah, U.S.A.
Osman, Marjorie. Unley Park, S. Australia.
Ottsen, Dr Ernst. Virchow Hospital, Berlin, Germany.
Oxenham, Nurse 'Mickey'. St John's Hospital, Johannesburg, Tvl., S.
    Africa.
Pace, Mary. Flippin, Ark., U.S.A.
Pache, 2/Lt. Ernest. 9th Replacement Bn, Camp MacArthur, Waco,
    Tex., U.S.A.
Palmer, Margaret. Schumpert Memorial Sanitorium, Shreveport, La.,
    U.S.A
Paltridge, Staff Nurse Bessie. Woodman's Point, W. Australia.
Panzeri, Lorenzo. Como, Italy.
Pardiny, Elizabeth. Charleroi, Pa., U.S.A.
Parikh, J. C. Delhi, India.
Parish, Lila. Boston, Mass., U.S.A.
Parr, Eric. Auckland, N.Z.
Parris, Phyllis. Victoria Coffee Palace. Melbourne, Vic., Australia.

Parsons, Mary. Rotunda Hospital, Perth, W. Australia.
Partridge, Edith. Milwaukee, Wis., U.S.A.
Partridge, Len. Toronto, Ont., Canada.
Pascale, Vincenzo. Rome, Italy.
Pasquini, Lieut. Luigi. 2nd Regt, Sardinian Grenadiers, Cavazuccherina, Italy.
Passelegue, Lieut. Georges. 206th Regt, 75th Artillery Coy, Reims, France.
Passerini, Nurse Lidia. 'Il Corallo' Military Hospital, Leghorn, Italy.
Pattaloung, Pluem Na. Pattaloung, Thailand.
Patterson, Dulcie. Auckland, N.Z.
Patterson, Sgt. Howard. 149 F.A. Rainbow Divn, Bad-Nuhenahr, Germany.
Patterson, Lawrence A. Brantford, Ont., Canada.
Patterson, Ruth. East Malvern, Vic., Australia.
Paulsen, Nurse Hanna. Harstad, Norway.
Paulson, G. B. San Francisco, Calif., U.S.A.
Pavanati, Linda. Ariano, Italy.
Paviotti, Signalman Umberto. 3rd Telegraph Coy, Trentino, Italy.
Paynter, Evelyn. West Echuca, Vic., Australia.
Pearce, Doreen. Southampton, England.
Pearce, Lillian. Wellington., N.Z.
Pearce, Nurse Miriam. Exhibition Building Emergency Hospital. Adelaide, S. Australia.
Pearman-White, George. Alice, C.P., S. Africa.
Pedersen, Alma. Kelstrupmark, Denmark.
Pedersen, Haakon. Nedgaard, Norway.
Pedroni, Angelina. Gussago, Italy.
Pellegri, Silvio. Parma, Italy.
Peltrera, Cesira Vittoria. Venice, Italy.
Perpich. Libia. Trieste, Italy.
Perradt, Molly. Mountain View, Pretoria, S. Africa.
Perry, Elizabeth. Haughton Institute, Va., U.S.A.
Persdotter, Maria. Mora, Sweden.
Persson, Ebba. Lund, Sweden.
Perssonn Gunvor. Skåne, Sweden.
Persson, Nils Lorents. Baskemölla, Sweden.
Pessoa, Vasco Silva. Amadora, Portugal.
Petrie, Annie. Sandstone School, Riversdale, N.Z.
Pettersson, Signaller Gustav. Heavy Field Artillery Regt, Stockholm, Sweden.
Pettigrew, May. Rufton, N.Z.
Petzel, Ada. Decatur, Ill., U.S.A.
Pfeiffer, Julie. Stuttgart, Germany.

Phillips, Choc. Tulsa, Okla., U.S.A.

Phillips, Gunner John. Royal Garrison Artillery, Villers-Bretonneux, France.

Phillips, Lydia. Twist Street School Emergency Hospital, Johannesburg, Tvl., S. Africa.

Pian, Alma. Piazza Armerina, Sicily.

Picard, Herbert. Birchton Rue, P.Q., Canada.

Picavet, Gunner Albert. 2nd Field Artillery Regt, Grenoble, France.

Pickett, Irma. Auckland, N.Z.

Picon, Jose Garcia. Badajoz, Spain.

Pieper, Otto. Rio de Janeiro, Brazil.

Pierallini, Anna Maria. Verona, Italy.

Pierantoni, Lucia. Verona, Italy.

Pierce, Mary. Attleboro, Mass., U.S.A.

Pigay, Andreina. Turin, Italy.

Piggin, Ethel. Nottingham, England.

Pilotti, Dionigi. Cremona, Italy.

Pimentel, Fernando Souza. Lisbon, Portugal.

Pineau, Edouard. Angoulême, France.

Pini, Tina. Grosseto, Italy.

Pinto, Jose Teixeira. Porto, Portugal.

Pinto Coelho, Maria. Mondiser de Basto, Portugal.

Pintor, Lieut. Mario. 87th Infantry Regt, Dossobuno, Italy.

Piona, Rina. Verbania-Intra, Italy.

Pirini, Manlio. Cesano Maderno, Italy.

Pirovano, Angela. Monza, Italy.

Pitcaithley, Al. Beatrice, Nebr., U.S.A.

Pitcher, Ernest. Alfred Hospital, Melbourne, Vic., Australia.

Pitzolu, Fortunato. Bolotana, Sardinia.

Plush, Edna. Hyde Park, Adelaide, S. Australia.

Poer, J. Ermin. Lebanon, Ind., U.S.A.

Poirier, Elsie. Trinidad, Colo., U.S.A.

Poland, Hope. Elvaston, Ill., U.S.A.

Poll, Jantje. Delft, Holland.

Pollard, Senior Nurse Winifred. Christchurch Hospital, N.Z.

Pollino, Pietro. Velletri, Italy.

Polo, Aurora. Madrid, Spain.

Pond, Pte. Benjamin. Bedfordshire Regiment, Ladyguard Camp, Felixstowe, England.

Ponnuswamy, C. R. Madras, India.

Popham, Hattie. Barons, Alta., Canada.

Poos, Gesina Maria. Nijmegen, Holland.

Del Portillo, Hector. San Francisco/Mazatlan, Mexico.

Poulter, Elizabeth. Port Elizabeth, C.P., S. Africa.

Post, Meta. Koonibba Mission Station, S. Australia.
Pozderovic, Enver. Gorazde, Yugoslavia.
Pozzesi, Alina. Milan, Italy.
Pradere, Marguerite. Dayton, Nev., U.S.A.
Prasad, Rajendra. Calcutta, India.
Pratesi, Sgt-Pilot Vincenzo. No 282 Squadron, Catania, Sicily.
Pratt, Pte. Billie. 4th Scottish Military Hospital, Glasgow, Scotland.
Pratt, Emily. Malvern, Natal, S. Africa.
Pratt, 2/Lt. Oliver. 6th Development Bn., Camp Meade, Md., U.S.A.
Preston, Katherine. Glen Williams, Ont., Canada.
Prevoteau, Sgt. Roger. 8th Infantry Regt, Lunéville, France.
Price, J. W. Merredin, W. Australia.
Prinsloo, Wesselim. Daggafontein, Tvl, S. Africa.
Pritchard, Josephine. Bloemfontein, O.F.S., S. Africa.
Pritchett, William. Kenbridge, Va., U.S.A.
Provini, Umberto. Turin, Italy.
Pugnaire, Nurse Marguerite. No 53 Military Hospital, Marseilles, France.
Purdie, Laura. Dunedin, N.Z.
Puryear, E. H. Richmond, Va., U.S.A.
Putman, Emma. Modesto, Calif., U.S.A.
Puttick, Hilda. Pietermaritzburg, Natal, S. Africa.
Quigley, Catharine. Palatka, Fla., U.S.A.
Quinn, Blanche. Blackville, N.B., Canada.
Raddatz, Chester. Milwaukee, Wis., U.S.A.
Rafael, Maria Fernanda. Cape St Vincent, Cape Verde Is.
Rahim, Ibrahim. Singapore.
Raimondi, Sapper Lino. 40th Supply Coy, 1st Engineers Regt, Bermo.
   Lomellino, Italy.
Ramaker, Clara. Milwaukee, Wis., U.S.A.
Ramsay, Nurse Mildred. Victoria Hospital, Winnipeg, Man., Canada.
Ramstad, Nancy. Namsos, Norway.
Rankine, Rachel. Bournville, Birmingham, England.
Ransom, Alice. Byrock, N.S.W., Australia.
Rath, Father Ern Jan. Den Dungen, Holland.
Rath, Cpl. Harold. 126 Field Artillery, H.M.S. *Kashmir.*
Rath, William. Adelaide, S. Australia.
Rathbone, Ruth, Carnforth, England.
Rautensparger, Ellinor. Coburg, Germany.
Ravasio, Vittorino. Villanuova sul Clisi, Italy.
Read, E. J. Nottingham Road, Natal, S. Africa.
Read, Harold. Lok Kan Rubber Estate, Nr. Brunei, Borneo.
Reams, Ruth. Richmond, Va., U.S.A.
Rech, Margarete. Ehrenbreitstein, Germany.
Reddano, Eileen. Essendon, Melbourne, Vic., Australia.

Redondo, Valentin. Mexico City.
Redshaw, Lila. Te Kowhai, N.Z.
Reed, Agnes. Bloemfontein, O.F.S., S. Africa.
Reichstein, Flo. Booleroo Whim, S. Australia.
Reid, Nurse Maude. Camp Beauregard, Alexandria, La., U.S.A.
Reid, Minnie. Coronation, Alta., Canada.
Reinbach, N. A. Cape Town, C.P., S. Africa.
Rentschler, Katie. Hamilton, Ohio, U.S.A.
Renz, Martha. Stuttgart, Germany.
Resmini, Maria. Treviglio, Italy.
Retief, Pieter. Lichtenburg, Tvl., S. Africa.
Reuch, Anna. Siegen, Germany.
Reutersvärd, Elsa. Uddevalla, Sweden.
Rhodes-Harrison, W. Bloemfontein General Hospital, O.F.S., S. Africa.
Richey, Homer. Starkville, Miss., U.S.A.
Richley, Frances. Kahibah, N.S.W., Australia.
Riddell, Leith. Wellington, N.Z.
Riddle, Alexander. South Shields, England.
Rielly, Ida. Auckland, N.Z.
Rijsbeek, Klaas. Wildervank, Holland.
Risendahl Petersen, Danine. Grindste, Denmark.
Riva, Laura. Valdagno, Italy.
Robba, Irene. Brisbane, Queensl., Australia.
Roberts, Alice. Oakland, Calif., U.S.A.
Roberts, Arthur. Penrith, N.S.W., Australia.
Roberts, Cecile. Durrington, England.
Roberts, Frances. Oshkosh, Wis., U.S.A.
Robertson, Carol. Quebec, P.Q., Canada.
Robertson, Clifton. Penniman, Va., U.S.A.
Robertson, Florence. Green Island, N.Z.
Robertson, Mina. Harrismith, O.F.S., S. Africa.
Robinson, Pte. Arthur. H.M.A.S., *Boonah*: Durban–Adelaide.
Robinson, Eldon. Arcola, Sask., Canada.
Robinson, Myrtle Mary. Heywood State School Hospital, Vic., Australia.
Robinson, Richard. St Louis, Mo., U.S.A.
Robson, Ethel. Coventry, England.
Roche, Elizabeth. Dunedin, N.Z.
Roche, Mary Agnes. Blackpool, England.
Rogers, Scout Douglass. Grahamstown, C.P., S. Africa.
Rogers, Pearl. Finis Creek, N.C., U.S.A.
Rognså, Nicolai. Sjövegan, Norway.
Rohlfing, Esther. Berger, Mo., U.S.A.
Roland, Goldena. Hannibal, Mo., U.S.A.
Roland, William. Hannibal, Mo., U.S.A.

Roller, Katharine. Stuttgart, Germany.
Rollins, Nurse Hazel. Fort Sam Houston, Tex., U.S.A.
Romagnolo, Pasquale. Ischitella Garganico, Italy.
Ronco, Alfredo. Genoa, Italy.
Ronning, Haakon. Skjeberg, Norway.
Rosaro, Angela. Zbaraz, Poland.
Rose, Ruth. Augusta, Ga., U.S.A.
Ross, Lillian. Whiritoa, N.Z.
Rossi, Celina. Turin, Italy.
Roth, Fritz. Cologne, Germany.
Roussin, Ray. Portland, Me., U.S.A.
Roux, Elizabeth. Murraysburg, C.P., S. Africa.
Rovira, Joaquin Collia. Alicante, Spain.
Rowe, A. L. Sydney, N.S.W., Australia.
Rowlands, William. Hays, Pa., U.S.A.
Rudström, John. Eksjö, Sweden.
Ruediger, Wilma. Gleiwitz, Germany.
Reuhl, Ray. Milwaukee, Wis., U.S.A.
Rummells, Amanda. Nichols, Ia., U.S.A.
Rush, Claude. Stradbroke, England.
Rush, Edmund. Rowhegan, R.I., U.S.A.
Russell, Patricia. Newmarket, England.
Rutherford, Agnes. Caulfield, Vic., Australia.
Rutledge, Laura. Vancouver, B.C., Canada.
Ryan, Nurse Dorothy. Victoria Hospital, Winnipeg, Man., Canada.
Sachs, Marga. Hamburg, Germany.
Sage, Esther. Goodland, Ind., U.S.A.
Saggers, S. H. Tambellup, W. Australia.
Sagvik, Dagfinn. Finnøy, Norway.
Sahinagic, Aisa. Gorazde, Yugoslavia.
Saija, Nicolò. Messina, Sicily.
Sainsbury, Laurel. Melbourne, Vic., Australia.
St Leger, Sister Claire. Summit Hospital, Cape Town, S. Africa.
St Pierre, Sgt-Major L. Bramshott Camp, England.
Sala, José Borrell. Segur, Spain.
Salb, Elsie. West Allis, Wis., U.S.A.
Salerno, Lila. Alfred Hospital, Melbourne, Australia.
Salter, Annie. Te Awamutu, N.Z.
Sanchez, Pedro. Buenos Aires, Argentina.
Sangiorgi. Pte. Guglielmo. Santa Chiara Hospital, Padua, Italy.
Sannino, Mario. Alba, Italy.
Santavicca, Elizabeth. Crofton, Pa., U.S.A.
Satterthwaite, Allan. Auckland, N.Z.

Saunders, Nurse Eunice. Mount Sinai Hospital, Milwaukee, Wis., U.S.A.

Sawyer, Rose. Hackney (East London), England.

Saylor, Dorothy. Norristown, Pa., U.S.A.

Scaetta, Lieut. Cesare. Hospital Vittorino de Feltre, Rome, Italy.

Scellier, Robert. Paris, France.

Schäfer, Lina. Zuffenhausen, Germany.

Schaible, Nurse Eleanor. Protestant Deaconess Hospital, Indianapolis, Ind., U.S.A.

Schillings, Amelie. Kirchherten, Germany.

Schley, Mabel. Milwaukee, Wis., U.S.A.

Schmidt, Ernst. Königszelt, Germany.

Schmitz, Aenne. Koblenz, Germany.

Schmitz, Grete. Koblenz, Germany.

Schöck, Gabriele. Freiburg, Germany.

Scholler, Erna. Stuttgart, Germany.

Schouland, Sapper F. W. Cape Fortress Engineers, Simonstown Barracks, C.P., S. Africa.

Schoyen, Gustav. Høyanger, Norway.

Schrik, Elizabeth. Emmen, Holland.

Schröder, Dr. Walter. Brandenburg City Hospital, Germany.

Schroeder, Veronica. St Louis, Mo., U.S.A.

Schultz, Rev. A. Josef. Shedden, Ont., Canada.

Schutzler, Miss J. W. Cape Town, C.P., S. Africa.

Scotland, Duncan. Dundee, Scotland.

Scott, Berta. Masterton, N.Z.

Scott, William. Columbia, S.C., U.S.A.

Seaban, Hilda. Montreal, P.Q., Canada.

Seacombe, Tilly. Deptford (South London), England.

Seager, Aline. Christchurch, N.Z.

Seal, Gertie. Leicester, England.

Sealey, Helen. Portland, Oreg., U.S.A.

Seckel, Ernst. Enschede, Holland.

Secone, Francesco. Spoleto, Italy.

Seeber, Pauline. Fonthill, Ont., Canada.

Sefverblad, Carl. Maria Hospital, Stockholm, Sweden.

Seifert, Elizabeth. St Louis, Mo., U.S.A.

Seip, Kathleen. Dallarnil, Vic., Australia.

Selakovich, Mary. Leadville, Colo., U.S.A.

Sennett, Norman. Lytton Quarantine Hospital, N.S.W., Australia.

Servadei, Arnaldo. Cesena, Italy.

Serventi, Cpl. Mario. 44th Infantry Regt, Silvano d'Orba, Italy.

Shackleton, W. A. Que Que, S. Rhodesia.

Shapiro, Ruth. Milwaukee, Wis., U.S.A.

Sharp, Hilda. Auckland, N.Z.
Sharpe, Leah. Carlton, Vic., Australia.
Sharpe, Lillie. Waverly, Va., U.S.A.
Shaw, Adeleine. Otiria Junction, N.Z.
Shaw, Bertha. South Porcupine, Ont., Canada.
Shaw, Evelyn. Phoenix, Ariz., U.S.A.
Sheaff, Eva. Rockford, Ill., U.S.A.
Sheehan, Doreen. Brompton, S. Australia.
Shell, Dorothy. Sydney, N.S.W., Australia.
Shinen, Vera. Los Angeles, Calif., U.S.A.
Short, Mary. Manilla, N.S.W., Australia.
Shuman, Pelagia. Huron, S. Dak., U.S.A.
Sias, Luigina. Ghilarsa, Sardinia.
Sidentz, Martha. South Bend, Ind., U.S.A.
Siksec, Marie. Ain Temouchent, Algeria.
Silvestri, Giulio. Rome, Italy.
Simansky, Capt Nicholas. 1st Russian Infantry Division, French Army
    of the East, nr Lake Ohrid, Macedonia.
Simeoni, Jole. Legnano, Italy.
Simpson, Marion. Fife, Scotland.
Simpson, Sarah. Belhelvie, Scotland.
Sinclair, Irene. Georgetown, Ont., Canada.
Sjöberg, Johan. Filipstad, Sweden.
Skillingstad, Ebbe. Naerøy, Norway.
Slee, Addie. Rushworth, Vic., Australia.
Slemmer, J. Le Roy, Phoenixville, Pa., U.S.A.
Sloan, Nellie. Tonopah, Nev., U.S.A.
Smelser, Marshall. Rockford, Ill., U.S.A.
Smidt, Dorris. Westonia, W. Australia.
Smith, Berenice. Winnipeg, Man., Canada.
Smith, Eric. Christchurch, N.Z.
Smith, Frances. Coventry, England.
Smith, Jody. Suffolk. Va., U.S.A.
Smith, Kathleen. Bardoe, W. Australia.
Smith, Nurse Louise. Ramona Hospital, San Bernardino, Calif., U.S.A.
Smith, Signalman Roger. U.S. Army Signal Corps, Fort Leavenworth,
    Kansas, U.S.A.
Smuts, Jan. Ermelo, Tvl., S. Africa.
Snowdon, Linda. Montreal. P.Q., Canada.
Sodre da Motta, Elvira. Olinda, Brazil.
Soh, Karen. Singapore.
Solberg, Aslaug. Naustdal, Norway.
Solinas, Francesco. Sennarolo, Sardinia.
Solomon, Dorothy. East Perth, W. Australia.

Sørensen, Peder. Ollerup, Denmark.
Sorge, Naval Cadet Herbert. Marine College, Flensburg, Germany.
Sossoman, Mary. South Bend, Ind., U.S.A.
Spangler, P. K. Longmont, Colo., U.S.A.
Spark, Annabella. Bieldside, Scotland.
Sperber, Joe. Kimberley, C.P., S. Africa.
Spicer, Gay. Apple Grove, Va., U.S.A.
Stackwood, J. R. Christchurch, N.Z.
Stacpoole, May. Napier, N.Z.
Stahl, Antonius. Barnflair, Holland.
Stainer, Alice. Helensburgh, N.S.W., Australia.
Starke, Jean. Coleman, Wis., U.S.A.
Starkey, Frank. Sydney, N.S.W., Australia.
Stavish, Marion. Ralph, Pa., U.S.A.
Steffens, Elsa. Hamburg, Germany.
Stegehuis, Hermina. Twekkelo, Holland.
Steicke, Victor. Mount Barker, W. Australia.
Stein, Lawrence. St Louis, Mo., U.S.A.
Stein, Simone. Comtois, France.
Stephens, A. B. Landsborough, Queensl., Australia.
Stephenson, Beatrice. Christchurch. N.Z.
Steppler, Frances. Morden, Man., Canada.
Sterr, Louise. Lomira, Wis., U.S.A.
Stevenson, Mary. Fletching, England.
Stevenson, Ruby. Penn's Grove, N.J., U.S.A.
Stewart, J. H. Karamea, N.Z.
Stirling, Naomi. Edgecombe, Vic., Australia.
Stoffel, Otto. Beuren-by-Irmenach, Germany.
Stoll, Harry. Milwaukee, Wis., U.S.A.
Stoll, Lillian. Jamaica, L.I., U.S.A.
Stolz, Johann. Komati River, Tvl., S. Africa.
Straating, Antje. Groningen, Holland.
Strain, Mary. Armadale State School Emergency Hospital, Melbourne, Vic., Australia.
Stritzingen, Claire. Norristown, Pa., U.S.A.
Struthers, A. H. Christchurch, N.Z.
Stuart, Veronica. Christchurch, N.Z.
Stubbe, Dr Hans. Blackboy Hill Camp, Perth, W. Australia.
Sturgeon, Pauline. Kirksville, Mo., U.S.A.
Stuttaford, Wallace. Notting Hill (London), England.
Sullivan, Aileen. Fargo, N. Dak., U.S.A.
Sulski, Julia. Bethal High School, Tvl., S. Africa.
Sumitomo, Uichi. Tokyo, Japan.
Summers, Dorothy. Carmangay, Alta., Canada.

Suque, Codina. Madrid, Spain.
Svenningsen, Marie. Arendal, Norway.
Svensson, Carolina. Löderup, Sweden.
Svensson, Frida. Kyrkhult, Sweden.
Swan, James. Petersham, N.S.W., Australia.
Swan, John. Harwich, England.
Swan, Robert. Stepney (East London), England.
Swancott, Charles. Willoughby, N.S.W., Australia.
Swanstrom, Mildred. Pecatonica, Ill., U.S.A.
Sweeting, Constance. St Albans, England.
Taillefer, Rita. Worcester, Mass., U.S.A.
Takahashi, Yoshihiro. Tokyo, Japan.
Talbot, Margaret. Bethlehem, Pa., U.S.A.
Tavis, Anna Mae. Boulder, Colo., U.S.A.
Taylor, Annie. Regina, Sask., Canada.
Taylor, Doris. Penzance, England.
Taylor, Florence. Jamestown, N. Dak., U.S.A.
Taylor, Lawrence. Greeley, Colo., U.S.A.
Taylor, Nurse Margaret. 2nd New Zealand General Hospital, Walton-on-Thames, England.
Tazewell, Stephen. Cootamundra, N.S.W., Australia.
Teague, Bernard. Wairoa, N.Z.
Teasdale, Frances. Longwood, N.Z.
Temple, Rebecca. Hopewell, Va., U.S.A.
Tennyson, 2/Lt. Alfred. 11th Bn. Depot Brigade Non-Coms School, Camp Devens, Mass., U.S.A.
Thamm, Xenia. Burra, S. Australia.
Theodorovich, Emma. Coutts, Alta., Canada.
Tholholte, Johan. Münster, Germany.
Thomas, Dr George. Tung Wa Hospital, Hong Kong.
Thomassen, Bertrand. Kirkenss, Norway.
Thomasson, Arthur. Lynchburg, Va., U.S.A.
Thompson, Doris. Casino, N.S.W., Australia.
Thompson, Florence. Dunedin, N.Z.
Thompson, Grace. Beaconsfield, N.S.W., Australia.
Thomson, Iris. Christchurch, N.Z.
Thomson, Lance. Melbourne, Vic., Australia.
Thomson, Lois. Hastings, N.Z.
Thomson, Pte. William. 47th Reinforcement Bn., N.Z.E.F., Featherston Camp, N.Z.
Thorn, Captain Albert. 'A' Company Machine Gun Battalion, 30th Canadian Division, Mt Kemmel, France.
Thornander, D. W. Westonia, W. Australia.
Thornton, Lillian. Springfield, Colo., U.S.A.

Thorpe, Nurse Mary Jane. West Riding Asylum, Wakefield, England.
Thunell, Marie. Avalon, Pittsburgh, Pa., U.S.A.
Thwaite, Anne. Liverpool, England.
Tiedjems, Goldie. Phillips, Wis., U.S.A.
Tilman, Mary. Emmett, Idaho, U.S.A.
Timms, Les. Melbourne, Vic., Australia.
Tiozzo, Byba. Venice, Italy.
Titman, Ida. Belvidere, Ill., U.S.A.
Tobin, William. Worcester, Mass., U.S.A.
Todd, Aircraftman Claude. Stamford, England.
Todesco, Enrica. Milan, Italy.
Tödt, Marie. Kiel, Germany.
Tokle, Arne. Honningsvaag, Norway.
Tommascella, Antonio. Caneva, Italy.
Toone, Hilda. Leicester, England.
Töpler, Margot. Dortmund, Germany.
Torelli, Mardella. Vienna, Austria.
Torp, Harald, Eidsberg, Norway.
Torricelli, Maria. Milan, Italy.
Traverso, Catherine. Marseilles, France.
Trembley, Francis. Naples, N.Y., U.S.A.
Treves, Nurse Silvia. Camp Hospital 0110, Marsan, Italy.
Trueta, Dr José. Madrid, Spain.
Trülsen, Günther. Rendsburg, Germany.
Tseung, Fat Im. Causeway Bay, Hong Kong.
Tucker, Pte Arthur. R.A.S.C. Bristol, England.
Turner, Elsie. Plenty, Sask., Canada.
Turner, Emma. Vivian, La., U.S.A.
Turner, Harry. Blackboy Hill Camp, Perth, W. Australia.
Turner, Susan. Petersburg, Va., U.S.A.
Ubbink, Maria. Gaast, Holland.
Ulfsnaes, Nordgren. Vannavalen, Norway.
Underhill, George. Sterling Bank, Mille Roches, Ont., Canada.
Underwood, Lenore. Enderline, N. Dak., U.S.A.
Upton, Daisy. Coalville, England.
Usher, Eleanor, Lusaka, N. Rhodesia.
Utt, Nurse Nettie, Terre Haute, Ind., U.S.A.
Valdes, Josefina. Mexico City.
Valentine, Helen. Bessemer, Pa., U.S.A.
Valerio, Thomas. Bloomfield, Pittsburgh, Pa., U.S.A.
Valle, Gina. Rome, Italy.
Vallini, Pte Antonio. 8th Company, Air Technicians, Turin, Italy.
Van Beekum, Student Nurse Margaretha. Vlaardings Hospital, Hof-
    singel, Vlaardingen, Holland.

Van der Byl, Zoë. Brackenfel, C.P., S. Africa.

Van der Harst, Olga. Goes, Holland.

Van der Wart, Peter. Voorburg, Holland.

Van der Merwe, Police-Constable F. J. De Aar, C.P., S. Africa.

Van Geuns, Dr Richard. Cape Town–Malmesbury–Darling, C.P., S. Africa.

Van Mook, Hendrikus. Losser, Holland.

Van Niekirk, Hester. Excelsior, O.F.S., S. Africa.

Van Schowen, Petronella. Haarlem, Holland.

Van Veldhuizen, Geurtje. Wolfheze, Holland.

Van Winkle, Nurse Pearl. Camp Oglethorpe, Ga., U.S.A.

Van Wyk, A. A. London 33, W. Tvl., S. Africa.

Varola, Ambrogio. Florence, Italy.

Vaught, Quartermaster 1st Class John. U.S.N.A.C., Miami, Fla., U.S.A.

Vecchia, Orlando. Lecce, Italy.

Vegter, Geert. Nieuw Weerdingen, Holland.

Verges, Dolores. Arenys de Mar, Spain.

Vermaak, Marthinus. Roberts Heights, Pretoria, Tvl., S. Africa.

Vernitis, Ann. Sheatown, Pa., U.S.A.

Versini, Violet. Pietermaritzburg, Natal, S. Africa.

Veum, Karoline. Vassbygdi, Norway.

Vicenzotto, Tersilla. Marina di Pisa/Padua, Italy.

Vieillard, Gunner Pierre. 82nd Heavy Artillery Regt, Esnes, France.

Viladanes, Pepita. Sans (Barcelona), Spain.

Vimpany, Marjorie. Hanover, C.P., S. Africa.

Vitarelli, Anthony. Waterbury, Conn., U.S.A.

Voight, Louis. Chicago, Ill., U.S.A.

Voillery, Charles. Puligny-Montrachet, France.

Volkers, Willem. Zwolle, Holland.

Vowell, Christopher. Christchurch, N.Z.

Wahlström, Anna. Umeå, Sweden.

Walker, Dr Gordon. Gormanston, Tasmania.

Walker, John. Walmer, C.P., S. Africa.

Walker, Mary. Madras General Hospital, India.

Wall, Ivy. Okangai, N.Z.

Waller, Cyril. Malvern College, Worcester, England.

Waller, Florence. Papanui, N.Z.

Wälles, Nurse Geertruida. Academic Hospital, Groningen, Holland.

Wallwin, Gladys. Barons, Alta., Canada.

Walsh, James. Dolerin Island, Placentia Bay, NF.

Walsh, Kathleen. Auckland, N.Z.

Walters, Lottie. Boulder, W. Australia.

Walz, Rose. St Louis, Mo., U.S.A.

Ward, Charles. Sunderland, England.

Ward, Teckla. Rockport, N.B., Canada.
Wärring, Ingeborg. Hälsinborg, Sweden.
Wäsche, Nurse Erna. Brunswick City Hospital, Germany.
Wäsche, Günther. Harzrand, Germany.
Wassung, Ernestine. Mossel Bay, C.P., S. Africa.
Waters, Winifred. St Albans, England.
Watkins, Clem. Snaresbrook, England.
Watson, Ethel. Toledo, Ohio, U.S.A.
Watson, Sydney. Anniston. Ala., U.S.A.
Waugh, Ann. Salem, Mass., U.S.A.
Wayne, Claude. Forest Lodge, Sydney, N.S.W., Australia.
Wayne, Ruth. Thames, N.Z.
Weaver, Mary. Midco, Mo., U.S.A.
Weaver, Ruth. Bethlehem, Pa., U.S.A.
Webster, Cdr. George, R.N. H.M.S. *Hyacinth*, Saldanha Bay, C.P., S. Africa.
Wedlog, Hans. Sunnmøre, Norway.
Weeden, Lois. Osceola, Nebr., U.S.A.
Weiley, W. R. Grafton, N.S.W., Australia.
Weinhold, Lucille. Milwaukee, Wis., U.S.A.
Weinstock, Fannie. Elwood, Nebr., U.S.A.
Welch, Euphimia. Montreal, P.Q., Canada.
Welfing, Simone. Pontaillac, France.
Wellbeloved, Grace. Ladybrand, O.F.S., S. Africa.
Weman, Gunnar. Stockholm, Sweden.
Wessel, Hendrikus. Uithoorn, Holland.
Wessner, Ellen. Stuttgart, Germany.
West, Charles. Spartanburg, S.C., U.S.A.
West, Gladys. Castleton, Kans., U.S.A.
West, Isabella. Dunedin, N.Z.
Westell, Lillian. Dresden, Ont., Canada.
Weyl, Henri. Enschede, Holland.
Wheeler, Edith. South Paris, Me., U.S.A.
Wheeler, Magdalene. South Bend, Ind., U.S.A.
Whelchel, James. Avant, Okla., U.S.A.
Whitcher, Dorothy. Coldstream, C.P., S. Africa.
White, Clara. Cambridge, Mass.
White, Edward, Hatfield, Pretoria, Tvl., S. Africa.
White, Evelyn. Kimberley, C.P., S. Africa.
White, Julia. Saint John, N.B., Canada.
White, Marion. St Joseph, Mo., U.S.A.
White, Mattye. Paces, Va., U.S.A.
Whiteway, Cicely. Southampton, England.
Whittaker, Nurse Alice. Auckland, N.Z.

Wickard, Nurse Harriet. Mercy Hospital, Hamilton, Ohio, U.S.A.
Wiggins, Peggy. Cleveland, Miss., U.S.A.
Wiggins, Sylvia. Cleveland, Miss., U.S.A.
Wigstrand, Rudolf. Stockholm Provisional Hospital, Sweden.
Wilford, Agnes. Barnsley, England.
Wilhelm, Seaman Karl. Wilhelmshaven Naval Hospital, Germany.
Wilkes, Laura Maria. Willenhall, England.
Wilkinson, Jean. Port Adelaide, S. Australia.
Wilkinson, Scout Robert. Sydenham Troop, Christchurch, N.Z.
Williams, Alex. Volksrust, Tvl., S. Africa.
Williams, Dr Park Pearl. Barada, Nebr., U.S.A.
Williamson, Charles. Melbourne, Vic., Australia.
Williamson, Thomas. Awakevi, N.Z.
Willis, Alice. Stonewall, Man., Canada.
Willock, Ronald. Montreal, P.Q., Canada.
Wilmot, Sally. Pretoria, Tvl., S. Africa.
Wilson, Bernard. Stepney (East London), England.
Wilson, Cecil. Pueblo, Colo., U.S.A.
Wilson, Dorothy. Hinsdale, Ill., U.S.A.
Wilson, Nurse Louise. Camp McLellan, Anniston, Ala., U.S.A.
Wilson, Nurse Marjorie. Pilot Mound, Man., Canada.
Wilson, Nurse Mary. Royal County Fever Hospital, York, England.
Wilson, Thomas. Reno, Nev., U.S.A.
Winek, Brita. Stockholm, Sweden.
Winter, Perce. Toowoomba. Queensl., Australia.
Wise, Iris. Port Elizabeth, C.P., S. Africa.
Wishart, Alethea. Port Elizabeth, C.P., S. Africa.
Wittgens, Maria. Milan, Italy.
Womack, Prentise. Auburn, Ky., U.S.A.
Wong, Robert. Singapore.
Wood, Connie. Kimberley, C.P., S. Africa.
Wood, G. T. Kendal, England.
Woodfin, Ruth. Chester, Va., U.S.A.
Woodhouse, Margaret. Larkhill, England.
Woodland, Percy. Haywards Heath, England.
Woodworth, Frances. Weedsport, N.Y., U.S.A.
Woolfard, Magdalena. Hanover, C.P., S. Africa.
Wright, Sapper Frederick. Maitland Hospital, Cape Town, S. Africa.
Wright, T. B. Grahamstown, C.P., S. Africa.
Wubbolts, Gerard. Delfzijl, Holland.
Yates, Kathleen. Matatiele, C.P., S. Africa.
Yost, Baker 2nd Class Orval, U.S.N. Yerba Buena Island, Calif., U.S.A.
Young, L/Cpl. George. 33rd M. G. Bn, St Quentin, France.
Youngberg, Margaret. Salida, Colo., U.S.A.

Zahn, Alice. Milwaukee, Wis., U.S.A.
Zambotto, Chiara. Verona, Italy.
Zamora, Dr Juan. Malànquilla   Facinas, Spain; Gibraltar.
Zanchettin, Luigi. Hospital Dante Alighieri, Rome, Italy.
Zanettin, Giovanni. Cembra, Italy.
Zannini, Antonio. Milan, Italy.
Zanoni, Adriana. Cavi di Lavagna, Italy.
Zappa, Giuseppe. Monza, Italy.
Zebellin, Pte. Ernesto. 3rd Signals Regt, Murmansk, Russia.
Zehendner, Anna. Bayreuth, Germany.
Zettler, Pte. George. S.A.T.C., St Xavier College, Cincinnati, Ohio,
U.S.A.
Ziel, Ruby. Rockford, Ill., U.S.A.
Zullini, Bruno. Cittanova d'Istria, Italy.